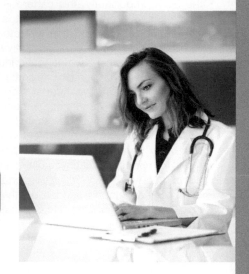

Advances and Challenges in Critical Care

Editors

SHYOKO HONIDEN
JONATHAN M. SINER

CLINICS IN
CHEST MEDICINE

www.chestmed.theclinics.com

September 2015 • Volume 36 • Number 3

ELSEVIER

1600 John F. Kennedy Boulevard • Suite 1800 • Philadelphia, Pennsylvania, 19103-2899

http://www.theclinics.com

CLINICS IN CHEST MEDICINE Volume 36, Number 3
September 2015 ISSN 0272-5231, ISBN-13: 978-0-323-39557-1

Editor: Patrick Manley
Developmental Editor: Casey Jackson

Clinics in Chest Medicine (ISSN 0272-5231) is published quarterly by Elsevier Inc., 360 Park Avenue South, New York, NY 10010-1710. Months of issue are March, June, September, and December. Periodicals postage paid at New York, NY and additional mailing offices. Subscription prices are $345.00 per year (domestic individuals), $556.00 per year (domestic institutions), $165.00 per year (domestic students/residents), $380.00 per year (Canadian individuals), $690.00 per year (Canadian institutions), $470.00 per year (international individuals), $690.00 per year (international institutions), and $230.00 per year (international and Canadian students/residents). International air speed delivery is included in all Clinics subscription prices. All prices are subject to change without notice. **POSTMASTER:** Send address changes to Clinics in Chest Medicine, Elsevier Health Sciences Division, Subscription Customer Service, 3251 Riverport Lane, Maryland Heights, MO 63043. **Customer Service: Telephone: 1-800-654-2452** (U.S. and Canada); **1-314-447-8871** (outside U.S. and Canada). **Fax: 1-314-447-8029. E-mail: journalscustomerservice-usa@elsevier.com (for print support); journalsonlinesupport-usa@elsevier.com (for online support).**

Reprints. For copies of 100 or more of articles in this publication, please contact the Commercial Reprints Department, Elsevier Inc., 360 Park Avenue South, New York, NY 10010-1710. Tel.: 212-633-3874; Fax: 212-633-3820; E-mail: reprints@elsevier.com.

Clinics in Chest Medicine is covered in *MEDLINE/PubMed (Index Medicus), Current Contents/Clinical Medicine, EMBASE/Excerpta Medica, Science Citation Index,* and *ISI/BIOMED.*

Contributors

EDITORS

SHYOKO HONIDEN, MSc, MD
Assistant Professor of Medicine, Section of
Pulmonary, Critical Care, and Sleep Medicine,
Yale University School of Medicine; Director of
Simulation for Internal Medicine; Associate
Program Director, Pulmonary and Critical Care
Medicine, New Haven, Connecticut

JONATHAN M. SINER, MD
Assistant Professor of Medicine, Section of
Pulmonary, Critical Care, and Sleep Medicine,
Department of Internal Medicine, Yale
University School of Medicine; Medical
Director, Medical Intensive Care Unit,
Yale-New Haven Hospital, New Haven,
Connecticut

AUTHORS

DARRYL ABRAMS, MD
Assistant Professor, Division of Pulmonary,
Allergy and Critical Care, Columbia University
College of Physicians and Surgeons,
New York, New York

MARY BAKER, MD
Pulmonary/Critical Care Fellow, Division of
Pulmonary and Critical Care Medicine,
Department of Internal Medicine, Indiana
University; Charles Warren Fairbanks Center
for Medical Ethics, IU Health Methodist
Hospital, Indianapolis, Indiana

PETER BENTZER, MD, PhD
Centre for Heart Lung Innovation; Division of
Critical Care Medicine, St. Paul's Hospital,
University of British Columbia, Vancouver,
British Columbia, Canada; Department of
Anesthesiology and Intensive Care,
Lund University, Lund, Sweden

GABRIEL T. BOSSLET, MD, MA
Assistant Professor of Clinical Medicine,
Division of Pulmonary and Critical Care
Medicine, Department of Internal Medicine,
Indiana University; Charles Warren Fairbanks
Center for Medical Ethics, IU Health Methodist
Hospital, Indianapolis, Indiana

DANIEL BRODIE, MD
Associate Professor, Division of Pulmonary,
Allergy and Critical Care, Columbia University

College of Physicians and Surgeons,
New York, New York

GEOFFREY R. CONNORS, MD
Assistant Professor of Medicine, Section of
Pulmonary, Critical Care and Sleep Medicine,
Department of Internal Medicine, Yale
University School of Medicine, New Haven,
Connecticut

WASSIM H. FARES, MD, MSc
Pulmonary Vascular Disease Program,
Pulmonary, Critical Care, and Sleep
Medicine, Department of Internal Medicine,
Yale School of Medicine, New Haven,
Connecticut

STEVEN A. FUHRMAN, MD
Division of Pulmonary and Critical Care
Medicine, Sentara Norfolk General Hospital,
Sentara eICU, Sentara Medical Group, Norfolk,
Virginia

RYAN HADLEY, MD
Clinical Assistant Professor of Medicine,
Division of Pulmonary and Critical Care
Medicine, University of Michigan Health
System, Ann Arbor, Michigan

DAVID N. HAGER, MD, PhD
Director, Medical Progressive Care Unit;
Associate Director, Medical Intensive Care
Unit; Assistant Professor of Medicine, Johns
Hopkins University, Baltimore, Maryland

JEFFREY A. HASPEL, MD, PhD
Assistant Professor, Division of Pulmonary, Critical Care and Sleep Medicine, Department of Internal Medicine, Washington University School of Medicine, St Louis, Missouri

JASON J. HEAVNER, MD
Section of Pulmonary, Critical Care, and Sleep Medicine, Department of Internal Medicine, Yale School of Medicine, New Haven, Connecticut

SHYOKO HONIDEN, MSc, MD
Assistant Professor of Medicine, Section of Pulmonary, Critical Care, and Sleep Medicine, Yale University School of Medicine; Director of Simulation for Internal Medicine; Associate Program Director, Pulmonary and Critical Care Medicine, New Haven, Connecticut

MICHAEL H. HOOPER, MD, MSc
Assistant Professor of Pulmonary and Critical Care Medicine, Eastern Virginia Medical School, Norfolk, Virginia

ROBERT HYZY, MD
Professor of Medicine, Division of Pulmonary and Critical Care Medicine, University of Michigan Health System, Ann Arbor, Michigan

CYRUS A. KHOLDANI, MD
Pulmonary Vascular Disease Program, Pulmonary, Critical Care, and Sleep Medicine, Department of Internal Medicine, Yale School of Medicine, New Haven, Connecticut

MELISSA P. KNAUERT, MD, PhD
Assistant Professor, Section of Pulmonary, Critical Care and Sleep Medicine, Department of Internal Medicine, Yale University School of Medicine, New Haven, Connecticut

MARIN H. KOLLEF, MD
Pulmonary and Critical Care Division, Washington University School of Medicine, St Louis, Missouri

VICKI R. LEBLANC, PhD
Associate Professor, Faculty of Dentistry, University of Toronto; Associate Director and Scientist, Wilson Centre, Toronto, Ontario, Canada

CRAIG M. LILLY, MD, FCCM, FCCP, FACP
Professor of Medicine, Anesthesiology, and Surgery, UMass Memorial Medical Center, University of Massachusetts Medical School, Worcester, Massachusetts

JIM LUCE, MSW
Administrative Director of Palliative Care Services, Palliative Care, Indiana University Health, Indianapolis, Indiana

PAUL E. MARIK, MD, FCCM, FCCP, ABPNS
Professor of Pulmonary and Critical Care Medicine, Eastern Virginia Medical School, Norfolk, Virginia

PETER MARSHALL, MD, MPH
Assistant Professor of Medicine, Section of Pulmonary, Critical Care and Sleep Medicine, Department of Medicine, Yale School of Medicine, New Haven, Connecticut

JOHN McGINNISS, MD
Fellow, Pulmonary, Allergy and Critical Care Division, Hospital of the University of Pennsylvania, Philadelphia, Pennsylvania

DOMINIQUE PIQUETTE, MD, MSc, MEd, PhD
Staff Physician, Department of Critical Care Medicine, Sunnybrook Health Sciences Centre; Assistant Professor, University of Toronto, Toronto, Ontario, Canada

MARGARET A. PISANI, MD, MPH
Assistant Professor, Section of Pulmonary, Critical Care and Sleep Medicine, Department of Internal Medicine, Yale University School of Medicine, New Haven, Connecticut

JAMES A. RUSSELL, MD
Centre for Heart Lung Innovation; Division of Critical Care Medicine, St. Paul's Hospital, University of British Columbia, Vancouver, British Columbia, Canada

JONATHAN M. SINER, MD
Assistant Professor of Medicine, Section of Pulmonary, Critical Care, and Sleep Medicine, Department of Internal Medicine, Yale University School of Medicine; Medical Director, Medical Intensive Care Unit, Yale-New Haven Hospital, New Haven, Connecticut

SERGIO E. TREVINO, MD
Pulmonary and Critical Care Division,
Washington University School of Medicine,
St Louis, Missouri

KEITH R. WALLEY, MD
Centre for Heart Lung Innovation; Division of
Critical Care Medicine, St. Paul's Hospital,
University of British Columbia, Vancouver,
British Columbia, Canada

Contents

is equivalent, if not superior, to full-dose feeding. Parenteral nutrition has no proved benefit over enteral nutrition, which is the preferred route of nutritional support in intensive care unit patients with a functional gastrointestinal tract. Continuous enteral and parental nutrition inhibits the release of important enterohormones. These changes are reversed with intermittent bolus feeding. Whey protein, which is high in leucine, has a greater effect on insulin release and protein synthesis than does a soy- or casein-based enteral formula.

unproven. A focus on ARDS risk factor reduction and the development of tools predicting progression to ARDS have the potential to further reduce its incidence.

Interstitial lung disease (ILD) is a clinical syndrome of various etiologies and histopathologic categorization that, when clinically significant, impair respiratory function. Patients with ILD may develop critical illness from respiratory failure, nonpulmonary organ failure, or after surgical procedures. Additionally, the intensivist must be adept at recognizing exacerbation syndromes, which can complicate the disease course of some forms of ILD. This article discusses mechanical ventilation, noninvasive mechanical ventilation, exacerbation syndromes, and surgical concerns for patients with ILD who are critically ill.

Right heart failure is a clinical syndrome of various causes that commonly involves failure of the right ventricle (RV). The hemodynamic hallmark of the syndrome is increasing central venous pressure and worsening cardiac output with a rising RV end-diastolic pressure. When dealing with RV failure, clinicians must assess and optimize the intravascular volume state, support RV contractility, and address any pathologic elevations of afterload so that systemic perfusion is preserved. Despite these measures, there may still be a need to offer rescue interventions to the failing RV in carefully selected patients.

Recent research has identified promising targets for therapeutic interventions aimed at modulating the inflammatory response in sepsis. Herein, the authors describe mechanisms involved in the clearance of pathogen toxin from the circulation and potential interventions aimed at enhancing clearance mechanisms. The authors also describe advances in the understanding of the innate immune response as potential therapeutic targets. Finally, novel potential treatment strategies aimed at decreasing vascular leak are discussed.

Infections with multidrug-resistant organisms (MDROs) are common in critically ill patients and are challenging to manage appropriately. Strategies that can be used in the treatment of MDRO infections in the intensive care unit (ICU) include combination therapy, adjunctive aerosolized therapy, and optimization of pharmacokinetics with higher doses or extended-infusion therapy as appropriate. Rapid diagnostic tests could assist in improving timely appropriate antimicrobial therapy for MDRO infections in the ICU.

PROGRAM OBJECTIVE

The goal of the *Clinics in Chest Medicine* is to provide practitioners with state-of-the-art information that is clinically useful, concise, well referenced, and comprehensive.

TARGET AUDIENCE

All practicing physicians and healthcare professionals who provide patient care utilizing findings from *Chest Medicine Clinics of North America*.

LEARNING OBJECTIVES

Upon completion of this activity, participants will be able to:

1. Review ongoing issues in the ICU such as sleep loss, nutrition, infection management, and the integration of palliative care services.
2. Discuss the use and limitations of simulation-based medical education.
3. Recognize new and ongoing advances in sepsis research.

ACCREDITATION

The Elsevier Office of Continuing Medical Education (EOCME) is accredited by the Accreditation Council for Continuing Medical Education (ACCME) to provide continuing medical education for physicians.

The EOCME designates this enduring material for a maximum of 15 *AMA PRA Category 1 Credit*(s)™. Physicians should claim only the credit commensurate with the extent of their participation in the activity.

All other health care professionals requesting continuing education credit for this enduring material will be issued a certificate of participation.

DISCLOSURE OF CONFLICTS OF INTEREST

The EOCME assesses conflict of interest with its instructors, faculty, planners, and other individuals who are in a position to control the content of CME activities. All relevant conflicts of interest that are identified are thoroughly vetted by EOCME for fair balance, scientific objectivity, and patient care recommendations. EOCME is committed to providing its learners with CME activities that promote improvements or quality in healthcare and not a specific proprietary business or a commercial interest.

The planning committee, staff, authors and editors listed below have identified no financial relationships or relationships to products or devices they or their spouse/life partner have with commercial interest related to the content of this CME activity:

Darryl Abrams, MD; Mary Baker, MD; Peter Bentzer, MD, PhD; Gabriel T. Bosslet, MD, MA; Daniel Brodie, MD; Geoffrey R. Connors, MD; Wassim H. Fares, MD, MSc; Anjali Fortna; Steven A. Fuhrman, MD; David N. Hager, MD, PhD; Jeffrey A. Haspel, MD, PhD; Jason J. Heavner, MD; Shyoko Honiden, MSc, MD; Michael H. Hooper, MD, MSc; Robert Hyzy, MD; Cyrus A. Kholdani, MD; Melissa P. Knauert, MD, PhD; Vicki R. LeBlanc, PhD; Craig M. Lilly, MD, FCCM, FCCP, FACP; Jim Luce, MSW; Patrick Manley; Peter Marshall, MD, MPH; John McGinniss, MD; Palani Murugesan; Dominique Piquette, MD, MSc, MEd, PhD; Margaret A. Pisani, MD, MPH; Jonathan M. Siner, MD; Megan Suermann; Sergio E. Trevino, MD.

The planning committee, staff, authors and editors listed below have identified financial relationships or relationships to products or devices they or their spouse/life partner have with commercial interest related to the content of this CME activity:

Ryan Hadley, **MD** is a consultant/advisor for Boehringer Ingelheim GmbH.

Marin H. Kollef, **MD** is on the speakers' bureau for Merck & Co., Inc.

Paul E. Marik, **M.D., FCCM, FCCP, ABPNS** has given educational lectures sponsored by Abbott and Nestlé.

James A. Russell, **MD** founded Cyon Therapeutics, which has licensed intellectual property from the University of British Columbia related to PCSK9 in sepsis.

Keith R. Walley, **MD** founded Cyon Therapeutics, which has licensed intellectual property from the University of British Columbia related to PCSK9 in sepsis.

UNAPPROVED/OFF-LABEL USE DISCLOSURE

The EOCME requires CME faculty to disclose to the participants:

1. When products or procedures being discussed are off-label, unlabelled, experimental, and/or investigational (not US Food and Drug Administration [FDA] approved); and
2. Any limitations on the information presented, such as data that are preliminary or that represent ongoing research, interim analyses, and/or unsupported opinions. Faculty may discuss information about pharmaceutical agents that is outside of FDA-approved labelling. This information is intended solely for CME and is not intended to promote off-label use of these medications. If you have any questions, contact the medical affairs department of the manufacturer for the most recent prescribing information.

TO ENROLL

To enroll in the *Chest Medicine Clinics* Continuing Medical Education program, call customer service at 1-800-654-2452 or sign up online at http://www.theclinics.com/home/cme. The CME program is available to subscribers for an additional annual fee of USD $225.

METHOD OF PARTICIPATION

In order to claim credit, participants must complete the following:

1. Complete enrolment as indicated above.
2. Read the activity.
3. Complete the CME Test and Evaluation. Participants must achieve a score of 70% on the test. All CME Tests and Evaluations must be completed online.

CME INQUIRIES/SPECIAL NEEDS

For all CME inquiries or special needs, please contact elsevierCME@elsevier.com.

CLINICS IN CHEST MEDICINE

THE CLINICS ARE AVAILABLE ONLINE!
Access your subscription at:
www.theclinics.com

CLINICS IN CHEST MEDICINE

FORTHCOMING ISSUES

December 2015
Sarcoidosis
Robert Baughman and Dan Culver, Editors

March 2016
Cystic Fibrosis
Jon Koff, Editor

June 2016
Sepsis
Julie A. Bastarache and Eric Seeley, Editors

RECENT ISSUES

June 2015
Chest Imaging
David A. Lynch and Jonathan H. Chung,
Editors

March 2015
Nontuberculous Mycobacteria
Gwen A. Huitt and Charles L. Daley, Editors

December 2014
Acute Respiratory Distress Syndrome
Lorraine B. Ware, Julie A. Bastarache, and
Carolyn S. Calfee, Editors

RELATED INTEREST

Critical Care Clinics, Vol. 31, No. 2 (April 2015)
Telemedicine in the ICU
Richard W. Carlson and Corey Scurlock, Editors

Preface
Advances and Challenges in Critical Care Medicine

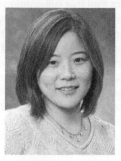 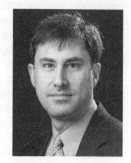

Shyoko Honiden, MSc, MD   Jonathan M. Siner, MD
Editors

Since the advent of modern critical care, the field has been marked by technological innovation and critical re-evaluation of accepted therapies. This evolution of critical care has allowed for technological development, improvements in supportive care, advances in education and quality improvement, as well as innovations in disease-specific management. In this issue of *Clinics in Chest Medicine*, we address several areas of modern critical care that characterize some of these new developments and highlight the challenges we still face. We specifically chose areas with recent novel developments, or alternatively common critical care topics that allowed for a fresh perspective based on recent data.

In the arena pertaining to ICU-based technologies, we focused on ECMO, therapeutic hypothermia, and telemedicine. While ECMO has become popularized recently as an emerging therapy for ARDS, the article in this issue focuses on several exciting new uses of ECMO. Similarly, targeted temperature management has become standard of care to improve neurologic outcomes after out-of-hospital cardiac arrest, but the article in this issue critically analyzes the literature related to novel indications that go beyond this accepted practice. Nationally, telemedicine continues to expand and providers now have a means of interacting remotely with care teams, patients, and families. The authors in this issue explain why telemedicine will continue to evolve and become

more integrated into future ICU operations far beyond the original conception of this technology.

Supportive care has been a mainstay of modern critical care, and while often overlooked, doing it properly is pivotal to improving patient outcomes. Nutrition has remained a challenge with a relative paucity of literature. The authors in this issue distill the current practice and outline future directions for this essential intervention. The ICU environment itself has received substantial attention in recent years, because it has implications on rest and sleep that in turn may impact development of ICU delirium as well as patient and family satisfaction. The article on sleep and circadian rhythms is an introduction to this rapidly growing area of critical care. Another key component of supportive care has been the advent of mobility programs for ICU patients. The authors outline the challenges of implementing a mobility program and provide a practical prescription for culture change. End-of-life planning is universally a challenge, and the authors provide a review of the benefits and barriers to palliative care involvement in the ICU and ways in which such care could be integrated and how outcomes might be tracked.

Quality improvement and education have become an essential component of modern critical care. Clinical decision-making is a commonly discussed topic in medical education, but adapting it for the critical care environment can be difficult. In this issue, the authors demonstrate one novel

Clin Chest Med 36 (2015) xv–xvi
http://dx.doi.org/10.1016/j.ccm.2015.07.002
0272-5231/15/$ – see front matter © 2015 Published by Elsevier Inc.

approach in which decision-making can be integrated into risk assessment. Diagnostic error has received increased attention by groups, including the Institute of Medicine. Understanding how adverse event reporting by medical providers can help address this nationwide problem is a focus of one of the articles. Finally, with work hour limitations and increasingly complex patients in the ICU, simulation-based education has been explored as a means of achieving educational goals that may not be easily addressed during traditional clinical training. The authors review the available evidence in support of simulation-based education and pose important questions to consider when planning this resource-intense mode of education.

Our final group of articles focuses on disease-specific management. Our basic understanding of interstitial lung disease has expanded substantially over the past 10 years. There is greater clarity about the distinguishing characteristics of many interstitial diseases that fall under the rubric of interstitial lung disease. The authors discuss the relevance of these advances in both therapy and disease pathogenesis and how this translates to care that is provided in the ICU environment. Right heart failure remains a morbid and challenging problem in the ICU. The article explores adjunctive measures and rescue interventions that may help offload the failing right ventricle. Despite the prevalence and importance of sepsis in the critically ill population, investigations for this disease have yielded many false starts. In the sepsis article, the authors return to the basics and explain why continued basic science research and understanding of pathophysiology are key to a more assured way forward. Finally, infections with multi-drug-resistant organisms have garnered attention in both the lay and the medical literature. The authors provide strategies that can be used to manage these infections in the ICU that may include combination therapy, adjunctive aerosolized treatment, and optimizing the pharmacokinetic properties of antibiotics using higher doses or extended infusions.

In summary, the field of critical care is rapidly changing, and we anticipate that this will continue, very likely in ways we may not anticipate today. Collectively, we have tried to highlight new aspects of ICU management that we feel might become increasingly relevant as our field develops. We thank all of our contributing authors for their thoughtful manuscripts and expertise. It has been a wonderful opportunity to work with talented colleagues. Additional thanks go to the very capable editorial staff at *Clinics in Chest Medicine* for their guidance and patience.

Shyoko Honiden, MSc, MD
Section of Pulmonary, Critical Care, and
Sleep Medicine
Yale University School of Medicine
333 Cedar Street
PO Box 208057
New Haven, CT 06520-8057, USA

Jonathan M. Siner, MD
Section of Pulmonary, Critical Care, and
Sleep Medicine
Department of Internal Medicine
Yale University School of Medicine
333 Cedar Street
PO Box 208057
New Haven, CT 06520-8057, USA

E-mail addresses:
shyoko.honiden@yale.edu (S. Honiden)
jonathan.siner@yale.edu (J.M. Siner)

Novel Uses of Extracorporeal Membrane Oxygenation in Adults

Darryl Abrams, MD, Daniel Brodie, MD*

KEYWORDS

- ECMO • ECCO$_2$R • ARDS • Lung transplantation • ECPR • Cardiogenic shock
- Pulmonary hypertension

KEY POINTS

- Extracorporeal carbon dioxide removal (ECCO$_2$R) may play an emerging role in the management of respiratory failure.
- Novel upper-body configurations help facilitate patient mobilization and are particularly well-suited to maintain physical conditioning in the pretransplant population.
- Extracorporeal cardiopulmonary resuscitation has the potential to improve neurologically intact survival from cardiac arrest. However, appropriate patient selection is a key factor in optimizing outcomes.
- In decompensated pulmonary hypertension, extracorporeal membrane oxygenation may serve as a bridge to recovery in patients with reversible processes or to transplantation for irreversible disease.
- More data are needed to define the optimal patient populations for extracorporeal support. Cost–benefit analyses should be undertaken.

INTRODUCTION

Extracorporeal membrane oxygenation (ECMO) has been available for decades as a supportive therapy for severe cardiopulmonary disease; however, its early use was marred by high complication rates and poor outcomes.[1,2] Advances in technology have led to improved complication rates[3] and an increasing amount of evidence suggesting a potential benefit in select forms of cardiac and respiratory failure has resulted in a notable increase in the use of ECMO.[4] As both cannulation technique and extracorporeal circuits evolve, there are an increasing number of indications for which ECMO may provide a benefit.[5] This article reviews these emerging indications and discusses potential future applications.

CONFIGURATIONS OF EXTRACORPOREAL MEMBRANE OXYGENATION

ECMO refers to an extracorporeal device that directly oxygenates and removes carbon dioxide from the blood. Deoxygenated blood is withdrawn

Funding Sources: None.
Conflicts of Interest: Dr D. Brodie previously received research support from Maquet Cardiovascular, including travel expenses for research meetings and compensation paid to Columbia University for research consulting. He is a member of the Medical Advisory Boards for ALung Technologies and Kadence. All compensation for these activities is paid to Columbia University. Dr D. Abrams has no conflicts of interest to report.
Division of Pulmonary, Allergy and Critical Care, Columbia University College of Physicians and Surgeons, PH 8E 101, New York, NY 10032, USA
* Corresponding author.
E-mail address: hdb5@cumc.columbia.edu

Clin Chest Med 36 (2015) 373–384
http://dx.doi.org/10.1016/j.ccm.2015.05.014

from a central vein through a drainage cannula via an external pump. The blood passes through an oxygenator, where gas exchange occurs across a semipermeable membrane, and is then reinfused into a central vessel. Venovenous ECMO refers to a circuit in which blood is both drained from and returned to a central vein. A venovenous configuration only supports gas exchange.[6] Venoarterial ECMO refers to a circuit in which blood is drained from a vein and reinfused into an artery. Venoarterial configurations can support impairments in both gas exchange and hemodynamics. Two of the major determinants of systemic oxygenation with the use of ECMO are the rate of extracorporeal blood flow and the fraction of oxygen in the gas compartment of the oxygenator.[7,8] Blood flow is determined predominantly by the size of the cannulae used for drainage, and, to a lesser extent, reinfusion. Larger cannulae are generally able to achieve higher blood flow rates, which results in a greater proportion of the cardiac output oxygenated by the ECMO circuit. The major determinant of carbon dioxide removal, by contrast, is the rate of gas flow through the gas compartment of the oxygenator (known as sweep gas), with extracorporeal blood flow rate, among other factors, having a less significant impact.[8] The intrinsic diffusion properties of the extracorporeal membrane and the contribution of the native lungs will also have a direct impact on gas exchange. Because oxygenator membranes are highly efficient at carbon dioxide removal, lower blood flow rates and, therefore, smaller cannulae may be used when the primary intention in using the device is extracorporeal carbon dioxide removal (ECCO$_2$R).[9] An alternative to venovenous and venoarterial configurations is an arteriovenous strategy, in which the patient's native cardiac output, instead of an external pump, generates the extracorporeal blood flow.[10] The blood flow rates are generally lower than what can be achieved with a mechanical pump, and, therefore, its use is predominantly restricted to ECCO$_2$R.

Venovenous ECMO configurations may consist of either a 2-site or single-site cannulation strategy. In a 2-site setup, the drainage cannula is typically placed into the inferior vena cava via the femoral vein and the reinfusion cannula is placed into the internal jugular vein with its tip near the junction between the superior vena cava and the right atrium (**Fig. 1**).[7] More recent advances in cannula design have led to the development of a bicaval, dual-lumen cannula that allows for both drainage and reinfusion through 1 cannula placed in the internal jugular vein (**Fig. 2**).[11] When properly positioned, which usually requires transesophageal and fluoroscopic guidance, the reinfusion jet of oxygenated blood is directed toward the

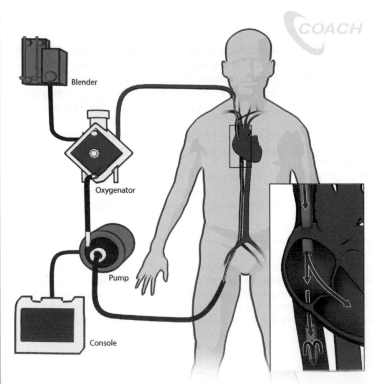

Fig. 1. Two-site venovenous extracorporeal membrane oxygenation. Venous blood is withdrawn from a central vein, pumped through an oxygenator, and reinfused into a central vein. *Inset*: When drainage and reinfusion ports are in close approximation, some portion of reinfused, oxygenated blood (*red arrow*) may be drawn back into the circuit without having entered the systemic circulation, known as recirculation (*purple arrow*). (Reprinted from CollectedMed.com; with permission.)

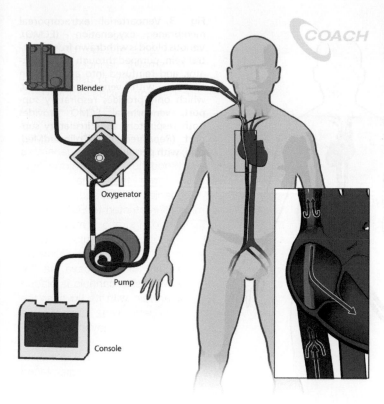

Fig. 2. Single-site venovenous extracorporeal membrane oxygenation (ECMO). Bicaval, dual-lumen cannulae allow for the institution of venovenous ECMO via a single venous access site. *Inset*: When the cannula is properly positioned, reinfused, oxygenated blood (*red arrow*) is directed toward the tricuspid valve, minimizing recirculation. (*Reprinted from* CollectedMed.com; with permission.)

Blender

Oxygenator

Pump

Console

tricuspid valve.[12] This approach precludes the need for cannulation of the femoral vein and may minimize the amount of recirculation, in which reinfused blood is drawn back into the circuit without passing through the systemic circulation.[13]

Venoarterial ECMO is accomplished traditionally with femoral venous drainage and femoral arterial reinfusion (**Fig. 3**).[5] However, this requires reinfused oxygenated blood to flow retrograde up the aorta. The reinfusion jet may encounter resistance from antegrade flow from the left ventricle if there is any residual native cardiac function, compromising the ability to supply oxygenated blood to the cerebral and coronary vascular beds when there is impaired native gas exchange and the blood being ejected from the left ventricle is poorly oxygenated (**Fig. 4**). There are 2 strategies that may overcome this limitation. A second reinfusion limb may be added to the femoral arterial reinfusion limb, via a "Y" connection, and inserted into an internal jugular vein (**Fig. 5**).[5,14] A portion of oxygenated blood is thereby returned to the native cardiac circulation and may improve oxygen delivery to the ascending aorta. This configuration, consisting of venous drainage and combined venous and arterial return, is referred to as venoarterial–venous ECMO.[14] A second strategy to improve

upper body oxygenation consists of internal jugular venous drainage and subclavian arterial reinfusion via an end-to-side graft.[15]

- Venovenous ECMO provides support for respiratory failure alone, whereas venoarterial ECMO provides both respiratory and hemodynamic support.
- Carbon dioxide removal requires lower blood flow rates and smaller cannulae than what is traditionally required for oxygenation.
- Delivery of oxygenated blood to the aortic arch and great vessels in venoarterial ECMO may be compromised by the combination of residual native cardiac output and impaired native gas exchange.

EMERGING INDICATIONS FOR EXTRACORPOREAL MEMBRANE OXYGENATION IN RESPIRATORY FAILURE
Acute Respiratory Distress Syndrome

Severe acute respiratory distress syndrome (ARDS) is the most commonly accepted indication for ECMO in respiratory failure, although the data supporting such use remains controversial.[4,6,16] ECMO has the potential to both correct

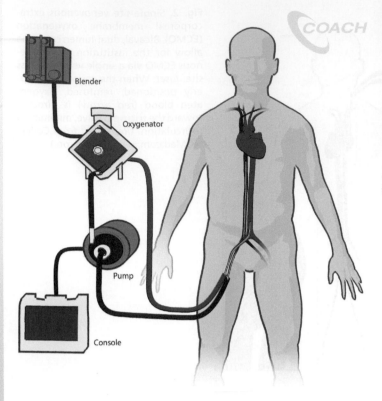

Fig. 3. Venoarterial extracorporeal membrane oxygenation (ECMO). Venous blood is withdrawn from a central vein, pumped through an oxygenator, and reinfused into an artery. In contrast with venovenous ECMO, which only provides respiratory support, venoarterial ECMO provides both respiratory and circulatory support. (*Reprinted from* CollectedMed. com; with permission.)

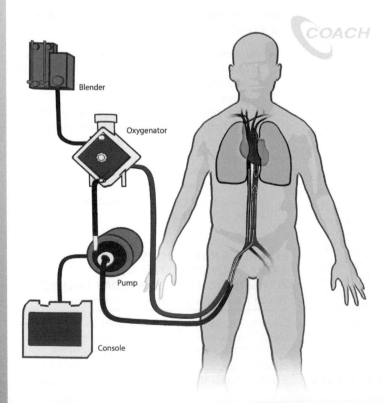

Fig. 4. Venoarterial extracorporeal membrane oxygenation in the setting of impaired native gas exchange. Blood flow reinfused retrograde into the aorta (*red arrow*) may encounter resistance from antegrade blood flow from residual native cardiac function (*purple arrow*). When there is impaired native gas exchange, oxygenation of the cerebral and coronary vascular beds may be compromised. (*Reprinted from* CollectedMed.com; with permission.)

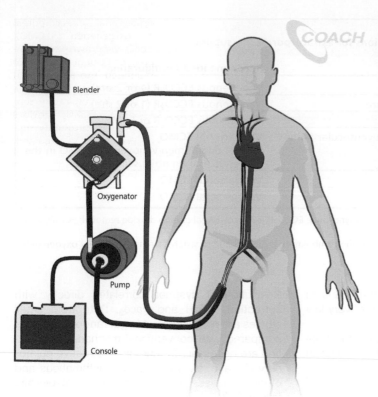

Fig. 5. Venoarterial venous extracorporeal membrane oxygenation (ECMO). The combination of femoral venoarterial ECMO, residual native cardiac function, and impaired native gas exchange may compromise oxygenation of the aortic arch and great vessels. This limitation may be overcome by returning a portion of the oxygenated blood to the native cardiac circulation with the addition of a second reinfusion limb in the internal jugular vein. (*Reprinted from* CollectedMed.com; with permission.)

life-threatening hypoxemia and facilitate a lung-protective ventilation strategy by correcting the acidemia and hypercapnia that may accompany low tidal volume ventilation in the setting of reduced respiratory system compliance.[17,18] A multicenter, randomized, clinical trial is underway to determine whether ECMO provides a survival advantage over standard of care conventional management in severe ARDS.[19] However, severe ARDS remains relatively uncommon.[20–22] Where ECMO is likely to have a greater impact is in its ability to facilitate lung-protective ventilation strategies beyond the currently accepted standard of care in less severe forms of ARDS (**Table 1**). Both animal data and post hoc analysis of a randomized clinical trial in humans suggest that tidal volumes and airway pressures lower than what were mandated in the ARMA trial may have additional benefit.[23,24] Permissive hypercapnia describes a strategy of allowing carbon dioxide to increase in the service of limiting ventilation. However, achieving very low tidal volumes—lower than the current standard of care—will be limited inevitably, at some point, by unacceptable levels of acidemia and hypercapnia; what might be termed "impermissible hypercapnia." ECCO$_2$R, which can be accomplished at low blood flow rates with smaller, potentially safer cannulae, can overcome this limitation to instituting a very lung-protective ventilation strategy. This concept was demonstrated in a study involving subjects with moderate to severe ARDS, in whom tidal volumes were reduced from 6 to 4 mL/kg predicted body weight and plateau airway pressures were reduced from 29 to 25 cm H$_2$O, with an associated decrease in inflammatory cytokines associated with lung injury.[25] ECCO$_2$R was used to correct the low pH (7.20) and high carbon dioxide levels (73.6 mm Hg) that accompanied the volume- and pressure-limited intervention. Post hoc analysis of a more recent study comparing ECCO$_2$R-assisted very low tidal volume ventilation (3 mL/kg predicted body weight) to standard of care lung-protective ventilation found that, in the subset of subjects with more severe hypoxemia, the ECCO$_2$R-assisted very low tidal volume group had more ventilator-free days (40.9 vs 28.2; $P = .033$).[26] Ultimately, more data are needed before such a strategy can be recommended. A multicenter, international, randomized, controlled trial comparing ECCO$_2$R-assisted very low tidal volumes to standard of care low tidal volume ventilation in the management of moderate to severe ARDS is in the planning phases.

Table 1
Potential and emerging considerations for extracorporeal life support

Indication	Recommended Configuration[a]
Moderate ARDS	Venovenous ECCO$_2$R (1 or 2 site)
Acute hypercapnic respiratory failure	Venovenous ECCO$_2$R (1 or 2 site)
Bridge to lung transplantation	Venovenous ECCO$_2$R or ECMO
Pulmonary hypertension with right ventricular failure	Venoarterial ECMO Bicaval dual-lumen venovenous ECMO in the presence of an atrial septal defect
Cardiogenic shock	Venoarterial ECMO
Cardiac arrest	Venoarterial ECMO

Abbreviations: ARDS, acute respiratory distress syndrome; ECCO$_2$R, extracorporeal carbon dioxide removal; ECMO, extracorporeal membrane oxygenation.
[a] Upper body configurations are preferred when ambulation is anticipated or when there is inadequate oxygen delivery to the aortic arch.

- An emerging role for ECCO$_2$R in ARDS is its ability to facilitate the application of very low tidal volume ventilation.
- Additional studies are needed to demonstrate the benefit of a very lung-protective ventilation strategy in ARDS.

Hypercapnic Respiratory Failure

The efficiency of carbon dioxide removal, along with an improved risk profile from smaller cannulae, may allow for an expansion of indications for ECCO$_2$R beyond ARDS. This is particularly relevant to patients with acute hypercapnic respiratory failure. In acute exacerbations of chronic obstructive pulmonary disease, noninvasive ventilation remains a mainstay of therapy for those with marked respiratory distress, hypercapnia, and excess work of breathing.[27] However, those who fail noninvasive ventilation and require intubation have mortality rates as high as 30%.[28] Invasive mechanical ventilation may be complicated by dynamic hyperinflation and increases in intrinsic positive end-expiratory pressure, ventilator-associated pneumonia and lung injury, and impaired ability to deliver aerosolized medications.[29–31] This particularly vulnerable population may benefit from ECCO$_2$R-assisted gas exchange, with the potential to minimize or eliminate the need for invasive mechanical ventilation, as has been demonstrated in several small studies.[32–34] In a prospective pilot study of 5 subjects with acute exacerbations of chronic obstructive pulmonary disease who required invasive mechanical ventilation in the context of uncompensated hypercapnic respiratory failure, the institution of ECCO$_2$R facilitated extubation within an average of 6.8 hours and ambulation within an average of 29.4 hours from the start of ECCO$_2$R.[32]

Resolution of dyspnea correlated directly with correction of pH and Paco$_2$. Data from small studies are promising, but larger randomized trials compared with conventional mechanical ventilation are necessary for chronic obstructive pulmonary disease, as well as status asthmaticus and other causes of hypercapnic respiratory failure.[35,36]

- Patients with acute hypercapnic respiratory failure are well-suited for extracorporeal support because of the efficiency with which ECCO$_2$R ameliorates hypercapnia and respiratory acidosis.
- A subset of patients with ECCO$_2$R-supported hypercapnic respiratory failure may be appropriate candidates for removal of invasive mechanical ventilation.

Bridge to Lung Transplantation

Patients requiring ECMO as a bridge to lung transplantation have historically had poor perioperative outcomes, particularly when ECMO is used as salvage therapy after invasive mechanical ventilation has already failed. These findings had led to ECMO being considered a relative contraindication to transplantation.[37] However, with the advent of improved circuitry with lower complication rates, more experience with its use, and institution of ECMO earlier in a patient's course, recent studies have demonstrated significantly improved posttransplant outcomes.[38–42] The use of upper-body configurations help to facilitate rehabilitation, including ambulation, which has the benefit of maintaining—or even improving—physical conditioning and, consequently, transplant candidacy.[11,15,43,44] For select patients, ECMO may provide sufficient gas exchange to allow for the removal of invasive mechanical ventilation, further facilitating mobilization while eliminating the risks associated with invasive mechanical ventilation.[41,44]

Although ECMO may serve as a bridging device to lung transplantation, in its current form there is no destination device available. For that reason, the only situation in which ECMO is absolutely contraindicated for respiratory failure is end-stage lung disease when transplantation will not be considered.[18]

- Recent data suggest that pretransplant use of ECMO may be associated with favorable posttransplant outcomes.
- An upper-body extracorporeal configuration facilitates active physical therapy, which helps to maintain or improve conditioning for those awaiting lung transplantation.

EMERGING INDICATIONS FOR EXTRACORPOREAL MEMBRANE OXYGENATION IN CARDIAC FAILURE
Cardiogenic Shock

ECMO is one of several percutaneous mechanical circulatory support strategies for cardiogenic shock, regardless of etiology. Although there are no randomized, controlled trials definitively demonstrating the efficacy of ECMO over other devices or medical therapy alone, observational data suggest a particular benefit to ECMO-assisted percutaneous coronary interventions (PCI) in myocardial infarction-associated cardiogenic shock versus PCI alone.[45–47] Likewise, in fulminant myocarditis complicated by cardiogenic shock, small case series have suggested a benefit to the addition of ECMO to conventional medical management.[48–51] Sepsis-associated cardiogenic shock, resulting from myocardial depression in the setting of severe sepsis, is also emerging as a potential target for venoarterial ECMO support.[50,51] More data are needed to determine whether ECMO in this setting confers a survival advantage.

Pulmonary Hypertension

Decompensated pulmonary hypertension (PH) with associated right ventricular failure is another area that may benefit from ECMO support. ECMO may serve as a bridge to recovery in the acute setting when there is a treatable cause of the decompensation, or it may provide support as a bridging therapy to lung transplantation in end-stage PH.[43,52] Venoarterial ECMO is ideally suited to support these patients because of its ability to unload the right ventricle and bypass the high-resistance pulmonary vasculature. In the

setting of an acute, potentially reversible decompensation, pulmonary vasodilators may be initiated or optimized. In the setting of irreversible PH, it may be preferable to titrate vasodilators down or off to divert blood preferentially through the lower resistance extracorporeal circuit, optimizing systemic oxygenation.[52]

Because ECMO for PH traditionally requires a venoarterial configuration to bypass the pulmonary vascular bed, such support may be associated with the complications of femoral arterial cannulation.[53,54] The development of several novel upper-body configuration strategies minimizes these risks and facilitates mobilization. Internal jugular venous drainage may be combined with subclavian arterial reinfusion via an end-to-side graft.[15,43] In patients with either an atrial septal defect or patent foramen ovale, a dual-lumen cannula may be placed via the internal jugular vein with the reinfusion jet directed across the atrial septal defect, thereby creating an oxygenated right-to-left shunt.[55] In those without a preexisting atrial septal defect, one may be created via a septostomy.[56,57] A third strategy involves drainage from the main pulmonary artery and reinfusion into the left atrium via sternotomy.[58]

- Venoarterial ECMO can unload the right ventricle while creating an oxygenated right-to-left shunt in decompensated PH.
- ECMO may support temporarily patients in PH crisis with a potentially reversible process.
- Novel upper-body configurations help to avoid complications associated with femoral arterial cannulation.

Extracorporeal Cardiopulmonary Resuscitation

Extracorporeal cardiopulmonary resuscitation (ECPR), referring to the use of extracorporeal support to restore circulation during cardiac arrest, is a rapidly expanding indication for venoarterial ECMO, although the practice seems to be outpacing the data supporting its use.[59–62] There are no randomized trials for ECPR; however, several propensity analyses of prospective observational studies suggest a benefit to ECPR over conventional resuscitative measures. In 1 such study of 46 subjects receiving ECPR compared with 46 subjects receiving conventional cardiopulmonary resuscitation (CPR) for witnessed in-hospital cardiac arrest, those receiving ECPR had a significantly higher rate of survival at discharge (32.6% vs 17.4%; $P < .0001$) and 1 year (hazard ratio, 0.53; $P = .006$).[59] In a propensity analysis of 406 subjects suffering in-hospital cardiac arrest, those receiving ECPR (n = 85) had a significantly higher

2-year neurologically intact survival (20.0% vs 5.0%; P = .002) than those receiving conventional CPR (n = 321).[61] Younger age, shorter duration of CPR, and subsequent cardiac intervention (PCI or cardiac surgery) were associated with more favorable neurologic outcomes in the ECPR group. The survival benefit of ECPR, if present, may extend to those suffering out-of-hospital cardiac arrest. A recent propensity analysis of subjects undergoing CPR for at least 20 minutes for out-of-hospital cardiac arrest of presumed cardiac origin showed that those who received ECPR had a significantly higher rate of neurologically intact 3-month survival than those not receiving ECMO (29.2% vs 8.3%; P = .018).[62]

The combination of ECMO and intra-arrest PCI may further increase the likelihood of survival when cardiac arrest is owing to an acute coronary syndrome. The feasibility of such a strategy was demonstrated in a nonrandomized study of 81 subjects receiving ECMO and emergency coronary angiography, with rates of return of spontaneous beating, 30-day survival, and favorable neurologic outcomes of 100%, 36%, and 33% in those receiving ECPR and intra-arrest PCI (n = 61).[63] In-hospital cardiac arrest and more rapid institution of ECMO correlated favorably with survival.

Although these results are promising, more rigorous data are needed to better define the role of ECPR in cardiac arrest. Patient selection is key.[64] Because of the extensive resources and specialization needed to implement ECMO properly, ECPR should be restricted to centers experienced in its use.[65] Likewise, there should be strict criteria for initiating and withholding ECPR, so as to minimize its use in patients unlikely to benefit.[66]

- Data increasingly supports the emerging role of ECMO in cardiopulmonary resuscitation.
- ECPR is associated with improved neurologically intact survival as compared with conventional CPR.
- Appropriate patient selection is an essential component of ECPR implementation to maximize benefit.

INTERHOSPITAL TRANSPORT ON EXTRACORPOREAL MEMBRANE OXYGENATION

Advanced therapies for cardiac or respiratory failure, including mechanical circulatory support and heart and lung transplantation, are often limited to highly specialized centers. This centralization of resources restricts their access for many patients who could benefit from these interventions

but are too unstable to transport. With advances in extracorporeal technology leading to more compact circuit components, ECMO is increasingly mobile, allowing patients to be cannulated at their hospital of origin and transported safely to specialized centers.[67–72]

EARLY MOBILIZATION ON EXTRACORPOREAL MEMBRANE OXYGENATION

Physical therapy is widely accepted as an intervention that can improve outcomes of critically ill patients, including those receiving mechanical ventilation.[73,74] Patients on ECMO may likewise benefit from early mobilization and physical rehabilitation.[44,75] The advent of compact circuits makes ECMO more amenable to patient mobilization in conjunction with reduced sedative use and upper-body configurations (although femoral cannulation does not preclude mobilization).[41,44,76] Physical therapy in lung transplant candidates is essential to avoid deconditioning, which can preclude transplantation.[39,42]

- Patient mobilization is improved by advances in ECMO circuitry and configuration strategies as well as reduced sedation.

EXTRACORPOREAL MEMBRANE OXYGENATION AS DESTINATION THERAPY

The intention of destination device therapy is to provide long-term mechanical support of end-stage organ failure in patients who are not candidates for transplantation. A major limitation to the more widespread use of ECMO is its inability to function as a destination device and the need for ongoing management within an intensive care setting. In its current form, it may serve as a bridge to recovery, ventricular assist device, or heart transplant in cardiac failure, but in respiratory failure it can only bridge a patient to recovery or lung transplantation. Patients with irreversible lung disease who are dependent on ECMO and are not transplant candidates have no viable options, making patient selection for ECMO support a particularly important decision.[66] With further advances in technology, there is hope for the development of a portable destination device, effectively an artificial lung, which would have major implications for the approach to both acute and chronic respiratory failure.

- There is currently no destination device available for end-stage lung disease.
- The development of a portable destination device would lead to a major paradigm shift in the management of respiratory failure.

COMPLICATIONS

As with any intervention, there should be a careful consideration of the risks and benefits of ECMO specific to its indications for use. The most commonly reported complications of ECMO include hemorrhage, thrombosis, hemolysis, and infection,[4,5] although these rates have been on the decline with advances in extracorporeal technology.[3]

ECONOMIC IMPACT OF EXTRACORPOREAL MEMBRANE OXYGENATION

There is a relative paucity of economic assessments of ECMO in cardiac and respiratory failure, with costs varying widely by health system, choice of device components, duration of support, and management strategies.[77–81] In a study from the United Kingdom of patients with severe acute respiratory failure randomized to consideration of ECMO versus conventional management, the average total costs per patient were £73,979 versus £33,435, respectively (cost of ECMO per quality-adjusted life-year, £19,252). A separate cost analysis from Portugal for H1N1-associated ARDS estimated a cost of €1370 per day of ECMO support in a single caregiver model. Given its resource-intensive nature, additional cost–benefit analyses will be necessary to help guide the appropriate use of this intervention, particularly as the list of indications expands and more physicians become experienced in its use.

ETHICAL IMPLICATIONS OF EXTRACORPOREAL MEMBRANE OXYGENATION

There are a host of ethical dilemmas that may arise with the institution of extracorporeal support.[66] The use of ECMO as bridge to lung transplantation without the existence of a destination device creates the possibility of a "bridge to nowhere" if a patient is no longer eligible for transplantation. ECPR, if used indiscriminately, could create the possibility of an expectation of ECMO with any cardiac arrest. Likewise, the approach discussing a patient's wishes with regard to cardiopulmonary resuscitation becomes complicated by the fact that venoarterial ECMO provides partial or full cardiopulmonary support and may constitute a form of continuous, ongoing resuscitation, calling into question the appropriateness and significance of a "do not resuscitate" order.[82] These ethical dilemmas, among others, will only become more common as ECMO use expands. Careful selection of patients before the initiation of ECMO and thoughtful discussions with patients and their surrogates may help to avoid or prepare for some of these situations.

SUMMARY

Advances in extracorporeal technology have resulted in a resurgence of ECMO for cardiopulmonary disease over the last several years. More efficient membrane oxygenators and novel cannulation strategies have broadened the indications for which ECMO may offer a benefit, including hypercapnic respiratory failure, cardiogenic shock, and cardiac arrest. Ultimately, more studies are needed to determine the appropriate use and clinical impact of ECMO on respiratory and cardiac failure.

REFERENCES

1. Zapol WM, Snider MT, Hill JD, et al. Extracorporeal membrane oxygenation in severe acute respiratory failure. A randomized prospective study. JAMA 1979;242(20):2193–6.
2. Morris AH, Wallace CJ, Menlove RL, et al. Randomized clinical trial of pressure-controlled inverse ratio ventilation and extracorporeal CO_2 removal for adult respiratory distress syndrome. Am J Respir Crit Care Med 1994;149(2 Pt 1):295–305.
3. Extracorporeal Life Support Organization Registry Report. US Complications January 2014. Available at: www.elso.org. Accessed April 14, 2014.
4. Paden ML, Conrad SA, Rycus PT, et al. Extracorporeal life support organization registry report 2012. ASAIO J 2013;59(3):202–10.
5. Abrams D, Combes A, Brodie D. Extracorporeal membrane oxygenation in cardiopulmonary disease in adults. J Am Coll Cardiol 2014;63(25 Pt A):2769–78.
6. Brodie D, Bacchetta M. Extracorporeal membrane oxygenation for ARDS in adults. N Engl J Med 2011;365(20):1905–14.
7. Agerstrand CL, Bacchetta MD, Brodie D. ECMO for adult respiratory failure: current use and evolving applications. ASAIO J 2014;60(3):255–62.
8. Schmidt M, Tachon G, Devilliers C, et al. Blood oxygenation and decarboxylation determinants during venovenous ECMO for respiratory failure in adults. Intensive Care Med 2013;39(5):838–46.
9. Abrams D, Brodie D. Emerging indications for extracorporeal membrane oxygenation in adults with respiratory failure. Ann Am Thorac Soc 2013;10(4): 371–7.
10. Bein T, Weber F, Philipp A, et al. A new pumpless extracorporeal interventional lung assist in critical hypoxemia/hypercapnia. Crit Care Med 2006;34(5): 1372–7.
11. Javidfar J, Brodie D, Wang D, et al. Use of bicaval dual-lumen catheter for adult venovenous

extracorporeal membrane oxygenation. Ann Thorac Surg 2011;91(6):1763–8 [discussion: 1769].

12. Javidfar J, Wang D, Zwischenberger JB, et al. Insertion of bicaval dual lumen extracorporeal membrane oxygenation catheter with image guidance. ASAIO J 2011;57(3):203–5.

13. Wang D, Zhou X, Liu X, et al. Wang-Zwische double lumen cannula-toward a percutaneous and ambulatory paracorporeal artificial lung. ASAIO J 2008; 54(6):606–11.

14. Biscotti M, Lee A, Basner RC, et al. Hybrid configurations via percutaneous access for extracorporeal membrane oxygenation: a single center experience. ASAIO J 2014;60(6):635–42.

15. Javidfar J, Brodie D, Costa J, et al. Subclavian artery cannulation for venoarterial extracorporeal membrane oxygenation. ASAIO J 2012;58(5):494–8.

16. Morris AH. Exciting new ECMO technology awaits compelling scientific evidence for widespread use in adults with respiratory failure. Intensive Care Med 2012;38(2):186–8.

17. Combes A, Brechot N, Luyt CE, et al. What is the niche for extracorporeal membrane oxygenation in severe acute respiratory distress syndrome? Curr Opin Crit Care 2012;18(5):527–32.

18. Abrams D, Brodie D. Extracorporeal circulatory approaches to treat ARDS. Clin Chest Med 2014; 35(4):765–79.

19. Assistance Publique - Hôpitaux de Paris. Extracorporeal membrane oxygenation for severe acute respiratory distress syndrome (EOLIA). ClinicalTrials.gov. Bethesda (MD): National Library of Medicine (US); 2000. Available at: http://clinicaltrials.gov/ct2/show/NCT01470703. NLM Identifier: NCT01470703. Accessed July 1, 2012.

20. Rubenfeld GD, Caldwell E, Peabody E, et al. Incidence and outcomes of acute lung injury. N Engl J Med 2005;353(16):1685–93.

21. Rubenfeld GD, Herridge MS. Epidemiology and outcomes of acute lung injury. Chest 2007;131(2):554–62.

22. Ranieri VM, Rubenfeld GD, Thompson BT, et al. Acute respiratory distress syndrome: the Berlin definition. JAMA 2012;307(23):2526–33.

23. Hager DN, Krishnan JA, Hayden DL, et al. Tidal volume reduction in patients with acute lung injury when plateau pressures are not high. Am J Respir Crit Care Med 2005;172(10):1241–5.

24. Frank JA, Gutierrez JA, Jones KD, et al. Low tidal volume reduces epithelial and endothelial injury in acid-injured rat lungs. Am J Respir Crit Care Med 2002;165(2):242–9.

25. Terragni PP, Del Sorbo L, Mascia L, et al. Tidal volume lower than 6 ml/kg enhances lung protection: role of extracorporeal carbon dioxide removal. Anesthesiology 2009;111(4):826–35.

26. Bein T, Weber-Carstens S, Goldmann A, et al. Lower tidal volume strategy (approximately 3 ml/kg) combined with extracorporeal CO_2 removal versus 'conventional' protective ventilation (6 ml/kg) in severe ARDS: the prospective randomized Xtravent-study. Intensive Care Med 2013;39(5):847–56.

27. Brochard L, Mancebo J, Wysocki M, et al. Noninvasive ventilation for acute exacerbations of chronic obstructive pulmonary disease. N Engl J Med 1995;333(13):817–22.

28. Chandra D, Stamm JA, Taylor B, et al. Outcomes of noninvasive ventilation for acute exacerbations of chronic obstructive pulmonary disease in the United States, 1998-2008. Am J Respir Crit Care Med 2012; 185(2):152–9.

29. Ai-Ping C, Lee KH, Lim TK. In-hospital and 5-year mortality of patients treated in the ICU for acute exacerbation of COPD: a retrospective study. Chest 2005;128(2):518–24.

30. Bekaert M, Timsit JF, Vansteelandt S, et al. Attributable mortality of ventilator-associated pneumonia: a reappraisal using causal analysis. Am J Respir Crit Care Med 2011;184(10):1133–9.

31. MacIntyre NR. Aerosol delivery through an artificial airway. Respir Care 2002;47(11):1279–88 [discussion: 1285–79].

32. Abrams DC, Brenner K, Burkart KM, et al. Pilot study of extracorporeal carbon dioxide removal to facilitate extubation and ambulation in exacerbations of chronic obstructive pulmonary disease. Ann Am Thorac Soc 2013;10(4):307–14.

33. Burki NK, Mani RK, Herth FJ, et al. A novel extracorporeal CO_2 removal system: results of a pilot study of hypercapnic respiratory failure in patients with COPD. Chest 2013;143(3):678–86.

34. Kluge S, Braune SA, Engel M, et al. Avoiding invasive mechanical ventilation by extracorporeal carbon dioxide removal in patients failing noninvasive ventilation. Intensive Care Med 2012;38(10): 1632–9.

35. Brenner K, Abrams D, Agerstrand C, et al. Extracorporeal carbon dioxide removal for refractory status asthmaticus: experience in distinct exacerbation phenotypes. Perfusion 2014;29(1):26–8.

36. Mikkelsen ME, Woo YJ, Sager JS, et al. Outcomes using extracorporeal life support for adult respiratory failure due to status asthmaticus. ASAIO J 2009;55(1):47–52.

37. Maurer JR, Frost AE, Estenne M, et al. International guidelines for the selection of lung transplant candidates. The International Society for Heart and Lung Transplantation, the American Thoracic Society, the American Society of Transplant Physicians, the European Respiratory Society. Transplantation 1998; 66(7):951–6.

38. George TJ, Beaty CA, Kilic A, et al. Outcomes and temporal trends among high-risk patients after lung transplantation in the United States. J Heart Lung Transplant 2012;31(11):1182–91.

39. Javidfar J, Brodie D, Iribarne A, et al. Extracorporeal membrane oxygenation as a bridge to lung transplantation and recovery. J Thorac Cardiovasc Surg 2012;144(3):716–21.

40. Toyoda Y, Bhama JK, Shigemura N, et al. Efficacy of extracorporeal membrane oxygenation as a bridge to lung transplantation. J Thorac Cardiovasc Surg 2013;145(4):1065–70.

41. Fuehner T, Kuehn C, Hadem J, et al. Extracorporeal membrane oxygenation in awake patients as bridge to lung transplantation. Am J Respir Crit Care Med 2012;185(7):763–8.

42. Hoopes CW, Kukreja J, Golden J, et al. Extracorporeal membrane oxygenation as a bridge to pulmonary transplantation. J Thorac Cardiovasc Surg 2013;145(3):862–7.

43. Abrams DC, Brodie D, Rosenzweig EB, et al. Upper-body extracorporeal membrane oxygenation as a strategy in decompensated pulmonary arterial hypertension. Pulm Circ 2013;3(2):432–5.

44. Abrams D, Javidfar J, Farrand E, et al. Early mobilization of patients receiving extracorporeal membrane oxygenation: a retrospective cohort study. Crit Care 2014;18(1):R38.

45. Sakamoto S, Taniguchi N, Nakajima S, et al. Extracorporeal life support for cardiogenic shock or cardiac arrest due to acute coronary syndrome. Ann Thorac Surg 2012;94(1):1–7.

46. Sheu JJ, Tsai TH, Lee FY, et al. Early extracorporeal membrane oxygenator-assisted primary percutaneous coronary intervention improved 30-day clinical outcomes in patients with ST-segment elevation myocardial infarction complicated with profound cardiogenic shock. Crit Care Med 2010; 38(9):1810–7.

47. Tsao NW, Shih CM, Yeh JS, et al. Extracorporeal membrane oxygenation-assisted primary percutaneous coronary intervention may improve survival of patients with acute myocardial infarction complicated by profound cardiogenic shock. J Crit Care 2012;27(5):530.e1–11.

48. Pages ON, Aubert S, Combes A, et al. Paracorporeal pulsatile biventricular assist device versus extracorporeal membrane oxygenation-extracorporeal life support in adult fulminant myocarditis. J Thorac Cardiovasc Surg 2009;137(1):194–7.

49. Asaumi Y, Yasuda S, Morii I, et al. Favourable clinical outcome in patients with cardiogenic shock due to fulminant myocarditis supported by percutaneous extracorporeal membrane oxygenation. Eur Heart J 2005;26(20):2185–92.

50. Fayssoil A, Nardi O, Orlikowski D, et al. Percutaneous extracorporeal membrane oxygenation for cardiogenic shock due to acute fulminant myocarditis. Ann Thorac Surg 2010;89(2):614–6.

51. Mirabel M, Luyt CE, Leprince P, et al. Outcomes, long-term quality of life, and psychologic assessment of fulminant myocarditis patients rescued by mechanical circulatory support. Crit Care Med 2011;39(5):1029–35.

52. Rosenzweig EB, Brodie D, Abrams DC, et al. Extracorporeal membrane oxygenation as a novel bridging strategy for acute right heart failure in group 1 pulmonary arterial hypertension. ASAIO J 2014;60(1):129–33.

53. Aziz F, Brehm CE, El-Banyosy A, et al. Arterial complications in patients undergoing extracorporeal membrane oxygenation via femoral cannulation. Ann Vasc Surg 2014;28(1):178–83.

54. Roussel A, Al-Attar N, Khaliel F, et al. Arterial vascular complications in peripheral extracorporeal membrane oxygenation support: a review of techniques and outcomes. Future Cardiol 2013;9(4): 489–95.

55. Javidfar J, Brodie D, Sonett J, et al. Venovenous extracorporeal membrane oxygenation using a single cannula in patients with pulmonary hypertension and atrial septal defects. J Thorac Cardiovasc Surg 2012;143(4):982–4.

56. Hoopes CW, Gurley JC, Zwischenberger JB, et al. Mechanical support for pulmonary veno-occlusive disease: combined atrial septostomy and venovenous extracorporeal membrane oxygenation. Semin Thorac Cardiovasc Surg 2012;24(3):232–4.

57. Camboni D, Akay B, Sassalos P, et al. Use of venovenous extracorporeal membrane oxygenation and an atrial septostomy for pulmonary and right ventricular failure. Ann Thorac Surg 2011;91(1):144–9.

58. Strueber M, Hoeper MM, Fischer S, et al. Bridge to thoracic organ transplantation in patients with pulmonary arterial hypertension using a pumpless lung assist device. Am J Transplant 2009;9(4): 853–7.

59. Chen YS, Lin JW, Yu HY, et al. Cardiopulmonary resuscitation with assisted extracorporeal life-support versus conventional cardiopulmonary resuscitation in adults with in-hospital cardiac arrest: an observational study and propensity analysis. Lancet 2008;372(9638):554–61.

60. Shin TG, Choi JH, Jo IJ, et al. Extracorporeal cardiopulmonary resuscitation in patients with inhospital cardiac arrest: a comparison with conventional cardiopulmonary resuscitation. Crit Care Med 2011; 39(1):1–7.

61. Shin TG, Jo IJ, Sim MS, et al. Two-year survival and neurological outcome of in-hospital cardiac arrest patients rescued by extracorporeal cardiopulmonary resuscitation. Int J Cardiol 2013;168(4): 3424–30.

62. Maekawa K, Tanno K, Hase M, et al. Extracorporeal cardiopulmonary resuscitation for patients with out-of-hospital cardiac arrest of cardiac origin: a propensity-matched study and predictor analysis. Crit Care Med 2013;41(5):1186–96.

63. Kagawa E, Dote K, Kato M, et al. Should we emergently revascularize occluded coronaries for cardiac arrest?: rapid-response extracorporeal membrane oxygenation and intra-arrest percutaneous coronary intervention. Circulation 2012;126(13):1605–13.

64. Lan C, Tsai PR, Chen YS, et al. Prognostic factors for adult patients receiving extracorporeal membrane oxygenation as mechanical circulatory support–a 14-year experience at a medical center. Artif Organs 2010;34(2):E59–64.

65. Cave DM, Gazmuri RJ, Otto CW, et al. Part 7: CPR techniques and devices: 2010 American Heart Association guidelines for cardiopulmonary resuscitation and emergency cardiovascular care. Circulation 2010;122(18 Suppl 3):S720–8.

66. Abrams DC, Prager K, Blinderman CD, et al. Ethical dilemmas encountered with the use of extracorporeal membrane oxygenation in adults. Chest 2014;145(4):876–82.

67. Javidfar J, Brodie D, Takayama H, et al. Safe transport of critically ill adult patients on extracorporeal membrane oxygenation support to a regional extracorporeal membrane oxygenation center. ASAIO J 2011;57(5):421–5.

68. Wallace DJ, Angus DC, Seymour CW, et al. Geographic access to high capability severe acute respiratory failure centers in the United States. PLoS One 2014;9(4):e94057.

69. Roch A, Hraiech S, Masson E, et al. Outcome of acute respiratory distress syndrome patients treated with extracorporeal membrane oxygenation and brought to a referral center. Intensive Care Med 2014;40(1):74–83.

70. Lee SG, Son BS, Kang PJ, et al. The feasibility of extracorporeal membrane oxygenation support for inter-hospital transport and as a bridge to lung transplantation. Ann Thorac Cardiovasc Surg 2014;20(1):26–31.

71. Raspe C, Ruckert F, Metz D, et al. Inter-hospital transfer of ECMO-assisted patients with a portable miniaturized ECMO device: 4 years of experience. Perfusion 2014;30(1):52–9.

72. Foley DS, Pranikoff T, Younger JG, et al. A review of 100 patients transported on extracorporeal life support. ASAIO J 2002;48(6):612–9.

73. Needham DM, Korupolu R. Rehabilitation quality improvement in an intensive care unit setting: implementation of a quality improvement model. Top Stroke Rehabil 2010;17(4):271–81.

74. Schweickert WD, Pohlman MC, Pohlman AS, et al. Early physical and occupational therapy in mechanically ventilated, critically ill patients: a randomised controlled trial. Lancet 2009;373(9678):1874–82.

75. Rehder KJ, Turner DA, Hartwig MG, et al. Active rehabilitation during extracorporeal membrane oxygenation as a bridge to lung transplantation. Respir Care 2013;58(8):1291–8.

76. Olsson KM, Simon A, Strueber M, et al. Extracorporeal membrane oxygenation in nonintubated patients as bridge to lung transplantation. Am J Transplant 2010;10(9):2173–8.

77. Peek GJ, Mugford M, Tiruvoipati R, et al. Efficacy and economic assessment of conventional ventilatory support versus extracorporeal membrane oxygenation for severe adult respiratory failure (CESAR): a multicentre randomised controlled trial. Lancet 2009;374(9698):1351–63.

78. Peek GJ, Elbourne D, Mugford M, et al. Randomised controlled trial and parallel economic evaluation of conventional ventilatory support versus extracorporeal membrane oxygenation for severe adult respiratory failure (CESAR). Health Technol Assess 2010;14(35):1–46.

79. Cavarocchi N, Wallace S, Hong E, et al. A cost-reducing extracorporeal membrane oxygenation (ECMO) program model: a single institution experience. Perfusion 2015;30(2):148–53.

80. Roncon-Albuquerque R Jr, Almeida V, Lopes M, et al. Cost analysis of miniaturized ECMO in H1N1-related ARDS managed by a single caregiver. Intensive Care Med 2014;40(6):910–1.

81. Borisenko O, Wylie G, Payne J, et al. The cost impact of short-term ventricular assist devices and extracorporeal life support systems therapies on the national health service in the UK. Interact Cardiovasc Thorac Surg 2014;19(1):41–8.

82. Meltzer EC, Ivascu NS, Fins JJ. DNR and ECMO: a paradox worth exploring. J Clin Ethics 2014;25(1):13–9.

Novel Uses of Targeted Temperature Management

John McGinniss, MD[a],*, Peter Marshall, MD, MPH[b],
Shyoko Honiden, MSc, MD[b]

KEYWORDS

- Targeted temperature management • Hypothermia • Cardiac arrest • Prognosis • Methodology
- Therapeutic hypothermia

KEY POINTS

- Compared with out-of-hospital cardiac arrest with ventricular tachycardia/ventricular fibrillation (VT/VF) as the initial rhythm, there is less benefit for targeted temperature management (TTM) after in-hospital cardiac arrest and for an initial rhythm of pulseless electrical activity/asystole.
- TTM has emerging evidence as a therapeutic modality for the critically ill patient with ischemia-reperfusion injury, refractory intracranial hypertension, and systemic inflammation.
- Maintaining normothermia may be as effective as deeper cooling in TTM. In addition, there is debate about the most effective method of TTM application as well as the optimal parameters for TTM.
- TTM is safe to use in a highly monitored setting in an experienced center. There seems to be an increased risk of pneumonia with TTM use, but no increased risk of bleeding or arrhythmia.
- TTM delays the ability of caregivers to accurately prognosticate in the comatose patient after cardiac arrest. The best estimates of prognosis take into consideration several of the following: patient factors, the clinical neurologic examination, neuroimaging, biomarkers, somatosensory-evoked potentials, and electroencephalogram.

INTRODUCTION
Historical Context and Current Practice

Over the past 200 years, purposefully lowering the body's temperature to improve health outcomes has evolved from anecdote to experimental therapy to widespread implementation. One of the first descriptions of medical hypothermia was by Russians in 1803, who would bury an individual to the neck in snow while trying for return of spontaneous circulation (ROSC).[1] This process of intentionally lowering a patient's core body temperature came to be known as therapeutic hypothermia (TH).

However, in 2011, a statement by 5 critical care societies found this term too vague, especially pertaining to appropriate temperature targets.[2] They reasoned that targeted temperature management (TTM) was a more specific term that emphasized the importance of protocols having 3 explicitly stated phases: induction, maintenance, and rewarming.

The first clinical trial of TTM in human cardiac arrest was by Benson and colleagues in 1959.[3] Despite finding a survival advantage of TTM, large-scale studies were not undertaken until the early 2000s, when 2 major prospective randomized

Disclosures: None.
[a] Pulmonary, Allergy & Critical Care Division, Hospital of the University of Pennsylvania, 3400 Spruce Street, 839 West Gates Building, Philadelphia, PA 19104, USA; [b] Section of Pulmonary, Critical Care and Sleep Medicine, Department of Medicine, Yale School of Medicine, 333 Cedar Street, New Haven, CT 06520-8057, USA
* Corresponding author.
E-mail address: john.mcginniss@uphs.upenn.edu

Clin Chest Med 36 (2015) 385–400
http://dx.doi.org/10.1016/j.ccm.2015.05.011
0272-5231/15/$ – see front matter © 2015 Elsevier Inc. All rights reserved.

controlled studies set the framework for modern application of TTM in out-of-hospital cardiac arrest (OHCA). The HACA (Hypothermia after Cardiac Arrest Study Group) reported a relative risk (RR) of 0.74 (95% confidence interval [CI]: 0.58–0.95) for mortality at 6 months after TTM to 32°C for 24 hours was applied for ventricular fibrillation (VF) arrest. The number needed to treat was 7 to save one life and 6 to achieve one favorable neurologic outcome.[4] A favorable neurologic outcome was defined as a 1 or 2 on the Pittsburgh Cerebral-Performance Category scale (**Box 1**).[5] This scale is the most used of the TTM outcomes literature. In the same issue of *New England Journal of Medicine*, Bernard and colleagues[6] found a higher likelihood of a good neurologic outcome defined as normal, mild, or moderate neurologic deficit, allowing discharge to home or short-term rehabilitation facility in the intervention group. These landmark studies changed how those with OHCA are managed and suggested that inducing moderate hypothermia could improve outcomes.

These 2 studies provided the evidence that led to the American Heart Association (AHA) rating TTM after VF OHCA for adults as a "class 1, level of evidence B" recommendation in 2010.[7] Perhaps in part helped by widespread adoption of post-cardiac arrest care that included TTM, OHCA outcomes have been improving. In 2014, the large CARES (Cardiac Arrest Registry to Enhance Survival) study reported an improvement in risk-adjusted survival in OHCA to hospital discharge from 5.7% in 2005 to 2006 to 7.2% in 2008 to 2009 and finally to 8.3% by 2012 to 2013, along with better neurologic outcomes of survivors.[8] In short, a patient with OHCA was 47% more likely to survive in 2011–2012 compared with 2005–2006.

Purpose of the Review

There are excellent comprehensive reviews on TTM.[9–11] The remainder of this review focuses on uncertainties intensivists face when making decisions regarding application of TTM to the adult patient other than for the class 1B application in OHCA. Selected landmark prospective randomized trials of TTM in these novel clinical situations are summarized in **Table 2**. The following clinical questions are addressed: Which patients might benefit from TTM? Which modality is best? At what temperature and for what duration should TTM be applied? What are the adverse events related to TTM and how can one monitor for them or prevent these complications? These questions are addressed in the context of emerging TTM evidence.

Targeted Temperature Management Mechanisms of Cellular Protection

Neurologic injury during cardiac arrest is a well-studied paradigm of ischemia-reperfusion injury. Classically described are 3 phases. Initially, lack of tissue perfusion results in primary cellular energy failure wherein anaerobic metabolism predominates, membrane potentials are lost, intracellular calcium accumulates, and excitatory neurotransmitters become abundant.[12] During the second phase (after ROSC), there is reperfusion injury. Here, injured, swollen mitochondria produce reactive oxygen species that cause direct cellular damage and activate pro-apoptotic pathways and intracellular proteases. During a delayed third phase, a pro-inflammatory state causes secondary cell injury.[10–12]

During ischemia-reperfusion, TTM reduces injury through multiple mechanisms. For every 1°C temperature drop, cerebral metabolism reduces 6%

Box 1
Cerebral performance category

Category

1	Good cerebral performance
	• Conscious, independent on ADL, IADL
	• Work full time
	• Minor neurologic impairment
2	Moderate cerebral disability
	• Conscious, independent ADL, IADL
	• Work part time
3	Severe cerebral disability
	• Conscious but dependent on others for ADL, IADL
4	Coma/vegetative state
	• Unconscious, unaware of surroundings
	• No cognition
5	Brain death
	• Unconscious
	• Traditional criteria by certified practitioners

Abbreviations: ADL, activities of daily living; IADL, instrumental activities of daily living.

Data from Blondin NA, Greer DM. Neurological prognosis in cardiac arrest patients treated with therapeutic hypothermia. Neurologist 2011;17:241–8.

to 10%; this reduces free radical production, calcium influx into cells, and mitochondrial injury and improves maintenance of cell membrane integrity.[10,11] In addition, inflammation during reperfusion and rewarming is dampened.[13] TTM also modulates the coagulation-fibrinolysis axis. Harmful microthrombi that occur during low-flow states are prevented by an anticoagulant effect during cooling along with less platelet activation; in parallel, however, fibrinolysis is reduced.[14]

Furthermore, TTM not only affects the CNS but also has wide reaching systemic effects (**Table 1**). The benefits of TTM must be balanced by the inherent risks when this therapy is considered.

QUESTION 1: WHICH INTENSIVE CARE UNIT PATIENTS WITH NEUROLOGIC INJURY SHOULD I COOL?

Nonshockable and In-Hospital Cardiac Arrest

The strongest evidence favoring TTM is in those with pulseless ventricular tachycardia (VT) or VF as the initial rhythm after cardiac arrest. In contrast, there is uncertain benefit of TTM in pulseless electrical activity (PEA)/asystole—the "nonshockable" rhythms.

In a prospective cohort analysis of OHCA patients, good neurologic outcome was seen in 39% of the total VT/VF cohort as opposed to only 16% of those presenting with PEA/asystole (P<.001).[15] Even after adjustment for treatment received, the odds of good neurologic outcome in VT/VF patients treated with TTM was increased (adjusted odds ratio [OR] 1.90; 95% CI: 1.18–3.06) compared with TTM-treated nonshockable rhythm patients (adjusted OR 0.71; 95% CI: 0.37–1.36).

A 2012 systematic review and meta-analysis of adults with OHCA with an initial nonshockable rhythm found no 6-month mortality benefit (RR 0.85; 95% CI: 0.65–1.11) or improved neurologic outcomes (RR 0.88; 95% CI: 0.71–1.08).[16] However a subanalysis of prospective, nonrandomized trials suggested reduced risk of in-hospital mortality with TTM (RR 0.86; 95% CI: 0.76–0.99) but no difference in neurologic outcome at discharge.[16] Therefore, benefit was seen in prospective, nonrandomized trials, but not in the randomized controlled trial (RCT) data or a large registry analysis. Accordingly, the intensive care unit (ICU) physician may apply TTM in this population knowing that an initial rhythm of PEA/asystole portends a poor prognosis, that TTM is unlikely to worsen outcomes, and if there are benefits, they are likely small based on the currently limited evidence.

As for those with IHCA, a large observational study found good outcomes for patients (both shockable and nonshockable rhythm) treated with TTM: 57% survived to hospital discharge and, of those, 41% had a good neurologic outcome.[17] Currently, the AHA guidelines suggest TTM should be considered for comatose survivors of IHCA as an IIB recommendation.[7]

Hepatic Encephalopathy

In the ICU, patients with acute liver failure (ALF), especially with severe (West Haven Grade III or IV) hepatic encephalopathy, are at very high risk of death by intracranial hypertension from cerebral edema. There is emerging evidence that TTM can mitigate this process. To date, there are retrospective studies and nonrandomized prospective data that support TTM in ALF as a bridge to transplantation.[18–20] Despite this being a high-risk population, data suggest TTM can be safely applied. In the authors' center, they have found TTM to be feasible and safe without increased bleeding or infection with a protocol that does not dictate routine use of invasive intracranial pressure (ICP) monitoring devices (McGinniss, unpublished data, 2014). The best use of TTM in the context of ALF with severe encephalopathy remains in highly specialized centers using TTM protocols with transplant capability. It is best thought of as an advanced, supportive technology to manage refractory intracranial hypertension while transplant evaluation is ongoing. There are no data to suggest benefit as a stand-alone therapy in ALF.

Acute Ischemic Stroke

Similar to hepatic encephalopathy, massive acute ischemic stroke (AIS) can be complicated by life-threatening cerebral edema that leads to herniation and death. Early interest in TTM for AIS arose from the observation that increased temperature during stroke was a poor prognostic sign.[21] Thereafter, the benefit of TTM was demonstrated in animals, preclinical models, and uncontrolled studies. Despite promising early data, a meta-analysis did not find that TTM during AIS improved neurologic outcomes or mortality, and in fact, suggested higher rates of pneumonia.[22]

To more definitively answer the question, 2 large randomized, multicenter, prospective clinical trials are underway comparing normothermia to hypothermia as an add-on therapy to tissue plasminogen activator: these are the Intravascular Cooling in the Treatment of Stroke 2/3 (ICTuS2/3, NCT01123161) and the Cooling Plus Best Medical Treatment versus Best Medical Treatment Alone for AIS (EuroHYP-1, NCT0183312) trial. Currently, TTM cannot be recommended in routine practice for AIS, but it may be considered salvage therapy for refractory ICP elevation after AIS.

Table 1
Physiologic effects of targeted temperature management

Organ System	Mechanism	Clinical Outcome	Monitoring
Cardiovascular	1. Spontaneous depolarization rate (sinus node included) 2. Myocardial contractility (EF down by 7% every 1°C) 3. Myocardial oxygen demand 4. SVR 5. Venous return with increased ANP	1. Atrial fibrillation 2. VF 3. Sinus bradycardia 4. Prolonged: PR, QRS, QT 5. Osborn waves (prominent J wave) with temperature <32°C	1. BP, HR 2. Systemic perfusion 3. QTc
Neurologic	1. Cerebral metabolism 2. Cerebral vasoconstriction 3. Protected blood-brain barrier integrity	1. ICP 2. Cerebral edema	1. EEG 2. Pupillary examination (neuromuscular blockers can interfere)
Pulmonary	1. CO_2 production 2. Tissue oxygen extraction	1. Hypoventilation	1. Monitor PCO_2 during ventilation to make sure not overventilating 2. Important to avoid hyperoxia after cardiac arrest
Hematological	1. Anticoagulant state 2. Fibrinolysis 3. Platelet activation	1. Bleeding	1. Coagulation studies 2. Clinical bleeding
Renal	1. Tubular dysfunction 2. Cellular shifts	1. Hypokalemia 2. Hypomagnesemia 3. Hypernatremia 4. Hypophosphatemia 5. Hypocalcemia 6. Cold diuresis	1. Chemistry 2. Urine output
Musculoskeletal/ dermatologic	1. Catecholamines released to oppose drop in body temperature	1. Shivering 2. Cutaneous vasoconstriction 3. Pressure ulcers	1. Clinical examination
Endocrine	1. Insulin release and sensitivity 2. Fat metabolism	1. Hyperglycemia 2. Circulating ketones	1. Glucose monitoring
Gastrointestinal	1. Gut motility 2. Hepatic dysfunction	1. Ileus 2. Risk of stress ulcer 3. Hepatic synthetic function 4. Hypoglycemia	1. LFT, INR 2. Monitor clinically for signs of enteral feeding intolerance and consider following gastric residuals
Immunologic	1. Risk of infection	1. Risk of secondary infection	1. High index of clinical suspicion of infection 2. Low threshold for empiric therapy
Pharmacologic	1. Delayed drug clearance	1. Drug toxicity 2. Drug-drug interactions	1. Measure serum levels when appropriate 2. Consult with pharmacist

Abbreviations: ANP, atrial natriuretic peptide; BP, blood pressure; EF, ejection fraction; HR, heart rate; INR, international normalized ratio; LFT, liver function tests; SVR, systemic vascular resistance.
    Data from Refs.[2,7,9–14]

Intracerebral Hemorrhage

TTM was used in a feasibility trial of patients with aneurysmal subarachnoid hemorrhage (SAH) complicated by refractory intracranial hypertension or cerebral vasospasm (CVS) requiring operative intervention. Patients were cooled to 33°C to 34°C until the increased ICP normalized, CVS resolved, or there was an intolerable side effect.[23] TTM was applied for a mean of 169 hours and 35.6% survived with good neurologic outcome, 16% were severely disabled, and 47.8% died. Although this was an uncontrolled case series, the outcomes at 1 year were better than historical data. They found patients younger than 60 years of age and those with CVS (as opposed to refractory ICP elevation) had better outcomes. Randomized trials reproducing these results are needed before TTM can be routinely recommended for the management of refractory intracranial hypertension or CVS in aneurysmal SAH.

A case series examining prolonged TTM for 8 to 10 days for large supratentorial ICH found a reduction in perihemorrhagic edema.[24] There are ongoing prospective, randomized clinical trials examining TTM after intracerebral hemorrhage: these include the Targeted Temperature Management after Intracerebral Hemorrhage (TTM-ICH, NCT01607151) and the Cooling in Intracerebral Hemorrhage (CINCH, ISRCTN2899995) studies. It is hoped that these studies will clarify the role of TTM in ICH.

Traumatic Brain Injury

There has been interest in using TTM as a means to attenuate secondary neurologic injury after traumatic brain injury (TBI). Early trials had mixed results.[25,26] A recent well-designed prospective RCT did not find any benefit of TTM in nonpenetrating TBI even with early application.[27] A *Cochrane Review* noted that studies of low methodological quality generally found improved neurologic outcomes and survival, but studies with higher methodological quality and good allocation concealment found no benefit to TTM.[28] Thus, TTM cannot be routinely recommended for secondary neurologic protection after TBI and should be considered only on a case-by-case basis for management of refractory intracranial hypertension.

QUESTION 2: WHICH INTENSIVE CARE UNIT PATIENTS WITH NONNEUROLOGIC INJURY SHOULD I COOL?
Acute Myocardial Infarction

Because TTM mitigates ischemia-reperfusion neurologic injury after OHCA, there has been interest in myocardial preservation after myocardial

infarction. Proponents have theorized that TTM will improve myocardial demand, tissue ischemia, and reperfusion injury to heart muscle, especially when combined with modern cardiac interventional care.

Clinical trials using TTM in ST-elevation myocardial infarction (STEMI) patients failed to show definite benefit. An early belief was that reaching a core temperature of less than 35°C before reperfusion was needed to have any effect on infarct size.[29] A 2014 RCT by Erlinge and colleagues[30] found that despite all TTM patients reaching goal temperature before percutaneous coronary intervention, there was only a 13% reduction in infarct size detected on cardiac MRI at 4 days, which was ultimately not statistically significant.

Current data in acute myocardial infarction (AMI) rely on surrogate outcomes such as infarct size on imaging and do not assess patient-centered outcomes such as mortality, symptoms, or quality of life. Future studies using clinical outcomes will have to demonstrate benefit before TTM can be recommended. Currently, applying TTM to STEMI patients is not prudent.

Sepsis

The discussion to this point has focused on conditions whereby time of onset (and mechanism) of injury is relatively well defined. Commonly encountered clinical situations in the ICU, such as sepsis and acute respiratory distress syndrome (ARDS), have more divergent tempo and pathways of injury. Can these entities derive benefit from TTM? Central to both sepsis and ARDS pathophysiology is a complex cascade of inflammatory responses to an insult that damages bystander normal tissue and fuels organ dysfunction.

TTM to 32°C in a rat model of induced invasive pneumococcal pneumonia has shown promise.[31] Hypothermic animals had no change in bacterial load in the lung, trended toward less bacteremia, and had less seeding of end organs. There was also less lung injury (based on bronchoalveolar lavage protein and interleukin-1 [IL-1] levels), reduced oxygen consumption, and increased ATP levels in the hypothermic rats. Other investigators, using a cecal ligation model to stimulate peritoneal sepsis in rats, found that animals cooled to 34°C had improved survival, lower serum creatinine, and preservation of adaptive increases in oxygen delivery usually observed in sepsis.[32]

In humans, an RCT studying TTM during sepsis used surface cooling to maintain normothermia in patients presenting with septic shock and fever.[33] They found that TTM was safe and that it aided in shock reversal with reductions in early vasopressor requirements. Fourteen-day mortality was lower compared with the control group, but there was no effect on overall ICU mortality or hospital mortality at hospital discharge. To date, this has been the only RCT investigating TTM use among septic shock patients. Although the data suggest TTM may help improve vascular tone and oxygen consumption and reduce inflammation, results need to be replicated in future studies. Thus, despite tantalizing preclinical animal models, TTM cannot currently be recommended for routine application in patients with septic shock.

Acute Respiratory Distress Syndrome

TTM has been beneficial in animal models of lung injury. A recent study of TTM to 32°C in rats with ARDS from ventilator-induced lung injury (ventilated at 18 mL/kg) noted reduced neutrophil recruitment, IL-6 levels, and histopathological injury.[34] In humans, however, data have been sparse. An early proof of concept trial in 1993 studied 19 patients with ARDS from sepsis. Those assigned to TTM at 32°C to 35°C had improvements in mortality (100% in the usual care group to 67% in the TTM arm), a reduction in A-a gradient, and preserved O_2 extraction.[35] Nonetheless, these results were obtained before modern ARDS care with low tidal volume ventilation (as evidenced by the 100% mortality in the control arm), which questions its relevance to the current ARDS population.

There has also been interest in studying the effect of TTM on respiratory mechanics. A study of mechanically ventilated patients after OHCA found those receiving TTM had decreased P_{CO_2} and decreased length of mechanical ventilation (7.3 vs 10.7 days, $P = .04$).[36] There was a nonstatistically significant trend toward improved Pa_{O_2}/Fi_{O_2} ratio.

It is likely that TTM reduces inflammation in the injured lung and may improve lung mechanics and gas exchange. Despite this, there is insufficient evidence to support the use of TTM in ARDS as an adjunct or salvage therapy. The current data do, however, provide a rationale for future human randomized trials.

Meningitis

TTM was studied in acute bacterial meningitis with the rationale that adjunctive TTM might reduce inflammation causing tissue damage.[37] Safety implications (**Table 2**) from one trial argue strongly against the use of TTM in bacterial meningitis.

Contrast-Induced Nephropathy

Contrast-induced nephropathy (CIN) is a common problem, especially in patients with chronic kidney disease. Few interventions have proven beneficial in reducing the incidence of CIN. In one RCT, TTM was attempted as a therapeutic modality in addition to the standard-of-care fluid management. There was no harm in the TTM arm, but no clinical benefit either.[40] Therefore, TTM should not be used to help prevent CIN given a lack of efficacy.

Traumatic Cardiac Arrest

As opposed to the above medical applications of TTM with mild cooling to 32°C to 34°C, there is a group of investigators interested in cooling patients to 10°C.[41] Deep cooling, known as emergency preservation and resuscitation (EPR), is being examined for patients suffering cardiac arrest after traumatic exsanguination. The hypothesis is that, in some cases, TTM to this extreme using a direct flush of cold saline into the aorta will preserve organs while allowing surgeons enough time to restore hemostasis. This direct flush of cold saline into the aorta has been done in pig and dog models with success, and there is a US Food and Drug Administration–approved clinical feasibility trial, the EPR for Cardiac Arrest from Trauma (EPR-CAT, NCT01042015), which will begin to enroll human trauma patients.

QUESTION 3: HOW SHOULD I COOL CRITICALLY ILL PATIENTS?
Surface Versus Endovascular

The critical care clinician has a variety of options when it comes to the modality (**Table 3**) of inducing hypothermia.[42,43] Endovascular cooling can be done by cold saline infusion or by an endovascular device. Cold saline can quickly reduce core temperature and is easy to use; however, low core temperature cannot be sustained with cold saline alone.[44]

Endovascular cooling may cause less shivering (and therefore, less need for sedatives and paralytics) by preferentially cooling the core. A single-center randomized trial in sudden cardiac arrest (including both IHCA and OHCA) found equivalent levels of neuron-specific enolase—a surrogate plasma marker for neuronal injury—and equivalent survival and neurologic outcomes.[45] The invasive device better maintained goal temperature but caused more clinical bleeding (44% vs 18%). A further risk to consider related to endovascular devices is an increased risk of deep vein thrombosis.[46]

Intranasal Induction

An intranasal device is another induction option: a catheter placed into the nasal passage vaporizes

Table 2
Selected meta-analysis and randomized controlled trials of targeted temperature management in novel clinical situations

Study	Patients	Design	Method of TTM	Outcome	Comment
OHCA: Nonshockable rhythm					
Bernard et al,[38] 2012	N: 163 Inclusion: OHCA, PEA/asystole on initial rhythm, age >14, SBP > 90 (can be on epinephrine drip) with prehospital IV cooled saline by EMS Control: Same criteria, ED initiated IV saline	Single-center, prospective, randomized trial	Mode: Intravenous cooled saline (EMS or ED) to hospital surface cooling Duration: 24 h Goal temperature: 32°C–34°C Rewarming: Active at 0.25°C/h to 0.5°C/h	Efficacy: 1. No difference in favorable outcome at discharge (to home or to rehabilitation) (P = .50) Safety: Not reported	No benefit of TTM started prehospital for OHCA from a nonshockable rhythm.
Myocardial infarction					
Erlinge et al,[29] 2013	N: 197 Inclusion: STEMI to undergo PCI, age 18–75, symptoms <6 h Control: Usual STEMI care	Pooled analysis of 2 RCTs (ICE-IT and RAPID MI-ICE)	Mode: IV chilled saline and endovascular cooling Duration: 6 h Goal temperature: <35°C Rewarming: Not reported	Efficacy: 1. TTM reduced infarct size relative to LV at risk by SPECT (P = .049). Effect increased for those with temperature <35°C before intervention Safety: Not reported	Reaching TTM before intervention may reduce infarct size.
Erlinge et al,[30] 2014	N: 120 Inclusion: STEMI to undergo PCI, age 18–75, symptoms <6 h Control: Usual STEMI care	Multicenter, multicountry prospective RCT	Mode: Chilled saline and endovascular cooling Duration: 1 h after reperfusion Goal temperature: 33°C Rewarming: Passive	Efficacy: 1. No change in infarct size relative to LV at risk (by cardiac MRI at 4 d) (P = .15) 2. No deaths in either group Safety: No difference in infection, arrhythmia, reinfarction, bleeding, or stroke	The highest quality study to date in AMI. TTM caused a delay of 9 min in door-to-balloon time. No change in infarct size was seen. Secondary analyses suggested there may be less CHF post-MI and improvement in the anterior MI infarct size.

(continued on next page)

Table 2
(continued)

Study	Patients	Design	Method of TTM	Outcome	Comment
Neurologic emergencies					

Wan et al,[22] 2014	N: 252 patients from 6 RCTs
	
	Inclusion:
	  Adults with AIS with symptoms ranging from 6 to 24 h
	
	Control:
	  Thrombolytic therapy when indicated, one study included hemicraniectomy
		Meta-analysis of 6 prospective RCTs from 2004 to 2014	Mode:
			  2 surface based, 2 endovascular, 2 IV chilled saline
			Duration:
			  Four studies for 24 h, one study 48 h, one study 10.5 h
			Goal temperature:
			  Four studies cooled to 33°C, 2 studies to 35°C
			Rewarming:
			  0.04–0.5°C/h
				Efficacy:
				1. No difference in mortality ($P = .70$)
				2. No difference in favorable neurologic outcome ($P = .46$)
				Safety:
				  RR for pneumonia of 3.3 ($P = .003$). No difference in intracranial hemorrhage, DVT, or atrial fibrillation
					This meta-analysis did not find any benefit in neurologic outcomes or mortality in the 6 included studies. They found increased incidence of pneumonia. When they analyzed the depth of TTM and rewarming speeds, neither were associated with better outcomes.

Todd et al,[39] 2005	N: 1001
	
	Inclusion:
	  Adult patients with acute aneurysmal SAH no more than 14 d before open surgical clipping. They had World Federation of Neurological Surgeon score of 1–3 (good-grade patients)
	
	Control:
	  Surgery without TTM
		Multicenter, prospective RCT	Mode:
			  Intraoperative surface cooling
			Duration:
			  Intraoperative, duration not specified
			Goal temperature:
			  33°C by placement of first clip
			Rewarming:
			  Passive
				Efficacy:
				1. No difference in 90-d mortality (6% in each group)
				2. No difference in Glasgow Outcome Score of 1 (good outcome) ($P = .32$)
				Safety:
				  5% of TTM patients had bacteremia compared with 3% in normothermia ($P = .05$)
					There was no difference in neurologic outcomes or mortality for intraoperative TTM for aneurysmal SAH. This study is limited by short application of TTM and uncontrolled rewarming. Higher incidence of bacteremia was noted.

Clifton et al,[27] 2011	N: 232 Inclusion: Adults 16–45 with nonpenetrating brain injury, not responsive to instruction. Control: Usual care	Multicenter, prospective, RCT, 1:1 concealed allocation	Mode: IV saline, then surface cooling Duration: 35°C during the trauma assessment, then 33°C for 48 h Goal temperature: 33°C Rewarming: 0.5°C/h	Efficacy: 1. No difference in poor neurologic outcome (severe disability, vegetative state, death) ($P = .67$) 2. No difference in mortality ($P = .52$) Safety: No increased bleeding, arrhythmia, infection	Early application of TTM for severe TBI did not result in improved neurologic outcomes in this well-designed trial.
Septic shock					
Schortgen et al,[33] 2012	N: 200 Inclusion: ICU patients with presumed infection, shock needing vasopressors, mechanical ventilation, and fever >38.3°C Control: No control of fever	Multicenter, prospective, RCT, 1:1 allocation	Mode: External cooling Duration: 48 h Goal temperature: Normothermia 36.5°C–37°C Rewarming: Passive	Efficacy: 1. More patients had a 50% reduction in vasopressors with TTM at 12 h ($P<.001$). Not significant at 48 h 2. More patients had shock reversal in the ICU with TTM ($P = .021$) 3. The TTM group had reduced 14-d mortality ($P = .013$) but this was not significant at ICU ($P = .26$) or hospital discharge ($P = .51$) Safety: No difference in acquired infection	This study suggests that TTM to maintain normothermia in septic shock patients with fever was safe, improved early hemodynamics and early mortality. These effects diminished after 48 h.

(continued on next page)

Table 2
(continued)

Study	Patients	Design	Method of TTM	Outcome	Comment
Meningitis					
Mourvillier et al,[37] 2013	N: 98 Inclusion: Community-acquired bacterial meningitis with GCS <8 Control: Usual care	Multicenter, prospective, open-label study	Mode: 4°C cold saline Duration: 48 h Goal temperature: 32°C–34°C Rewarming: Passive	Efficacy: 1. There was higher mortality in the TTM group (P = .04). After adjustment for age, GCS, shock on admission, mortality, HR 1.76 (P = .10) Safety: No difference in pneumonia, hemorrhage, arrhythmia	This trial was stopped early for concern of excess mortality in the TTM arm. After adjustment, this effect was no longer statistically significant.
Contrast-induced nephropathy					
Stone et al,[40] 2011	N: 128 Inclusion: CKD (creatinine clearance 20–50 mL/min) getting >50 mL of iodinated contrast Control: IV hydration	1:1 allocation, prospective RCT	Mode: Endovascular cooling device Duration: Before procedure and 3 h afterward Goal temperature: 33°C–34°C Rewarming: 1°C/h	Efficacy: 1. There was no difference in incidence of a >25% increase in creatinine postcontrast (P = .59) Safety: Similar mortality, MI, arrhythmia, bleeding, dialysis, rehospitalization between groups	TTM in addition to IV hydration is safe but ineffective for CIN prevention.

Abbreviations: CKD, chronic kidney disease; DVT, deep vein thrombosis; ED, emergency department; EMS, emergency medical services; GCS, Glasgow Coma Scale; HR, hazard ratio; ICE-IT, Intravascular Cooling Adjunctive to Percutaneous Coronary Intervention; IV, intravenous; LV, left ventricle; MI, myocardial infarction; RAPID MI-ICE, Rapid Intravascular Cooling in Myocardial Infarction as Adjunctive to Percutaneous Coronary Intervention; SPECT, single-photon emission computed tomography.

an inert, volatile coolant, allowing rapid cooling of the nasal passage, then the brain, followed by the rest of the body. In a feasibility trial called PRINCE, investigators used this device during OHCA in the prehospital setting and found a faster time to goal (34°C) temperature—102 versus 282 minutes.[47] This study was not powered to detect survival or neurologic outcome so a larger study for OHCA and intra-arrest cooling, the PRINCESS study (NCT01400373), is ongoing. Currently, this device is only used as a means to rapidly initiate TH and is not recommended for maintenance of hypothermia.

Use of Adjunctive Agents: Inhaled Xenon

Xenon is a noble gas that is a noncompetitive antagonist of the glutamate *N*-methyl-D-aspartate receptor. This property makes it an attractive agent for neuroprotection by attenuating the excitotoxic injury common in the post-cardiac arrest syndrome (PCAS) and other secondary neurologic injuries. In VT/VF OHCA, patients receiving TTM combined with Xenon had no difference in complication rates, experienced lower heart rates, reduced norepinephrine needs, and lowered troponin-T serum concentrations compared with those receiving TTM alone.[48] Larger studies will be needed to confirm the safety of inhaled Xenon and prove its efficacy.

Overall, in terms of choosing the modality of TTM, there are no clear efficacy data to guide the intensivist in deciding between endovascular and surface modalities. The decision to choose surface versus endovascular cooling should be based on the local expertise and general risks and benefits regarding indwelling intravascular devices. The intravascular device likely puts patients at higher risk of catheter-related adverse events (ie, infection and bleeding), but allows the patient to be examined freely and would be less intrusive should procedures need to be done. Intranasal and inhaled Xenon should be considered investigational. Cold saline should be used adjunctively if rapid induction is desired.

QUESTION 4: WHAT ARE THE PRACTICAL CONSIDERATIONS FOR TARGETED TEMPERATURE MANAGEMENT USE?
Timing of Targeted Temperature Management

A prospective, randomized trial of patients with OHCA from VF and without VF were randomized to receive prehospital 4°C normal saline, up to 2 L, as soon as possible after ROSC.[49] This intervention reduced the time to goal 34°C by about 1 hour; however, neurologic outcomes and survival were unchanged. Another smaller study of prehospital induction of TTM in nonshockable rhythms also found no difference in outcomes.[38]

Time to Goal Temperature

A small study found that each hour delay to goal temperature conferred a 30% increased chance of worse neurologic outcome.[50] It is difficult to reconcile this observation with the finding that initiation of cooling prehospitalization does not improve clinical outcomes.[49] To complicate this picture, a retrospective cohort study analyzing time to goal temperature and OHCA outcomes found patients with an unfavorable neurologic outcome had a faster time to goal than those with good neurologic outcome.[51] This study was retrospective but suggests more severely injured patients are easier to cool because of impaired thermoregulation. Most protocols suggest rapid induction of TTM to goal temperature, and the authors agree that this should be done until higher quality evidence proves otherwise.

Depth of Cooling

In a large international, multicenter RCT comparing 33°C versus 36°C in OHCA of presumed cardiac cause, there was no difference in survival or neurologic outcomes.[52] Another recent study found that TTM to 33°C or 36°C after OHCA resulted in similar IL-6 levels and other inflammatory cytokines when measured for up to 72 hours after rewarming.[53] These studies call into question the old adage, "colder is better" when it comes to cooling in OHCA, or other applications. Controlling temperature and prevention of hyperthermia may be the most important aspects of TTM.

Duration and Rewarming

An animal study in cardiac arrest found slow rewarming at 0.5°C to 1°C per hour improved cardiovascular and neurologic outcomes compared with rewarming at 2°C per hour.[54] There have been sparse data in humans, however. An observational study did not find a benefit to active versus passive rewarming approach.[55] Another study noted fever within 36 hours after the rewarming phase portended higher mortality and worse neurologic outcomes.[56]

Most experts recommend fast induction, sustained TTM at goal for 12 to 36 hours (or until clinical improvement, particularly for noncardiac arrest scenarios), and controlled rewarming.[7] They additionally agree that sustained TTM for more than 36 hours will increase the infection risk and other adverse events.

Table 3
Comparison of cooling devices

Parameter	Internal		External				Inhaled
	Endovascular/Catheter Devices	Infused Cool Crystalloid (4°C)	Hydrogel Coated Water-Circulating Pads	Water Circulating Cooling Blankets/Pads	Conducting Gel Pads	Ice Packs	Intranasal Induction
Core cooling rate (°C/h)	2.0–5.0	2.5–3.5	1.5–2.0	1.0–1.5	2.6–3.5	1.0	1.1–1.4
Relative cost[a]	++++	−−	+++	+	+	−−	++
Controlled rewarming possible	Yes	N/A (induction)	Yes	Yes	No	No	N/A (induction)
Advantages	• Fast rate of cooling; reliable maintenance and rewarming • Tolerable in conscious patients (eg, stroke, MI)	• Fast rate of cooling • Easily accessible • Adjunct to other methods	• Easy to use; fast rate of cooling; reliable rewarming	• Targeted neck cooling possible; inexpensive compared with disposable devices	• Fastest surface cooling device • Easy to use • Portable, can be used prehospital	• Easy; inexpensive	• Easy to use • Can initiate in field • Preferential brain cooling • Adjunct to other methods
Disadvantages	• Requires central access → may cause delays & add risk • Risk of catheter-related thrombosis, infections, bleeding	• Cannot use to maintain temperature • Cannot use to control rewarming	• Slight risk of skin lesions if prolonged use	• Labor intensive for nurses • Two blankets required	• No temperature feedback • Difficult to keep temperature stable	• Risk of skin lesions and burns • Unreliable maintenance & rewarming • Comparatively slower	• Adverse effects to nasal area (epistaxis, periorbital gas emphysema) • Potential aspiration of coolant into lungs • Gradient between tympanic and core temperatures
Examples	Thermoguard XP (Zoll), InterCool RTx (Phillips)	LR, NSS	Arctic Sun 2000, 5000	Blanketrol III	Flex.Pad	N/A	RhinoChill

[a] Per manufacturers: Cincinnati Sub-Zero Company for Blanketrol III©, Medivance for Arctic Sun 5000©; BeneChill for RhinoChill©; EMCools for Flex.Pad©; Zoll for Thermoguard xP©, and Alsius Catheters© (Icy Catheter & Cool Line); Phillips for IntreCool RTx© (Accutrol Catheter).
Data from Refs.[42–47]

QUESTION 5: IS TARGETED TEMPERATURE MANAGEMENT SAFE? HOW SHOULD I MONITOR TARGETED TEMPERATURE MANAGEMENT PATIENTS?

Infection

Most patients undergoing TTM are in the ICU, are intubated, and have indwelling catheters that already increase their risk of infection. Review of randomized trials using TTM for any indication found no increased prevalence of overall infection but risk of pneumonia was increased (RR 1.44; 95% CI: 1.10–1.90).[57]

Patients should be monitored closely while receiving TTM with a low threshold to obtain cultures and start antibiotics given they have a blunting of the usual signs and symptoms of infection. Sepsis should be suspected if a patient's hemodynamics decompensate while on TTM. A retrospective study suggested that patients treated with early systemic antibiotics within 1 week during TTM after OHCA had improved survival.[58] Despite this limited observation, routine administration of prophylactic antibiotics for possible pneumonia cannot be recommended and needs further study. Proven ventilator-associated pneumonia prevention measures should be adhered to.

Bleeding

Another concern in TTM application is induced coagulopathy. A recent meta-analysis in OHCA found a nonstatistically significant trend toward increased overall bleeding in patients receiving TTM, but no difference in major bleeding.[59]

Electroencephalogram Monitoring

Osborn waves or J waves has a characteristic upright deflection beginning at the end of the QRS complex and continuing into the early ST segment that occurs during hypothermia—both accidental and during TTM. There is a weak correlation between amplitude of the J wave and degree of hypothermia.[60]

A study of ECG changes for TTM patients found prolonged PR and QTc intervals, lower heart rate, and shortened QRS intervals.[61] None of these, including prolonged QTc, were associated with poor outcomes. Even in the myocardial infarction TTM literature, there was no increased incidence of atrial or ventricular arrhythmias.[29,30]

Electrolyte Monitoring

A pH less than 7.20 on initiation of TTM correlates with poor neurologic outcomes in OHCA.[62] Hyperglycemia on initiation of TTM also seems to be an independent risk factor for mortality in OHCA and is common during TTM due to worsened insulin resistance. Thus, attentive glucose control should be standard practice.[63,64] During rewarming, however, clinicians need to be aware of potential hypoglycemia because the hypothermia-induced insulin resistance is reversed.

Renal tubular function is diminished and, with induction and maintenance of TTM, there is a cold diuresis with polyuria.[65] Along with the kaliuresis, potassium shifts intracellularly and may result in significant hypokalemia (see **Table 1**). Potassium along with magnesium, calcium, and phosphorus needs close monitoring.

Prognostication

Despite improved survival in OHCA and to some extent for other disease states where TTM is used, many patients still face poor neurologic outcomes. The use of sedatives, paralytics, and anticonvulsants in the setting of delayed drug metabolism caused by TTM renders conventional means of assessing prognosis less reliable.[5] The widely used American Academy of Neurology 2006 guidelines for prognostication for comatose survivors of cardiac arrest was made before the widespread use of TTM.[66] A recent report of OHCA survivors who received TTM found 78% regained consciousness within 48 hours after rewarming, 11% from 48 to 72 hours, and 11% after 72 hours—suggesting there is a subset of patients who will have good neurologic recovery even if they awaken after 3 days post-rewarming.[67]

To date, the neuroimaging literature for prognostication is heterogeneous with no clear best practice. A review found CT and diffusion-weighted MRI detected structural brain injury from anoxia and protocols that were combined with the clinical examination seemed to perform best.[68]

A multimodal evaluation using clinical assessment of brainstem reflexes and myoclonus, electroencephalogram (EEG) reactivity, and a neuron-specific enolase level great than 33 ug/L had the high positive predictive value for mortality and poor neurologic outcome.[69] The European Resuscitation Council and the European Society of Intensive Care Medicine concluded, based on the limited evidence, that absent or extensor motor response 72 hours after ROSC, absent corneal or pupillary reflexes, and bilateral absence of N20 wave of short-latency somatosensory-evoked potential (SSEP) were the most robust predictors of poor outcome.[70] They also stated that myoclonus, EEG, and CT/MRI were useful in the evaluation of the comatose postarrest patient.

Currently, there is no consensus on the best algorithm for prognostication, but a multimodal approach integrating clinical examination, EEG, SSEP, neuroimaging and, if available, neuron-specific enolase serum levels therefore seems most promising. It is best to err on the side of caution and delay decisions about withdrawal of care in the setting of uncertainty until at least 72 hours after normothermia has been achieved.[5]

SUMMARY

TTM has an established role in treating the PCAS in OHCA for VT/VF with less certain benefit in PEA/asystole and IHCA. It is a reliable salvage modality for conditions causing intracranial hypertension, and the evidence for use in other disorders characterized by systemic inflammation or local ischemia-reperfusion injury is evolving. Questions remain as to the optimal parameters for TTM application, ideal monitoring, and best prognostication protocols for the comatose patient after TTM.

REFERENCES

1. Varon J, Acosta P. Therapeutic hypothermia: past, present, and future. Chest 2008;133:1267–74.
2. Nunnally NE, Jaeschke R, Bellingan GJ, et al. Targeted temperature management in critical care: a report and recommendations from five professional societies. Crit Care Med 2011;39:1113–25.
3. Benson DW, Williams GR, Spencer FC, et al. The use of hypothermia after cardiac arrest. Anesth Analg 1959;38:423–8.
4. The Hypothermia After Cardiac Arrest Study Group. Mild hypothermia to improve the neurological outcome after cardiac arrest. N Engl J Med 2002; 346:549–56.
5. Blondin NA, Greer DM. Neurological prognosis in cardiac arrest patients treated with therapeutic hypothermia. Neurologist 2011;17:241–8.
6. Bernard SA, Gray TW, Buist MD, et al. Treatment of comatose survivors of out-of-hospital cardiac arrest with induced hypothermia. N Engl J Med 2002; 346:557–63.
7. Peberdy MA, Callaway CW, Neumar RW, et al. Part 9: post-cardiac arrest care: 2010 American Heart Association Guidelines for Cardiopulmonary Resuscitation and Emergency Cardiovascular Care. Circulation 2010;122:S768–86.
8. Chan PS, McNally B, Tang F, et al. Recent trends in survival from out-of-hospital cardiac arrest in the United States. Circulation 2014;130:1876–82.
9. Perman SM, Goyal M, Neurman RW, et al. Clinical applications of targeted temperature management. Chest 2014;145:386–93.
10. Scirica BM. Therapeutic hypothermia. Circulation 2013;127:244–50.
11. Delhaye C, Mahmoudi M, Waksman R, et al. Hypothermia therapy: neurological and cardiac benefits. J Am Coll Cardiol 2012;59:197–210.
12. Poldermann KH. Mechanisms of action, physiological effects, and complications of hypothermia. Crit Care Med 2009;37:S186–202.
13. Bisschops LA, van der Hoeven JG, Mollnes TE, et al. Seventy-two hours of mild hypothermia after cardiac arrest is associated with a lowered inflammatory response during rewarming in a prospective observational study. Crit Care 2014;18:546–53.
14. Gong P, Zhang MY, Zhao H, et al. Effect of mild hypothermia on the coagulation-fibrinolysis system and physiological anticoagulants after cardiopulmonary resuscitation in a porcine model. PLoS One 2013;8:e67476.
15. Dumas F, Grimaldi D, Zuber B, et al. Is hypothermia after cardiac arrest effective in both shockable and nonshockable patients?: Insights from a large registry. Circulation 2011;123:877–86.
16. Kim YM, Yim HW, Jeong SH, et al. Does therapeutic hypothermia benefit adult cardiac arrest patients presenting with non-shockable rhythms?: A systematic review and meta-analysis of randomized and non-randomized studies. Resuscitation 2012;83:188–96.
17. Dankiewicz J, Schmidbauer S, Nielsen N, et al. Safety, feasibility, and outcomes of induced hypothermia therapy following in-hospital cardiac arrest—evaluation of a large prospective registry. Crit Care Med 2014;42:2537–45.
18. Jalan R, Damink SW, Deutz NE, et al. Moderate hypothermia for uncontrolled intracranial hypertension in acute liver failure. Lancet 1999;354:1164–8.
19. Jalan R, Damink SW, Deutz NE, et al. Moderate hypothermia in patients with acute liver failure and uncontrolled intracranial hypertension. Gastroenterology 2004;127:1338–46.
20. Raschke RA, Curry SC, Rempe S, et al. Results of a protocol for the management of patients with fulminant liver failure. Crit Care Med 2008;36:2244–8.
21. Reith J, Jørgensen HS, Pedersen PM, et al. Body temperature in acute stroke: relation to stroke severity, infarct size, mortality and outcome. Lancet 1996;347:422–5.
22. Wan YH, Nie C, Wang HL, et al. Therapeutic hypothermia (different depths, durations, and rewarming speeds) for acute ischemic stroke: a meta-analysis. J Stroke Cerebrovasc Dis 2014;23:2736–47.
23. Seule MA, Muroi C, Mink S, et al. Therapeutic hypothermia in patients with aneurysmal subarachnoid hemorrhage, refractory intracranial hypertension, or cerebral vasospasm. Neurosurgery 2009;64:86–92.
24. Staykov D, Wagner I, Volbers B, et al. Mild prolonged hypothermia for large intracerebral hemorrhage. Neurocrit Care 2013;18:178–83.
25. Marion DW, Penrod LE, Kelsey SF, et al. Treatment of traumatic brain injury with moderate hypothermia. N Engl J Med 1997;20:540–6.

26. Clifton GL, Miller ER, Choi SC, et al. Lack of effect of induction of hypothermia after acute brain injury. N Engl J Med 2001;344:556–63.

27. Clifton GL, Valadka A, Zygun D, et al. Very early hypothermia induction in patients with severe brain injury (the National Acute Brain Injury Study: Hypothermia II): a randomised trial. Lancet Neurol 2011; 10:131–9.

28. Sydenham E, Roberts I, Alderson P. Hypothermia for traumatic head injury. Cochrane Database Syst Rev 2009;(2):CD001048.

29. Erlinge D, Götberg M, Grines C, et al. A pooled analysis of the effect of endovascular cooling on infarct size in patients with ST-elevation myocardial infarction. EuroIntervention 2013;8:1435–40.

30. Erlinge D, Götberg M, Lang I, et al. Rapid endovascular catheter core cooling combined with cold saline as an adjunct to percutaneous coronary intervention for the treatment of acute myocardial infarction [CHILL-MI]. J Am Coll Cardiol 2014;63:1857–65.

31. Beurskens CJ, Aslami H, Kuipers MT, et al. Induced hypothermia is protective in a rat model of pneumococcal pneumonia associated with increased adenosine triphosphate availability and turnover. Crit Care Med 2012;40:916–26.

32. Léon K, Pichavant-Rafini K, Quéméner E, et al. Oxygen transport during experimental sepsis: effect of hypothermia. Crit Care Med 2012;40:912–8.

33. Schortgen F, Clabault K, Katsahian S, et al. Fever control using external cooling in septic shock: a randomized controlled trial. Am J Respir Crit Care Med 2012;185:1088–95.

34. Aslami H, Kuipers MT, Beurskens CJ, et al. Mild hypothermia reduces ventilator-induced lung injury, irrespective of reducing respiratory rate. Transl Res 2012;159:110–7.

35. Villar J, Slutsky AS. Effects of induced hypothermia in patients with septic adult respiratory distress syndrome. Resuscitation 1993;26:183–92.

36. Karnatovskaia LV, Festic E, Freeman WD, et al. Effect of therapeutic hypothermia on gas exchange and respiratory mechanics: a retrospective cohort study. Ther Hypothermia Temp Manag 2014;4:88–95.

37. Mourvillier B, Tubach F, va de Beek D, et al. Induced hypothermia in severe bacterial meningitis. JAMA 2013;310:2174–83.

38. Bernard SA, Smith K, Cameron P, et al. Induction of prehospital therapeutic hypothermia after resuscitation from nonventricular fibrillation cardiac arrest. Crit Care Med 2012;40:747–53.

39. Todd MM, Hindman BJ, Clarke WR, et al. Mild intraoperative hypothermia during surgery for intracranial aneurysm. N Engl J Med 2005;352:135–45.

40. Stone GW, Vora K, Schindler J, et al. Systemic hypothermia to prevent radiocontrast nephropathy (from the COOL-RCN randomized trial). Am J Cardiol 2011;108:741–6.

41. Tisherman SA. Salvage techniques in traumatic cardiac arrest: thoracotomy, extracorporeal life support, and therapeutic hypothermia. Curr Opin Crit Care 2013;19:594–8.

42. Hoedemaekers CW, Ezzahti M, Gerritsen A, et al. Comparison of cooling methods to induce and maintain normo- and hypothermia in intensive care unit patients: a prospective intervention study. Crit Care 2007;11:R91.

43. Tømte Ø, Drægni T, Mangschau A, et al. A comparison of intravascular and surface cooling techniques in comatose cardiac arrest survivors. Crit Care Med 2011;39:443–9.

44. Polderman KH, Rijnsburger ER, Peerdeman SM, et al. Induction of hypothermia in patients with various types of neurological injury with use of large volumes of ice-cold intravenous fluid. Crit Care Med 2005;33:2744–51.

45. Pittl U, Schratter A, Desch S, et al. Invasive versus non-invasive cooling after in- and out-of-hospital cardiac arrest: a randomized trial. Clin Res Cardiol 2013;102:607–14.

46. Simosa HF, Petersen DJ, Agarwal SK, et al. Increased risk of deep venous thrombosis with endovascular cooling in patients with traumatic head injury. Am Surg 2007;73:461–4.

47. Castrén M, Norberg P, Svensson L, et al. Intra-arrest transnasal evaporative cooling: a randomized prehospital, multicenter study (PRINCE: pre-ROSC intranasal cooling effectiveness). Circulation 2010; 122:729–36.

48. Arola OJ, Laitio RM, Roine RO, et al. Feasibility and cardiac safety of inhaled xenon in combination with therapeutic hypothermia following out-of-hospital cardiac arrest. Crit Care Med 2013;41:2116–24.

49. Kim F, Nichol G, Maynard C, et al. Effect of prehospital induction of mild hypothermia on survival and neurological status among adults with cardiac arrest. JAMA 2014;311:45–52.

50. Wolff B, Machill K, Schumacher D, et al. Early achievement of mild therapeutic hypothermia and the neurological outcome after cardiac arrest. Int J Cardiol 2009;133:223–8.

51. Haugk M, Testori C, Sterz F, et al. Relationship between time to target temperature and outcome in patients treated with therapeutic hypothermia after cardiac arrest. Crit Care 2011;15:R101.

52. Nielsen N, Wetterslev J, Cronberg T, et al. Targeted temperature management at 33°C versus 36°C after cardiac arrest. N Engl J Med 2013;369:2197–206.

53. Bro-Jeppesen J, Kjaergaard J, Wanscher M, et al. The inflammatory response after out-of-hospital cardiac arrest is not modified by targeted temperature management at 33°C or 36°C. Resuscitation 2014; 85:1480–7.

54. Lu X, Ma L, Sun S, et al. The effects of the rate of postresuscitation rewarming following hypothermia

on outcomes of cardiopulmonary resuscitation in a rat model. Crit Care Med 2014;42:e106–13.

55. Bouwes A, Robillard LB, Binnekade JM, et al. The influence of rewarming after therapeutic hypothermia on outcome after cardiac arrest. Resuscitation 2012;83:996–1000.

56. Bro-Jeppesen J, Hassager C, Wanscher M, et al. Post-hypothermia fever is associated with increased mortality after out-of-hospital cardiac arrest. Resuscitation 2013;84:1734–40.

57. Geurts M, Macleod MR, Kollmar R, et al. Therapeutic hypothermia and the risk of infection: a systematic review and meta-analysis. Crit Care Med 2014;42:231–42.

58. Davies KJ, Walters JH, Kerslake IM, et al. Early antibiotics improve survival following out-of hospital cardiac arrest. Resuscitation 2013;84:616–9.

59. Stockmann H, Krannich A, Schroeder T, et al. Therapeutic temperature management after cardiac arrest and the risk of bleeding: systematic review and meta-analysis. Resuscitation 2014;85:1492–503.

60. Omar HR, Camporesi EM. The correlation between the amplitude of Osborn wave and core body temperature. Eur Heart J Acute Cardiovasc Care 2014. http://dx.doi.org/10.1177/2048872614552057.

61. Lam DH, Dhingra R, Conley SM, et al. Therapeutic hypothermia-induced electrocardiographic changes and relations to in-hospital mortality. Clin Cardiol 2014;37:97–102.

62. Ganga HV, Kallur KR, Patel NB, et al. The impact of severe acidemia on neurological outcome of cardiac arrest survivors undergoing therapeutic hypothermia. Resuscitation 2013;84:1723–7.

63. Kim SH, Choi SP, Park KN, et al. Association of blood glucose at admission with outcomes in patients treated with therapeutic hypothermia after cardiac arrest. Am J Emerg Med 2014;32:900–4.

64. Sah Pri A, Chase JG, Pretty CG, et al. Evolution of insulin sensitivity and its variability in out-of-hospital cardiac arrest (OHCA) patients treated with hypothermia. Crit Care 2014;18:586.

65. Raper JD, Wang HE. Urine output changes during postcardiac arrest therapeutic hypothermia. Ther Hypothermia Temp Manag 2013;3:173–7.

66. Wijdicks EF, Hijdra A, Bassetti CL, et al. Practice parameter: prediction of outcome in comatose survivors after cardiopulmonary resuscitation (an evidence-based review). Neurology 2006;67:203–10.

67. Gold B, Puerta L, Davis SP, et al. Awakening after cardiac arrest and post resuscitation hypothermia: are we pulling the plug too early? Resuscitation 2014;85:211–4.

68. Hahn DK, Geocadin RG, Greer DM. Quality of evidence in studies evaluating neuroimaging for neurological prognostication in adult patients resuscitated from cardiac arrest. Resuscitation 2014;85:165–72.

69. Oddo M, Rossetti AO. Early multimodal outcome prediction after cardiac arrest in patients treated with hypothermia. Crit Care Med 2014;42:1340–7.

70. Sandroni C, Cariou A, Cavallaro F, et al. Prognostication in comatose survivors of cardiac arrest: an advisory statement from the European Resuscitation Council and the European Society of Intensive Care Medicine. Intensive Care Med 2014;40:1816–31.

ICU Telemedicine Solutions

Steven A. Fuhrman, MD[a], Craig M. Lilly, MD[b,c,d],*

KEYWORDS

- Telemedicine • Intensive care unit • eICU • Virtual medicine • Tele-ICU

KEY POINTS

- Intensive care unit (ICU) telemedicine programs have improved patient safety practices by standardizing best-practice processes and achieving high rates of adherence through real-time collaboration.
- ICU telemedicine programs provide an effective solution to the problem of alarm fatigue and provide immediate management by off-site Critical Care experts.
- ICU telemedicine programs are one remedy for physician and nursing staffing shortages.
- ICU telemedicine programs can improve the financial performance of health care systems that standardize processes and engage in population management.
- ICU telemedicine–associated reporting solutions and real-time intervention are increasingly being used to improve ICU quality metrics, including those that are publicly reported.

INTENSIVE CARE UNIT TELEMEDICINE SOLUTIONS

In April, 1924, *Radio News*[1] teased that a "radio doctor" may someday bring virtual medical care directly to patients. In that decade, house calls were common and twice-daily hospital rounds a mainstay of patient evaluation and treatment so the construct probably seemed nonsensical. However, the increasing need for high-quality subspecialty care and advances in telecommunication technology have now transformed that prescient fantasy of 1924 into an achievable and increasingly common[2] approach to getting the right expertise to the right patient at the right time.

This article focuses on critical care services that are provided via telemedicine. It describes the evolution of the technology and the ways that telemedicine tools are supporting the practices of critical care professionals.

The potential for telecommunications technology to make information available where and when it is needed was explored nearly 40 years ago by a group that provided real-time intensive care unit (ICU) consultation using television.[3,4] The failure of this attempt to use telecommunication tools without informatics support stifled the development of ICU telemedicine. Clinicians learned that television consultation that relied on verbal descriptions of clinical information is

Disclosures: None.
[a] Division of Pulmonary and Critical Care Medicine, Sentara Norfolk General Hospital, Sentara eICU, Sentara Medical Group, Raleigh 306, Norfolk, VA 23507, USA; [b] Department of Medicine, UMass Memorial Medical Center, University of Massachusetts Medical School, 281 Lincoln Street, Worcester, MA 01605, USA; [c] Department of Anesthesiology, UMass Memorial Medical Center, University of Massachusetts Medical School, 281 Lincoln Street, Worcester, MA 01605, USA; [d] Department of Surgery, UMass Memorial Medical Center, University of Massachusetts Medical School, 281 Lincoln Street, Worcester, MA 01605, USA
* Corresponding author. University of Massachusetts Medical School, UMass Memorial Medical Center, 281 Lincoln Street, Worcester, MA 01605.
E-mail address: craig.lilly@umassmed.edu

Clin Chest Med 36 (2015) 401–407
http://dx.doi.org/10.1016/j.ccm.2015.05.004

inefficient and prone to errors of omission and interpretation. Since then, advances and integration of health information technology have led to the wide adoption of ICU telemedicine. Reports from a 1997 intervention provided proof of concept for a critical care delivery construct in which off-site intensivists could deliver care that was superior to usual care.[5] The maturation of the tools and refinement of the interactions among bedside clinicians and off-site intensivists led to reports from Norfolk, Virginia, of an ICU telemedicine program implementation in the year 2000 that was associated with less mortality and shorter length of stay (LOS).[6]

These studies led to the commercialization of enabling health information and telecommunications technologies.[7,8] The adoption of ICU telemedicine was increasingly driven by the evolving shortage of critical care–trained physicians that was accurately predicted by Angus and Kelley.[9] During the first decade of the growth of ICU telemedicine, services were most commonly delivered by a team of professionals located at an off-site telemedicine center. Initial reports were promising because program implementation was associated with lower ICU mortality and ICU LOS.[2,8,10] One key element of these reports was that access to high-quality critical care services was increased through workforce leveraging that allowed each telemedicine intensive care specialist to support many more patients than was possible with geographically restricted staffing models.

These early reports were followed by studies of ICU telemedicine program implementations with mixed results, including studies that were not associated with significantly reduced mortality or LOS.[11–13] One conclusion was that simply making telemedicine tools available is not sufficient to guarantee improved outcomes. Several investigators prominently cited poor integration and acceptance of the telemedicine program in the conventional work flow of the ICU as one explanation for limited impact. The recognition that both implementation and outcomes were heterogeneous led to analyses of combined studies.[10,13] These reports also generated mixed results because some could not distinguish a lack of effect because of inadequate sample size.[10,14] Moreover, lack of information about specific processes that were changed by this complex intervention made it difficult to identify characteristics and process changes that predict association with better outcomes. A subsequent large multi-center study showed that workstation-assisted remote intensivist case review, improved adherence to ICU best practices, reduced response times to alarms, interprofessional rounding, and

real-time use of performance measures were characteristics of ICU telemedicine programs that were significantly associated with larger reductions in mortality and LOS.[15]

Three common factors have emerged that prompt transitions from traditional ICU staffing models to those that integrate ICU telemedicine: (1) enhanced patient safety; (2) a workforce solution; and (3) improved outcomes through population management, standardization of the process of care, and reporting solutions that improve ICU management.

PATIENT SAFETY

The most common primary driver for the earliest wave of adoption of an ICU telemedicine program was patient safety. An influx of patients presenting to hospital emergency departments with critical illness and injuries[16] increased the number of at-risk patients at a time when workforce growth was limited by a lack of physicians who were trained in critical care,[9] the restriction of duty hours for physicians in training,[17] and nursing workforce shortages.[18]

Further, the advent of sparsely tested and expensive bedside monitors resulted in new risks for patients. One widely adopted strategy to limit labor costs was to replace telemetry staff with monitoring systems that alerted bedside staff at central monitoring stations. The unintended consequence of relying on monitoring systems with high false-positive alarm rates was that some alerts were missed because most were not actionable.[19–24] Increased rates of failure to rescue have defined the alarm-fatigue crisis that is a target of current national patient safety efforts.[25]

ICU telemedicine professionals who provide real-time evaluation of physiologic alerts, filter false-positive signals, and triage true-positive alarms are one effective remedy for alarm fatigue.[26] A community hospital 10-bed ICU with an average APACHE IV (Acute Physiology and Chronic Health Evaluation) score of 50 to 60 generates as many as 100,000 alerts for physiologic instability per year. Most alerts are attended to by bedside nurses, but several true-positive events per patient per day are not recognized by the bedside team in a time that is considered safe. On average, video evaluation by an off-site critical care professional resulted in more than 1 intervention per ICU per day that was recorded in the medical record as involving a major change to the care plan. Telemedicine interventions for higher-acuity populations are more frequent despite the availability of more bedside resources; however, delays in bedside attendance to true-positive alerts are more common among the lower-acuity ICU patients. ICU telemedicine support applies both technology-based alerting and professional review to augment the situational awareness of the bedside staff. Studies that evaluate alerts have also documented that, without ICU telemedicine support, bedside nursing response to 90% of alarms for physiologic instability within 3 minutes of their onset occurs in only 45% of ICUs, whereas, with ICU telemedicine support, 71% report achieving this benchmark (P<.001).[27] ICUs with reported response times to physiologic alerts of less than 3 minutes had significantly shorter ICU LOS compared with those reporting longer response times.[15] Delays in response for unstable patients were clustered at times when nurses were helping colleagues, had new or more than 1 unstable patient, were retrieving or preparing medications, or were engaged in change-of-shift communication. One study documented that nurses only responded to 80% of true-positive alerts for impending physiologic instability without prompting from an off-site provider.[26] Teamwork around alarm management is a key element of safer ICU care that is part of an ICU telemedicine program.

A large multicenter study that analyzed the characteristics of 56 ICUs and changes in processes of critical care delivery in relation to outcomes after an ICU telemedicine implementation identified critical care specialist case involvement, short response times to alerts and alarms, interprofessional rounding, and the use of real-time feedback on adherence to performance measures as factors that were associated with larger improvements in survival and LOS.[15] Case reviews by critical care specialists that focus on care plan implementation are thought to improve outcomes because they help to ensure the completeness of volume resuscitation, timeliness of infection source control measures, early administration of antimicrobials, efficient detection and effective management of hypoxemia, and achievement of high rates of adherence to consensus ICU best practices.[7,26] There is increasing evidence that intensivist review at the onset of physiologic instability is associated with improved outcomes.

INCREASED ACCESS TO EXPERTISE: A LEVERAGED WORKFORCE SOLUTION

The need for greater access to adult ICUs was accurately predicted based on the aging of the population[16] and the exponential increase in the use of critical care services as a function of age after adulthood. The implementation of an ICU telemedicine program that can provide a leveraged workforce solution is one effective means

of increasing access to high-quality ICU care.[28] The most common model leverages off-site board-certified critical care specialists to provide evaluation and management services to support nonspecialist bedside providers at times when bedside specialists are not on site. This model is most frequently applicable with reduced bedside specialist availability at night and on weekends but also has significant impact on the immediacy of evaluation and care as bedside specialists move to other geographies during their regular daytime responsibilities. The ICU telemedicine solution has also been effective for hospitals that do not have on-site critical care specialists.[15] In this model ICU telemedicine specialists support hospitalists by providing care plan reviews at the time of admission and real-time management and comanagement. Alternatively or concomitantly, nurse practitioners or physician assistants may be supported with after-hours supervision by the ICU telemedicine critical care specialist.[29] Telemedicine tools allow oversight, remove geographic barriers to specialist availability, and equip qualified specialists with organized clinical information and early-warning systems.

The efficiency of the off-site intensivist approach is related to the ability of the telemedicine ICU team to provide care for geographically dispersed patients. The team is configured based on patient volume, efficiency of communication with bedside providers, patient acuity, and the ability of the electronic infrastructure to capture and organize clinical information. At the time of this writing, an ICU telemedicine team with 1 intensivist can effectively care for as many as 150 ICU patients. The typical ICU telemedicine team partners 1 intensivist with 2 to 4 nurses and administrative personnel to provide evaluation and management services. The common work flow involves a methodical routine of surveillance that is typically patient by patient, often as a skill-based assessment organized by organ system that includes a review of best-practice adherence. Telemedicine review has achieved higher rates of best-practice adherence than bedside hardcopy checklists.[26,30] This routine may be interrupted by system-generated alerts for abnormal laboratory values, physiologic trends, or by bedside caregiver request; however, a striking preponderance of clinical events are detected by electronic early warning systems rather than requests from bedside providers.[26]

The ICU telemedicine model also has an impact by increasing bedside staff efficiency, job satisfaction,[31,32] and career longevity. Increased access to an intensivist has been viewed favorably by bedside nurses.[33] Immediate availability of an intensivist[34] who has few competing priorities, whether by telephone or video conference, reduces the time required to address questions raised by bedside caregivers, improves access to provider orders, and results in fewer disruptive calls to bedside physicians.[35,36] Nurses also recognize the value of help with urgent communication for unscheduled interventions by surgeons,[37] invasive cardiologists, radiologists, and other specialists. Implementation of an ICU telemedicine program has been associated with higher staff satisfaction scores in the domains of communication, work environment, and education.[38]

In community hospitals, greater access to the subspecialty expertise provided by an ICU telemedicine program allows higher-acuity patients to be served closer to home. In one independently audited study of 2 community hospitals the implementation of an ICU telemedicine program was associated with an average increase of 45% in case volume.[39] ICU telemedicine programs can also provide surge and disaster relief by providing ICU capacity in community hospitals.[40] Increased community hospital case revenue, from both volume and the retention of higher-acuity cases, is more than sufficient to cover the capital and operating costs of the ICU telemedicine services.[39] The availability of a leveraged workforce solution has fostered continued growth in ICU telemedicine programs, which supported 13% of nonfederal hospital adult intensive care unit beds in 2014.

IMPROVING EFFECTIVENESS: POPULATION MANAGEMENT, STANDARDIZATION, AND REPORTING

The changing landscape of health care has led to the latest wave of adoption of ICU telemedicine programs. Institutions have implemented ICU telemedicine programs so that they can improve effectiveness through standardization of care delivery practices and better manage the high costs of providing adult critical care.[41] ICU telemedicine programs enable population management by providing standardized actionable performance reports. The addition of real-time population management tools has been associated with higher rates of adherence to venous thromboembolism prophylaxis, cardioprotection, and stress ulcer prevention best practices compared with a checklist used during ICU rounds alone.[26,30] Higher rates of adherence to ICU best practices were associated with lower rates of preventable complications and accounted for 25% of the overall mortality and LOS improvements associated with implementation of the ICU telemedicine program.[26]

Real-time identification of cases that are nonadherent to safe practices and regulatory mandates

allows more rapid remediation. ICU telemedicine interventions are effective for an increasingly diverse set of regulatory mandates, including restraint documentation, monitoring pain and response to analgesics, agitation and delirium assessment and treatment, skin and fall risk assessment, and certification of inpatient status. Timely notification and discussion during interdisciplinary rounds has been a particularly helpful approach.[31] ICU telemedicine programs are also able to share deidentified clinical information, which allows meaningful comparisons of adherence to ICU best practices and tracking trends in practice and outcomes over time. Most measures that had low early rates of adherence had those rates increase over the first few years of reporting. High levels of adherence to best practices are routinely achieved by ICU telemedicine systems with leaders that focus on performance.

INTENSIVE CARE UNIT TELEMEDICINE STAFFING

The staff required to provide ICU telemedicine services is a function of the intensity of the services that are provided. ICU telemedicine services can be provided continuously or can start when bedside providers have left the ICU. First-call support is commonly provided when bedside intensivists have signed their service out to the ICU telemedicine intensivist. ICUs with very high acuity can benefit from continuous intensivist coverage to manage events that occur when the dedicated on-site team is rounding on or supporting other patients. Management by off-site team members or the interruption of rounds is required as frequently as every other day in a high-acuity 10-bed to 20-bed ICU.[26] Sites serving only lower-acuity services can opt for cost savings from adjusted hours of off-site intensivist service. In these models, during the daytime hours, the ICU telemedicine nurses provide their findings from task-oriented surveillance or alert-driven evaluations directly to the bedside team. Other sites, especially smaller or rural hospitals supported by providers with non-ICU daytime responsibilities, and those supported by nonspecialist hospitalist teams,[42] have found 24-hour-a-day, 7-days-a-week ICU telemedicine support to be desirable.

INTERMITTENT INTENSIVE CARE UNIT TELEMEDICINE

The continuous ICU telemedicine center approach involves recurrent routines of task-oriented or system-based patient review and electronic surveillance that result in need-based or alert-driven patient evaluation and management. When the trigger for evaluation is based on a time schedule or when telemedicine evaluation requires initiation by a bedside provider, the telemedicine approach is defined as intermittent or episodic.

The intermittent approach is well suited for consultation, to provide access to underserved geographies, and for high-risk comanagement decisions; for example, administration decisions for medications with significant side effects, such as thrombolytics.[43] Most often, either a portable telemedicine connection, either remotely controlled or manually transported to the patient, is enabled by an on-site caregiver to provide integration with the hospital information system and allow health information technology–supported patient evaluation by the remote specialist.[35] In some constructs, remote physicians may use telemedicine tools to round daily or even participate in multidisciplinary rounds.[44–46]

FINANCIAL CONSIDERATIONS

Implementing an ICU telemedicine program requires substantial financial commitment[47] and has been most successful for health care systems that leverage the technology to increase intensivist involvement in care plan creation and review, to generate and act on performance reports, to achieve high rates of adherence to consensus ICU best practices, to encourage the exchange of ideas at interprofessional rounds, and to ensure that alerts and alarms for physiologic instability are addressed within 3 minutes of their onset.[15] In addition to financial benefits derived from improved efficiency, health care systems have used ICU telemedicine programs to derive revenue from providing program services to other institutions and to increase the number of patient referrals to a tertiary medical center of the sponsoring health care system.[48]

Several health care systems that did not change[15] or did not measure these key behaviors[13] did not derive financial benefits from shorter LOS during the months following implementation of an ICU telemedicine program. Programs that have achieved the 20% reduction in adjusted ICU LOS have been able to use this additional capacity at rates of 85% or more, and that corresponds with an additional 800 cases per year for a 100-bed system that served 5000 patients annually before implementing an ICU telemedicine program. These health care systems are able to recover the $2 million to $10 million capital costs of program implementation in 2 to 3 years. The incremental annual revenue is $800,000 when each patient generates a profit of $1000 and is $8 million when each

case generates a $10,000 profit. The uptake of ICU telemedicine programs has been caused in part by the ability of programs to increase per-case hospital revenue, increase case volume, and reduce variable costs per case.

The value proposition for community hospitals that subscribe to ICU telemedicine services is based on increasing case volume or acuity. Audited financial reporting from 2 community hospitals that subscribed to ICU telemedicine services provided by an academic medical center documented an average 44% increase in case volume.[39] Community hospitals were able to retain more cases with sepsis, respiratory failure, toxin ingestion, and heart failure with shock. The average acuity for each of the diagnosis-related groups (DRGs) corresponding with these diagnoses was significantly higher after subscription to an ICU telemedicine service.[39] The financial costs of managing equivalent patients (same age, primary diagnosis, and APACHE acuity score) at a telemedicine-supported community hospital were lower than at a tertiary care medical center. On average, cases were managed at a $10,000 health care system cost saving and with improved patient and family satisfaction for care closer to their homes.[39] The New England Healthcare Institute estimated the statewide benefits of the adoption of ICU telemedicine to be $122 million for Massachusetts.[39] ICU telemedicine programs are increasingly adopted to enhance patient flow, and to provide high-quality care at less-costly locations.

Health care systems can leverage telemedicine ICU programs to provide off-hours specialist evaluation and management services and provide physicians who staff their centers with direct compensation. Although specialist physicians can use existing telemedicine technologies to provide consultative services to critically ill adults, few payers are currently allowing provider reimbursement. However, the landscape is rapidly evolving, and reimbursement for ICU telemedicine services has recently been summarized on a state-by-state basis in a frequently updated online format.[49]

SUMMARY

ICU telemedicine program implementation can have significant impact on ICU patient outcomes. A well-implemented program can standardize processes that improve patient safety and offer more immediate and more consistent expert review of both bedside alerting and alerting unique to the telemedicine center. Furthermore, an ICU telemedicine program is effective for providing rapidly available expertise across the 24-hour continuum and without regard to geography, thereby increasing access to high-quality adult critical care services. In addition, proper implementation of an ICU telemedicine program may be associated with health care system cost savings and with improved patient and family satisfaction.

REFERENCES

1. Gernsback H, Gernsback S, Dermott RW. The radio doctor - maybe. Radio News 1924;1406.

2. Lilly CM, Zubrow MT, Kempner KM, et al. Critical care telemedicine: evolution and state of the art. Crit Care Med 2014;42:2429–36.

3. Grundy BL, Jones PK, Lovitt A. Telemedicine in critical care: problems in design, implementation, and assessment. Crit Care Med 1982;10:471–5.

4. Grundy BL, Crawford P, Jones PK, et al. Telemedicine in critical care: an experiment in health care delivery. JACEP 1977;6:439–44.

5. Rosenfeld BA, Dorman T, Breslow MJ, et al. Intensive care unit telemedicine: alternate paradigm for providing continuous intensivist care. Crit Care Med 2000;28:3925–31.

6. Breslow MJ, Rosenfeld BA, Doerfler M, et al. Effect of a multiple-site intensive care unit telemedicine program on clinical and economic outcomes: an alternative paradigm for intensivist staffing. Crit Care Med 2004;32:31–8.

7. Lilly CM, Thomas EJ. Tele-ICU: experience to date. J Intensive Care Med 2010;25:16–22.

8. McCambridge M, Jones K, Paxton H, et al. Association of health information technology and teleintensivist coverage with decreased mortality and ventilator use in critically ill patients. Arch Intern Med 2010;170:648–53.

9. Angus DC, Kelley MA, Schmitz RJ, et al. Caring for the critically ill patient. Current and projected workforce requirements for care of the critically ill and patients with pulmonary disease: can we meet the requirements of an aging population? JAMA 2000;284:2762–70.

10. Wilcox ME, Adhikari NK. The effect of telemedicine in critically ill patients: systematic review and meta-analysis. Crit Care 2012;16:R127.

11. Thomas EJ, Lucke JF, Wueste L, et al. Association of telemedicine for remote monitoring of intensive care patients with mortality, complications, and length of stay. JAMA 2009;302:2671–8.

12. Morrison JL, Cai Q, Davis N, et al. Clinical and economic outcomes of the electronic intensive care unit: results from two community hospitals. Crit Care Med 2010;38:2–8.

13. Nassar BS, Vaughan-Sarrazin MS, Jiang L, et al. Impact of an intensive care unit telemedicine program on patient outcomes in an integrated health care system. JAMA Intern Med 2014;174:1160–7.

14. Young LB, Chan PS, Lu X, et al. Impact of telemedicine intensive care unit coverage on patient outcomes: a systematic review and meta-analysis. Arch Intern Med 2011;171:498–506.

15. Lilly CM, McLaughlin JM, Zhao H, et al. A multicenter study of ICU telemedicine reengineering of adult critical care. Chest 2014;145:500–7.

16. Angus DC, Shorr AF, White A, et al. Critical care delivery in the United States: distribution of services and compliance with Leapfrog recommendations. Crit Care Med 2006;34:1016–24.

17. Pastores SM, O'Connor MF, Kleinpell RM, et al. The Accreditation Council for Graduate Medical Education resident duty hour new standards: history, changes, and impact on staffing of intensive care units. Crit Care Med 2011;39:2540–9.

18. Bleich MR, Hewlett PO, Santos SR, et al. Analysis of the nursing workforce crisis: a call to action. Am J Nurs 2003;103:66–74.

19. Bell L. Monitor alarm fatigue. Am J Crit Care 2010;19:38.

20. Graham KC, Cvach M. Monitor alarm fatigue: standardizing use of physiological monitors and decreasing nuisance alarms. Am J Crit Care 2010;19:28–34 [quiz: 35].

21. Kenny PE. Alarm fatigue and patient safety. Pa Nurse 2011;66(3):22.

22. Cvach M. Monitor alarm fatigue: an integrative review. Biomed Instrum Technol 2012;46:268–77.

23. Christensen M, Dodds A, Sauer J, et al. Alarm setting for the critically ill patient: a descriptive pilot survey of nurses' perceptions of current practice in an Australian regional critical care unit. Intensive Crit Care Nurs 2014;30:204–10.

24. Funk M, Clark JT, Bauld TJ, et al. Attitudes and practices related to clinical alarms. Am J Crit Care 2014;23:e9–18.

25. National patient safety goals 2014. INTELECOM, 2014. Available at: http://uproxy.library.dc-uoit.ca/login?url=http://searchcenter.intelecomonline.net/marc.aspx?clip=MC_m223r16. Accessed September 16, 2014.

26. Lilly CM, Cody S, Zhao H, et al. Hospital mortality, length of stay, and preventable complications among critically ill patients before and after tele-ICU reengineering of critical care processes. JAMA 2011;305:2175–83.

27. Lilly CM, Fisher KA, Ries M, et al. A national ICU telemedicine survey: validation and results. Chest 2012;142:40–7.

28. Kruklitis RJ, Tracy JA, McCambridge MM. Clinical and financial considerations for implementing an ICU telemedicine program. Chest 2014;145:1392–6.

29. Carpenter DL, Gregg SR, Owens DS, et al. Patient-care time allocation by nurse practitioners and physician assistants in the intensive care unit. Crit Care 2012;16:R27.

30. Kahn JM, Gunn SR, Lorenz HL, et al. Impact of nurse-led remote screening and prompting for

evidence-based practices in the ICU*. Crit Care Med 2014;42:896–904.

31. Goran SF, Mullen-Fortino M. Partnership for a healthy work environment: tele-ICU/ICU collaborative. AACN Adv Crit Care 2012;23:289–301.

32. Young LB, Chan PS, Cram P. Staff acceptance of tele-ICU coverage: a systematic review. Chest 2011;139:279–88.

33. Chu-Weininger MY, Wueste L, Lucke JF, et al. The impact of a tele-ICU on provider attitudes about teamwork and safety climate. Qual Saf Health Care 2010;19:e39.

34. Nielsen M, Saracino J. Telemedicine in the intensive care unit. Crit Care Nurs Clin North Am 2012;24:491–500.

35. McNelis J, Schwall GJ, Collins JF. Robotic remote presence technology in the surgical intensive care unit. J Trauma Acute Care Surg 2012;72:527–30.

36. Groves RH Jr, Holcomb BW Jr, Smith ML. Intensive care telemedicine: evaluating a model for proactive remote monitoring and intervention in the critical care setting. Stud Health Technol Inform 2008;131:131–46.

37. Rincon F, Vibbert M, Childs V, et al. Implementation of a model of robotic tele-presence (RTP) in the neuro-ICU: effect on critical care nursing team satisfaction. Neurocrit Care 2012;17:97–101.

38. Romig MC, Latif A, Gill RS, et al. Perceived benefit of a telemedicine consultative service in a highly staffed intensive care unit. J Crit Care 2012;27:426. e9–16.

39. Fifer S, Everett W, Adams M, et al. Critical care, critical choices the case for tele-ICUs in intensive care. Cambridge (MA): New England Healthcare Institute; Massachusetts Technology Collaborative; 2010. p. 1–64.

40. Einav S, Hick JL, Hanfling D, et al. Surge capacity logistics: care of the critically ill and injured during pandemics and disasters: CHEST consensus statement. Chest 2014;146:e17S–43S.

41. Alsarraf AA, Fowler R. Health, economic evaluation, and critical care. J Crit Care 2005;20:194–7.

42. Labarbera JM, Ellenby MS, Bouressa P, et al. The impact of telemedicine intensivist support and a pediatric hospitalist program on a community hospital. Telemed J E Health 2013;19:760–6.

43. Silva GS, Schwamm LH. Use of telemedicine and other strategies to increase the number of patients that may be treated with intravenous thrombolysis. Curr Neurol Neurosci Rep 2012;12:10–6.

44. Marcin JP, Trujano J, Sadorra C, et al. Telemedicine in rural pediatric care: the fundamentals. Pediatr Ann 2009;38:224–6.

45. Vespa PM, Miller C, Hu X, et al. Intensive care unit robotic telepresence facilitates rapid physician response to unstable patients and decreased cost in neurointensive care. Surg Neurol 2007;67:331–7.

46. Vespa P. Robotic telepresence in the intensive care unit. Crit Care 2005;9:319–20.

47. Kumar G, Falk DM, Bonello RS, et al. The costs of critical care telemedicine programs: a systematic review and analysis. Chest 2013;143:19–29.

48. Whitten P, Holtz B, Nguyen L. Keys to a successful and sustainable telemedicine program. Int J Technol Assess Health Care 2010;26:211–6.

49. State telehealth laws and reimbursement policies: a comprehensive scan of the 50 states and the District of Columbia. California Health Care Foundation. Sacramento, CA: Mario Gutierrez; 2013. p. 1–184.

Controversies and Misconceptions in Intensive Care Unit Nutrition

Michael H. Hooper, MD, MSc*, Paul E. Marik, MD

KEYWORDS

- Nutrition • ICU nutrition • Critical care nutrition • Enteral nutrition • Parenteral nutrition
- Trophic feeding

KEY POINTS

- Nutritional support should be initiated early during every critical care admission. Starvation of patients is not acceptable.
- Parenteral nutrition has a limited role in ICU patients, being limited to those patients with a discontinuous gastrointestinal tract or those unable to tolerate even small volumes of enteral feed.
- Physical disability following critical illness is common and associated with loss of muscle mass and weakness. Protein provided as a continuous infusion, especially in high doses, suppresses muscle synthesis. Whey protein (high in leucine) promotes greater muscle synthesis compared with casein- or soy-based enteral formulas.
- Although clinical data are sparse, intermittent bolus feeding has numerous potential advantages over continuous feeding including preservation of muscle mass; preservation of intestinal, hepatic, and gallbladder function; and improved glycemic control.

INTRODUCTION

Many of the most effective interventions in critical care are not directed at the disease that led to critical illness, but rather provide physiologic support and prevent complications. Nutritional support is among these supportive measures and has advanced considerably over the past several decades. As the understanding of nutrition has grown, many nutritional formulas, supplements, delivery methods, and protocols have been created. These important developments allow the provision of essential calories and nutrients to patients in almost any clinical situation. Nutritional support is now considered an essential component of comprehensive intensive care unit (ICU) care.[1–3]

As understanding, tools, and methods have proliferated, new questions have arisen. Unanswered questions stirred controversy as clinicians and researchers have implemented and investigated novel strategies to benefit their patients. This article identifies the questions and controversies surrounding ICU nutrition, reviews the pertinent literature, and provides recommendations for critical care providers and investigators.

ANSWERS TO COMMON MISCONCEPTIONS IN INTENSIVE CARE UNIT NUTRITION
Starvation During Hospitalization Negatively Impacts Clinical Outcomes

It has been well established that delivering early enteral nutritional support reduces disease severity, diminishes complications, decreases length of stay in the ICU, and favorably impacts patient

Disclosures: Dr M.H. Hooper has no financial or other conflicts of interest to disclose. Dr P.E. Marik has given educational lectures sponsored by Abbott and Nestle corporations.
Eastern Virginia Medical School, Department of Internal Medicine, 825 Fairfax Avenue, Suite 410, Norfolk, VA 23507, USA
* Corresponding author.
E-mail address: hoopermh@evms.edu

Clin Chest Med 36 (2015) 409–418
http://dx.doi.org/10.1016/j.ccm.2015.05.013
0272-5231/15/$ – see front matter © 2015 Elsevier Inc. All rights reserved.

outcome.[4–11] Yet, a large proportion of ICU patients receive inadequate nutritional support.[11–14]

Although most physicians have witnessed patients survive critical illness despite prolonged periods without nutrition, this does not mean that those patients benefited (or were not harmed) by this approach. In the German Competence Network Sepsis (SepNet) point prevalence study, 10% of patients with sepsis received no nutrition and an additional 35% of patients were denied any enteral nutrition.[11] A study conducted in 18 ICUs in the United States and Canada revealed that 25% of mechanically ventilated patients were not given any artificial nutrition.[15] A lack of randomized controlled data proving that starvation is detrimental to critically ill patients likely is caused by the lack of equipoise from researchers and the questionable ethics of performing such an experiment. The observational data in support of providing nutritional support are robust. The Society of Critical Care Medicine and American Society of Parenteral and Enteral Nutrition guidelines[1] and the Canadian[3,16] and European guidelines[2] all recommend that enteral nutrition be started within 48 hours. Withholding nutrition has never been shown to be beneficial to patients. However, the optimal amount and best way to deliver nutrients to critically ill patients are controversial.

Enteral Nutrition Is Almost Never Contraindicated in Critically Ill Patients

Hemodynamic instability requiring vasopressor support is common in the critically ill population. It is known that the use of agents that induce vasoconstriction disproportionately decreases blood flow to the gastrointestinal (GI) tract. This observation has fueled speculation that enteral feeding in patients receiving vasopressors may have a causal relationship to the development of mesenteric ischemia. Enteral infusion of nutrients improves enteric blood flow, prevents structural and functional alterations of the gut barrier, maintains mucosal integrity, decreases enteric permeability, and improves local and systemic immune responsiveness. These effects are mediated by direct and indirect (ie, hormonal and neuronal) effects.[17–19] In endotoxic and septic shock animal models, enteral feeding improved blood flow to the hepatic artery, portal vein, superior mesenteric, and intestinal mucosa with improvement in hepatic and intestinal tissue oxygenation.[19–21] Clinical studies support the findings in animal models. Revelly and colleagues[22] evaluated patients requiring catecholamines 1 day after cardiac surgery. In this small group of patients, enteral feeding was associated with increased cardiac index, indocyanine green clearance, and glucose absorption. Gastric tonometry remained unchanged. Berger and colleagues[23] showed near normal measurements of intestinal absorption after enteral nutrition in hemodynamically unstable cardiac surgery patients. Improved mortality has been associated with early enteral nutrition in critically ill patients requiring vasopressors (34% vs 44%; $P<.001$).[24] In this study the benefits of early enteral nutrition were greatest in the sickest patients and those receiving multiple vasopressors.

The initiation of enteral nutrition is often delayed in patients receiving mechanical ventilation. In the German Competence Network Sepsis (SepNet) study mechanical ventilation was a strong predictor for the failure to provide enteral nutrition.[11] Artinian and colleagues[6] demonstrated a strong association between early enteral nutrition and decreased mortality.

Parenteral Nutrition Is Not Superior or Equivalent to Enteral Nutrition

The use of parenteral nutrition by the imprudent clinician may seem attractive. A simplistic understanding of nutrition defines the gut as simply a route by which one delivers protein, carbohydrates, and fats to the bloodstream for delivery to end organs and tissues. If viewed as nothing but another route to accomplish the same task, the parenteral route has the advantages of exact delivery of finely tuned proportions of nutritional components without the risk of aspiration, GI intolerance, ileus, or diarrhea.

Decades of scientific investigations have revealed risks to parenteral nutrition. Use of early enteral nutrition in critically ill patients is associated with improved outcomes.[4,6] It is now accepted that the enteral route is preferred for delivering nutritional support.[25] Consensus guidelines recommend enteral nutrition over parenteral nutrition in ICU patients.[1–3,16]

There are multiple reasons that the use of parenteral nutrition may be harmful, which seem to stem from two fundamental differences between enteral and parenteral nutrition: failure to deliver enteral nutrition denies the gut and liver direct exposure to nutritional components; and parenteral nutrition delivers nutrition directly into the systemic venous circulation and bypasses the hormonal and metabolic processes within the liver.

Enteral nutrition stimulates the release of a wide variety of hormones that play a crucial role in regulating gut function and metabolic pathways. The hormones secreted by the enteroendocrine cells include cholecystokinin (CCK), peptide YY, glucose-dependent insulinotropic polypeptide

1 (GIP-1), glucagon-like peptide (GLP-1), and peptides that inhibit dipeptidyl-peptidase-4.[26] In addition to playing a major role in insulin release, GLP-1 has a protective effect on the endothelium and brain, cardiovascular, and renal function.[26–31] The potential risks of parenteral nutrition are outlined in **Box 1**.

Because parenteral nutrition is associated with a myriad of potentially harmful effects, its use in critically ill patients has been controversial.[32,33] Recently, randomized controlled trials (RCTs) have been reported that improve understanding of this issue. The Early Parenteral Nutrition Completing Enteral Nutrition in Adult Critically Ill Patients (EPaNIC) study randomized 4640 ICU patients to early (within 48 hours) or late (after 8 days) parenteral nutrition.[34] For all outcomes analyzed, the early parental nutritional group did worse. The CALORIES study randomized 2400 ICU patients within 36 hours after admission to receive enteral or parenteral nutrition, which was continued for up to 5 days or until transition to exclusive oral feeding.[35] There was no difference in any outcome variable between groups. Almost all of the patients in the total parenteral nutrition arm of the CALORIES study were transitioned to enteral nutrition after 5 days of total parenteral nutrition; this nutritional strategy does not seem to have a scientific basis, seems illogical, and raises questions regarding the practicality and external validity of such an approach. A conclusion of equivalence between enteral and parenteral nutrition based on this approach is incorrect.

Importantly, patients in both groups were underfed receiving on average 3 g/kg protein over the 5-day period (0.5 g/kg/day) and 20 kcal/kg/day. This is significantly less protein and calories than the group of patients in the early parenteral nutrition group of the EPANIC study. Furthermore, most importantly, a clear dose–response relationship was evident in the EPaNIC study; paradoxically the more protein the patients received the worse the outcome.[36] This observation is supported by well-established physiologic principles discussed later in this article. Heidegger and colleagues[37] tested the benefit of 5 days of supplemental parental nutrition in ICU patients who by Day 3 did not meet their enteral caloric targets. By intention-to-treat analysis there was no difference in the risk of acquired infection, the primary outcome of this study.[38] It should be noted that the intervention group received a low dose of parenteral nutrition for a short period of time (5 days); approximately 8 cal/kg/day and 0.4 g/kg/day of protein. In summary, these data suggest that parenteral nutrition (short duration and low dose) has no proved benefit over enteral nutrition in critically ill patients. The administration of parenteral nutrition with a high protein content is likely harmful. It is likely that strict glycemic control and aseptic management are necessary to limit the harm associated with the use of an intravenous solution containing a high concentration of glucose through a central catheter.[39] In a nonresearch practice setting where attention to detail is not strictly followed, short duration and low-dose parenteral nutrition increases the complexity and resource requirements of care, has not been shown to improve outcomes, and may be associated with an increased likelihood of complications.

Box 1
Potential harmful effects of parenteral nutrition

Hyperglycemia: Increased gluconeogenesis and glycogenolysis[79,80]

Small bowel atrophy[81,82]

Hepatosteatosis and hepatocellular injury[83]

Atrophy of gastrointestinal-associated lymphoid tissue[84]

Bacterial translocation[85,86]

Altered bowel flora[85]

Increased intestinal permeability[81,82,85,87]

Impaired leukocyte chemotaxis, phagocytosis, and bacterial killing[88–90]

Refeeding syndrome[91]

Increased release of proinflammatory mediators[87]

Increased free radical formation[92]

Mandatory Use of Gastric Residual Volumes to Assess Tolerance of Enteral Nutrition Is Unnecessary

In critically ill patients requiring enteral nutritional support, common practice is to periodically measure the amount of residual volume within the stomach to guide subsequent enteral nutrition. Concern for intolerance of enteral feeds often leads clinicians to stop or reduce enteral feeding.[40,41] The causal connection between high gastric residual volumes and subsequent aspiration pneumonia or poor clinical outcomes is not supported by evidence. Published literature on the topic of gastric residual volumes demonstrates that measured volumes do not correlate well with the incidence of pneumonia or other complications.[42,43] Changing the cutoff volume in protocols is not protective of pneumonia or other complications.[44] A large multicenter French RCT failed to show any difference in clinical outcomes when comparing protocols with or without gastric residual monitoring.[45] The use of rigid feeding protocols based on gastric residual volumes leads to unnecessary interruption of nutritional support. Protocols based on clinical evidence of GI intolerance (abdominal distention, pain regurgitation, or vomiting) seem equally effective and are easier to follow.

OTHER CONTROVERSIES IN INTENSIVE CARE UNIT NUTRITION
The Optimal Dose: Trophic Versus Full Feeds

Although the timing of initiation of nutrition (early) and the route (enteral) are fairly settled questions, the amount of nutrition to provide remains controversial. Although some observational trials have suggested that feeding is correlated with improved outcomes in a dose-dependent fashion,[14] this finding is confounded by the ability of healthier patients to tolerate greater amounts of nutrition and the willingness of physicians to provide larger amounts of nutrition to healthier patients.[12,46,47] It has been assumed and is generally accepted that reaching caloric (about 25 kcal/kg/day) and protein targets (1.2 g–2.0/kg/day) improves patient outcomes. Indeed, the Society of Critical Care Medicine/American Society of Parenteral and Enteral Nutrition, the European Society of Parenteral and Enteral Nutrition, and the Canadian Clinical Practice Guidelines for Nutrition Support endorse these targets.[1–3] However, five recent RCTs strongly challenge this concept.[15,48–51] These studies compared trophic with full feeds,[48,49] hypocaloric with goal nutritional targets,[15,50] and a PepUp protocol.[15] All these studies demonstrated no benefit (or harm[50]) in the group of patients that received more calories and protein. The Initial Trophic vs. Full Enteral Feeding in Patients with Acute Lung Injury (EDEN) trial[49] is the largest study to date with follow-up of patients to 1 year and is worthy of further analysis. The EDEN trial randomized 1000 patients from the acute respiratory distress syndrome (ARDS) clinical trials network to either early trophic feeding or early full feeding during the first 6 days of critical illness. The trophic group received approximately 400 kcal of daily nutrition during the first 5 days versus approximately 1300 kcal in the full-feeding group. All patients received continuous feeding. There was no difference in ventilator-free days, 60-day mortality, or infectious complications. Additional follow-up showed continued outcome equivalence at 6 and 12 months.[52] GI intolerance was slightly worse in

the full-feeding group, although the absolute differences in GI intolerances were very low.

Although trophic feedings have been shown to have beneficial physiologic effects, including the preservation of intestinal epithelium, functioning of the intestinal brush border, and less bacterial translocation,[53] it is difficult to explain why full feeds are not more beneficial than trophic feeds. It has been postulated that anorexia is a normal physiologic response to severe illness, and that trophic feeding is sufficient to counteract the negative effects of starvation without subjecting patients to the potential unwanted side effects of GI intolerance and aspiration. Early in the course of critical illness, full feedings cannot be considered to be superior to trophic feedings and cause increased GI intolerance.

Continuous Versus Intermittent/Bolus

No mammalian species outside of the hospitalized environment eats continuously, but this has become a standard practice because of simplicity, convenience, and convention. Continuous enteral feeding of critically ill adults seems to be the standard of care around the world.[1] This is not physiologic and may be associated with complications and side effects. Experimental animal and human data have demonstrated the negative effects of continuous tube feeding on muscle synthesis, hepatic and intestinal structure and function, and multiple metabolic and endocrine effects when compared with intermittent/bolus feeding, as detailed next.

Insulin and the branched-chain amino acid, leucine, play a critical role in muscle synthesis by activating AKT/protein kinase B and mammalian target of rapamycin (mTOR), respectively.[54] Insulin and branch-chain amino acids independently increase muscle synthesis with the effects of both being additive.[55,56] Muscle catabolism is largely mediated by protein-ubiquination, which is mediated by action of forkhead box class O-1 after activation by inflammatory mediators. In health, skeletal muscle undergoes protein synthesis following a protein meal. Muscle breakdown (catabolism) occurs between meals with the net effect of stable muscle mass. However, in critically ill patients muscle breakdown exceeds muscle synthesis.[54] Skeletal muscle wasting leads to significant weakness in most ICU survivors.[57] A landmark study Herridge and colleagues[58] demonstrated that survivors of ARDS had marked functional disabilities that persisted for years after hospital discharge. Puthucheary and colleagues[54] demonstrated that critically ill patients lose 20% of their quadriceps femoris muscle mass within 10 days of their ICU stay. In humans a continuous infusion of amino acids leads to increased muscle synthesis; however, after 2 hours protein synthesis returns to baseline despite the continuation of the amino acid infusion.[59] In humans a bolus of whey protein (high in leucine) results in the pulsatile release of insulin; a pulsatile increase in intramuscular leucine concentration; and an increase in the synthetic rate of muscle, which peaks at 90 minutes and returns to baseline at 180 minutes.[60] Experimental studies that have compared the rate of muscle synthesis and breakdown in animals that received continuous versus intermittent feeds have demonstrated significantly increased intramuscular AKT and mTOR and increased muscle protein synthesis with bolus as compared with continuous feeding.[61] Puthucheary and colleagues[54] demonstrated that the degree of muscle wasting in critically ill patients was proportional to the amount of protein delivered (as a continuous infusion). These data suggest that when protein is provided as a continuous infusion (enterally or parenterally) it decreases protein synthesis. The greater the amount of protein provided the greater the suppressive effect. This provides a plausible physiologic explanation for the apparent harm of high-dose parenteral nutrition (and the dose–response effect described previously) and the lack of benefit (or harm) with the increased delivery of enteral calories and protein (given as a continuous infusion). In addition, whey-based protein (high in leucine) leads to significantly greater protein synthesis and less breakdown than casein- or soy-based protein.[62]

In addition to its effects on protein synthesis, continuous feeds have adverse metabolic effects with associated organ dysfunction. Following the ingestion of a meal several hormones including GLP-1, GIP, CCK, ghrelin, and peptide YY are secreted by the enteroendocrine cells lining the GI tract. These hormones serve complex roles regulating GI motility, gallbladder contraction, pancreatic function, and nutrient absorption.[26] Most of these gut hormones are secreted within minutes of nutrient ingestion, rise transiently, and fall back to basal levels after termination of feeding. This enterohormonal response to nutrition is almost completely absent following continuous tube feeding.[63–65] The incretins GIP and GLP-1 play an important role in preparing the pancreas to handle incoming nutrient load.[66] Both these hormones potentiate insulin secretion from the islet β cell in a glucose-dependent manner and account for up to 70% of insulin release. In an elegant set of experiments, Stoll and colleagues[65] studied the kinetics of GIP and GLP-1, insulin receptor phosphorylation, and GI function in neonatal pigs who received either continuous enteral feed or a polymeric formula given intermittently. In this study, blood GIP and GLP-1 levels and insulin receptor phosphorylation and phosphatidylinositol-3-kinase levels in liver and muscle were significantly reduced with continuous feeding as opposed to intermittent feeding. Ileal mass and villus height were significantly less with continuous as opposed to bolus feeds. Furthermore, insulin resistance, hepatic steatosis, and hepatic inflammation were greater with continuous feeding. Shulman and colleagues[67] demonstrated greater small intestinal mucosal weight and ileal mass in newborn pigs fed by bolus feeds as compared with continuous feeds. Furthermore, it has recently been appreciated that there are GLP-1 receptors on many organs and tissues including the brain, heart, kidney, and macrophages and that GLP-1 has neuroprotective, cardioprotective, renoprotective, and anti-inflammatory properties.[27–31,68]

Mashako and colleagues[63] measured CCK levels in children receiving continuous enteral nutrition, discontinuous tube feeding, and control subjects receiving normal alimentation. During continuous enteral feeding the CCK levels were similar to the preprandial levels of the control subjects; however, the postprandial CCK levels increased significantly in the patients receiving discontinuous oral feeding reaching levels similar to those of normal control subjects. In a prospective crossover study Jawaheer and colleagues[69] compared the effects of bolus versus continuous feed on gallbladder function in 15 infants. These authors demonstrated that continuous enteral feeding led to an enlarged noncontractile gallbladder. The gallbladder contraction index was 65% during bolus feeds. It is thus reasonable to hypothesize that continuous, rather than bolus, feeding is a major cause of distended, nonfunctioning gallbladders and acalculous cholecystitis in critically ill patients.

Based on these physiologic insights, the arbitrary convention of continuous feeding, together with data demonstrating that providing more protein and calories as a continuous infusion does not improve outcome (may be harmful), we suggest that it is logical to feed ICU patients by intermittent/bolus rather than continuous feeding. Furthermore, we propose that whey (rather than casein or soy) should be used as the predominant source of protein.

Because continuous tube feeding is considered the standard of care only a limited number of studies (with few patients) have been performed comparing continuous with bolus feeding. Although these studies did not evaluate the major end points of interest (muscle mass, ventilator-free days, mortality, delirium, and metabolic parameters) they have demonstrated that this approach is safe and feasible.[70–72] The largest study to date was performed in 164 trauma patients who were randomized to an intermittent feeding regimen (one-sixth of daily needs infused every 4 hours) or a continuous feeding regimen.[70] The intermittent feed was delivered via an enteral feeding pump over a 30- to 60-minute period of time. In this study there was no difference in the complication rate between groups (diarrhea and pneumonia), but the caloric goal was achieved earlier in the intermittent-fed patients. Serpa and colleagues[71] randomized 28 ICU patients to receive intermittent feeds given as 1-hour "bolus" every 3 hours or a continuous infusion. There was no difference in outcome between groups including the rate of aspiration and diarrhea. Maurya and coworkers[72] performed a small RCT comparing bolus with continuous feeds in 40 head-injured patients. Despite the fact the feeds were given as a bolus (with a 50-mL syringe) the risk of aspiration and diarrhea was similar between groups. In addition to the benefits of intermittent feeding noted previously, intermittent regimens represent a logistically simple method by which delivery of nutritional intake may continue uninterrupted despite the necessity for multiple procedures and diagnostics that traditionally require discontinuance of continuous enteral feeds.

Based on these data we recommend intermittent feeding over continuous feeding and believe that additional randomized, controlled studies comparing continuous with intermittent/bolus feeding are desperately needed. We currently have experience with feeding more than 400 patients by this method (detailed in **Fig. 1**); this technique has been very well tolerated with no evidence of an increase in the risk of aspiration or diarrhea. Compared with historical control subjects our data suggest that glycemic control improves with intermittent feeding. Furthermore, our nursing staff now prefer intermittent over continuous feeding. It is important to emphasize that the intermittent boluses are given using an enteral feeding pump over a period 20 to 40 minutes. Although the optimal amount of calories and protein that should be given using the intermittent "bolus" approach is unknown, we target 20 to 25 cal/kg/day and 1 g/kg/protein divided into six aliquots given every 4 hours. We initiate feeding using a 100-mL "bolus" of enteral formula and increase by 50 mL as tolerated by the patient to reach a goal at 48 hours. The gastric residual volume is checked before the next bolus only in those patients demonstrating evidence of enteral intolerance (abdominal distention, pain, nausea, vomiting). In patients demonstrating enteral intolerance we would reduce the volume of feeds (but do not stop feeding) and administer a prokinetic agent. In patients with diabetes we suggest the basal/bolus method of insulin administration; low-dose, long-acting together with a bolus of insulin (based on blood glucose level) with each bolus of enteral formula.

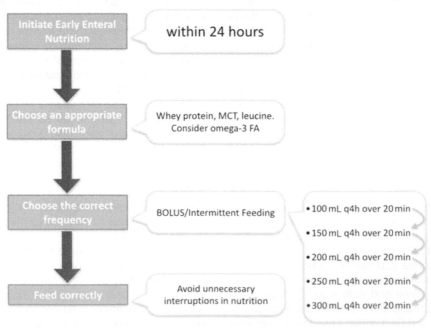

Fig. 1. Proposed bolus feeding algorithm for critically ill patients. MCT, medium chain triglycerides.

Use of Omega-3 Fatty Acids

Omega-3 (O-3) fatty acids have important anti-inflammatory and immunomodulating properties. In addition, O-3 fatty acids act synergistically with insulin and leucine to increase muscle synthesis.[73] The use of O-3 fatty acid supplemented enteral formulas in patients with sepsis and ARDS is currently very controversial. It should, however, be recognized that Paleolithic man subsided on a diet high in O-3 fatty acids (O-3/O-6 ratio of 1:1)[74] and that a diet high in O-3 fatty acids is cardioprotective[75]; it therefore seems illogical to propose the O-3 fatty acids may be harmful in critically ill patients. Three RCTs demonstrated that an enteral formula high in O-3 fatty acids improved oxygenation, the number of ventilator-free days, ICU length of stay, and mortality in patients with ARDS.[76] The OMEGA study was an RCT that randomized 272 adults within 48 hours of developing acute lung injury to receive twice-daily enteral supplementation with O-3 fatty acids or an isocaloric control.[77] Enteral nutrition was delivered separately from the study supplement. The study was stopped early for futility. The adjusted 60-day mortality was 25.1% and 17.6% in the O-3 and control groups, respectively. Several peculiarities of this study make the results difficult to interpret; nevertheless, this study has tempered the enthusiasm for the use of high concentrations of O-3 fatty acids in ARDS. A subsequent meta-analysis of O-3 fatty acids in ARDS did not demonstrate a survival advantage or a reduction in ventilator-free days or other secondary outcomes.[78] Nevertheless the use of O-3 fatty acids in ARDS is supported by a sound physiologic basis and prior experimental studies. Discarding or accepting therapies or treatments based on single studies has previously led to incorrect conclusions and we believe that the diverse, positive biologic effects of O-3 fatty acids combined with multiple prior positive studies suggest that further investigation is required to more definitively resolve this issue.

SUMMARY

We currently recommend a high-quality, peptide-based, whey-dominant nutritional supplement with an increased fat/carbohydrate ratio in critically ill patients. Inclusion of a structured lipid, such as O-3 fatty acids, is our current practice, despite conflicting data on their impact on outcomes in critically ill patients. A formula with these components has anti-inflammatory properties; promotes insulin and incretin release, which reduces the risk of hyperglycemia; and likely limits protein breakdown. We recommend that this formula be given as intermittent "boluses" rather than as a continuous infusion. Additional studies are desperately needed to clarify the best practice feeding frequency. All critically ill patients with a functional bowel should be fed early (within 24 hours of ICU admission) using the GI tract. A feeding tube placed in the stomach is recommended in those patients who cannot be fed orally. Parenteral nutrition should only be considered in patients with a discontinuous or absent bowel or those rare patients that are unable to tolerate even small volumes (trophic) of enteral nutrition.

REFERENCES

1. McClave SA, Martindale RG, Vanek VW, et al. Guidelines for the provision and assessment of nutrition support therapy in the adult critically ill patient: Society of Critical Care Medicine (SCCM) and American Society for Parenteral and Enteral Nutrition (A.S.P.E.N.). JPEN J Parenter Enteral Nutr 2009; 33(3):277–316.
2. Kreymann KG, Berger MM, Deutz NE, et al. ESPEN guidelines on enteral nutrition: intensive care. Clin Nutr 2006;25:210–23.
3. Heyland DK, Dhaliwal R, Drover JW, et al, Canadian Critical Care Clinical Practice Guidelines Committee. Canadian clinical practice guidelines for nutrition support in mechanically ventilated, critically ill adult patients. JPEN J Parenter Enteral Nutr 2003;27(5): 355–73.
4. Marik PE, Zaloga GP. Early enteral nutrition in acutely ill patients: a systematic review. Crit Care Med 2001;29(12):2264–70.
5. Lewis SJ, Egger M, Sylvester PA, et al. Early enteral feeding versus "nil by mouth" after gastrointestinal surgery: systematic review and meta-analysis of controlled trials. BMJ 2001;323(7316):773–6.
6. Artinian V, Krayem H, DiGiovine B. Effects of early enteral feeding on the outcome of critically ill mechanically ventilated medical patients. Chest 2006; 129(4):960–7.
7. Doig GS, Heighes PT, Simpson F, et al. Early enteral nutrition, provided within 24 h of injury or intensive care unit admission, significantly reduces mortality in critically ill patients: a meta-analysis of randomised controlled trials. Intensive Care Med 2009; 35(12):2018–27.
8. Doig GS, Heighes PT, Simpson F, et al. Early enteral nutrition reduces mortality in trauma patients requiring intensive care: a meta-analysis of randomised controlled trials. Injury 2011;42(1):50–6.
9. Barlow R, Price P, Reid TD, et al. Prospective multicentre randomised controlled trial of early enteral nutrition for patients undergoing major upper gastrointestinal surgical resection. Clin Nutr 2011;30(5): 560–6.

10. Osland E, Yunus RM, Khan S, et al. Early versus traditional postoperative feeding in patients undergoing resectional gastrointestinal surgery: a meta-analysis. JPEN J Parenter Enteral Nutr 2011;35(4): 473–87.

11. Elke G, Schädler D, Engel C, et al. Current practice in nutritional support and its association with mortality in septic patients: results from a national, prospective, multicenter study. Crit Care Med 2008; 36(6):1762–7.

12. Krishnan JA, Parce PB, Martinez A, et al. Caloric intake in medical ICU patients: consistency of care with guidelines and relationship to clinical outcomes. Chest 2003;124(1):297–305.

13. McClave SA, Sexton LK, Spain DA, et al. Enteral tube feeding in the intensive care unit: factors impeding adequate delivery. Crit Care Med 1999; 27(7):1252–6.

14. Alberda C, Gramlich L, Jones N, et al. The relationship between nutritional intake and clinical outcomes in critically ill patients: results of an international multicenter observational study. Intensive Care Med 2009;35(10):1728–37.

15. Heyland DK, Murch L, Cahill N, et al. Enhanced protein-energy provision via the enteral route feeding protocol in critically ill patients: results of a cluster randomized trial. Crit Care Med 2013; 41(12):2743–53.

16. Dhaliwal R, Cahill N, Lemieux M, et al. The Canadian critical care nutrition guidelines in 2013: an update on current recommendations and implementation strategies. Nutr Clin Pract 2014;29(1):29–43.

17. Siregar H, Chou CC. Relative contribution of fat, protein, carbohydrate, and ethanol to intestinal hyperemia. Am J Physiol 1982;242(1):G27–31.

18. Chou CC, Kvietys P, Post J, et al. Constituents of chyme responsible for postprandial intestinal hyperemia. Am J Physiol 1978;235(6):H677–82.

19. Gosche JR, Garrison RN, Harris PD, et al. Absorptive hyperemia restores intestinal blood flow during *Escherichia coli* sepsis in the rat. Arch Surg 1990; 125(12):1573–6.

20. Zaloga GP, Roberts PR, Marik P. Feeding the hemodynamically unstable patient: a critical evaluation of the evidence. Nutr Clin Pract 2003;18(4):285–93.

21. Kazamias P, Kotzampassi K, Koufogiannis D, et al. Influence of enteral nutrition-induced splanchnic hyperemia on the septic origin of splanchnic ischemia. World J Surg 1998;22(1):6–11.

22. Revelly JP, Tappy L, Berger MM, et al. Early metabolic and splanchnic responses to enteral nutrition in postoperative cardiac surgery patients with circulatory compromise. Intensive Care Med 2001;27(3): 540–7.

23. Berger MM, Berger-Gryllaki M, Wiesel PH, et al. Intestinal absorption in patients after cardiac surgery. Crit Care Med 2000;28(7):2217–23.

24. Khalid I, Doshi P, DiGiovine B. Early enteral nutrition and outcomes of critically ill patients treated with vasopressors and mechanical ventilation. Am J Crit Care 2010;19(3):261–8.

25. Zaloga GP. Parenteral nutrition in adult inpatients with functioning gastrointestinal tracts: assessment of outcomes. Lancet 2006;367(9516):1101–11.

26. Gutierrez-Aguilar R, Woods SC. Nutrition and L and K-enteroendocrine cells. Curr Opin Endocrinol Diabetes Obes 2011;18(1):35–41.

27. Phillips LK, Prins JB. Update on incretin hormones. Ann N Y Acad Sci 2012;1243(1):E55–74.

28. Muskiet MH, Smits MM, Morsink LM, et al. The gut-renal axis: do incretin-based agents confer renoprotection in diabetes? Nat Rev Nephrol 2014; 10(2):88–103.

29. Oyama JI, Higashi Y, Node K. Do incretins improve endothelial function? Cardiovasc Diabetol 2014; 13(1):21.

30. Yabe D, Seino Y. Incretin actions beyond the pancreas: lessons from knockout mice. Curr Opin Pharmacol 2013;13(6):946–53.

31. Nadkarni P, Chepurny OG, Holz GG. Regulation of glucose homeostasis by GLP-1. In: Glucose homeostatis and the pathogenesis of diabetes mellitus. Prog Mol Biol Trans Sci 2014;121:23–65.

32. Jeejeebhoy KN. Total parenteral nutrition: potion or poison? Am J Clin Nutr 2001;74(2):160–3.

33. Marik PE, Pinsky M. Death by parenteral nutrition. Intensive Care Med 2003;29(6):867–9.

34. Casaer MP, Mesotten D, Hermans G, et al. Early versus late parenteral nutrition in critically ill adults. N Engl J Med 2011;365(6):506–17.

35. Harvey SE, Parrott F, Harrison DA, et al. Trial of the route of early nutritional support in critically ill adults. N Engl J Med 2014;371(18):1673–84.

36. Casaer MP, Wilmer A, Hermans G, et al. Role of disease and macronutrient dose in the randomized controlled EPaNIC trial. Am J Respir Crit Care Med 2013;187(3):247–55.

37. Heidegger CP, Berger MM, Graf S, et al. Optimisation of energy provision with supplemental parenteral nutrition in critically ill patients: a randomised controlled clinical trial. Lancet 2013;381(9864): 385–93.

38. Marik P, Hooper M. Supplemental parenteral nutrition in critically ill patients. Lancet 2013;381(9879):1716.

39. Marik PE, Preiser JC. Toward understanding tight glycemic control in the ICU: a systematic review and metaanalysis. Chest 2010;137(3):544–51.

40. Rice TW, Swope T, Bozeman S, et al. Variation in enteral nutrition delivery in mechanically ventilated patients. Nutrition 2005;21(7–8):786–92.

41. Mentec H, Dupont H, Bocchetti M, et al. Upper digestive intolerance during enteral nutrition in critically ill patients: frequency, risk factors, and complications. Crit Care Med 2001;29(10):1955–61.

42. Pinilla JC, Samphire J, Arnold C, et al. Comparison of gastrointestinal tolerance to two enteral feeding protocols in critically ill patients: a prospective, randomized controlled trial. JPEN J Parenter Enteral Nutr 2001;25(2):81–6.

43. Montejo JC, Miñambres E, Bordejé L, et al. Gastric residual volume during enteral nutrition in ICU patients: the REGANE study. Intensive Care Med 2010;36(8):1386–93.

44. McClave SA, Lukan JK, Stefater JA, et al. Poor validity of residual volumes as a marker for risk of aspiration in critically ill patients. Crit Care Med 2005;33(2): 324–30 [meta-analysis or systematic review].

45. Reignier J, Mercier E, Le Gouge A, et al. Effect of not monitoring residual gastric volume on risk of ventilator-associated pneumonia in adults receiving mechanical ventilation and early enteral feeding: a randomized controlled trial. JAMA 2013;309(3): 249–56.

46. Arabi YM, Haddad SH, Tamim HM, et al. Near-target caloric intake in critically ill medical-surgical patients is associated with adverse outcomes. JPEN J Parenter Enteral Nutr 2010;34(3):280–8.

47. Patel JJ, Kozeniecki M, Biesboer A, et al. Early trophic enteral nutrition is associated with improved outcomes in mechanically ventilated patients with septic shock: a retrospective review. J Intensive Care Med 2014. [Epub ahead of print].

48. Rice TW, Mogan S, Hays MA, et al. Randomized trial of initial trophic versus full-energy enteral nutrition in mechanically ventilated patients with acute respiratory failure. Crit Care Med 2011; 39(5):967–74.

49. National Heart, Lung, and Blood Institute Acute Respiratory Distress Syndrome (ARDS) Clinical Trials Network, Rice TW, Wheeler AP, et al. Initial trophic vs full enteral feeding in patients with acute lung injury: the EDEN randomized trial. JAMA 2012; 307(8):795–803.

50. Arabi YM, Tamim HM, Dhar GS, et al. Permissive underfeeding and intensive insulin therapy in critically ill patients: a randomized controlled trial. Am J Clin Nutr 2011;93(3):569–77.

51. Charles EJ, Petroze RT, Metzger R, et al. Hypocaloric compared with eucaloric nutritional support and its effect on infection rates in a surgical intensive care unit: a randomized controlled trial. Am J Clin Nutr 2014;100(5):1337–43.

52. Needham DM, Dinglas VD, Bienvenu OJ, et al. One year outcomes in patients with acute lung injury randomised to initial trophic or full enteral feeding: prospective follow-up of EDEN randomised trial. BMJ 2013;346:f1532.

53. Hadfield RJ, Sinclair DG, Houldsworth PE, et al. Effects of enteral and parenteral nutrition on gut mucosal permeability in the critically ill. Am J Respir Crit Care Med 1995;152(5 Pt 1):1545–8.

54. Puthucheary ZA, Rawal J, McPhail M, et al. Acute skeletal muscle wasting in critical illness. JAMA 2013;310(15):1591–600.

55. Suryawan A, O'Connor PM, Bush JA, et al. Differential regulation of protein synthesis by amino acids and insulin in peripheral and visceral tissues of neonatal pigs. Amino Acids 2009;37(1):97–104.

56. O'Connor PM, Bush JA, Suryawan A, et al. Insulin and amino acids independently stimulate skeletal muscle protein synthesis in neonatal pigs. Am J Physiol Endocrinol Metab 2003;284(1):E110–9.

57. Stevens RD, Dowdy DW, Michaels RK, et al. Neuromuscular dysfunction acquired in critical illness: a systematic review. Intensive Care Med 2007; 33(11):1876–91.

58. Herridge MS, Tansey CM, Matté A, et al. Functional disability 5 years after acute respiratory distress syndrome. N Engl J Med 2011;364(14):1293–304.

59. Bohé J, Low JF, Wolfe RR, et al. Latency and duration of stimulation of human muscle protein synthesis during continuous infusion of amino acids. J Physiol (Lond) 2001;532(Pt 2):575–9.

60. Atherton PJ, Etheridge T, Watt PW, et al. Muscle full effect after oral protein: time-dependent concordance and discordance between human muscle protein synthesis and mTORC1 signaling. Am J Clin Nutr 2010;92(5):1080–8.

61. Gazzaneo MC, Suryawan A, Orellana RA, et al. Intermittent bolus feeding has a greater stimulatory effect on protein synthesis in skeletal muscle than continuous feeding in neonatal pigs. J Nutr 2011; 141(12):2152–8.

62. Pennings B, Boirie Y, Senden JMG, et al. Whey protein stimulates postprandial muscle protein accretion more effectively than do casein and casein hydrolysate in older men. Am J Clin Nutr 2011; 93(5):997–1005.

63. Mashako MN, Bernard C, Cezard JP, et al. Effect of total parenteral nutrition, constant rate enteral nutrition, and discontinuous oral feeding on plasma cholecystokinin immunoreactivity in children. J Pediatr Gastroenterol Nutr 1987;6(6):948–52.

64. Ledeboer M, Masclee AA, Biemond I, et al. Gallbladder motility and cholecystokinin secretion during continuous enteral nutrition. Am J Gastroenterol 1997;92(12):2274–9.

65. Stoll B, Puiman PJ, Cui L, et al. Continuous parenteral and enteral nutrition induces metabolic dysfunction in neonatal pigs. JPEN J Parenter Enteral Nutr 2012;36(5):538–50.

66. Drucker DJ. Enhancing the action of incretin hormones: a new whey forward? Endocrinology 2006; 147(7):3171–2.

67. Shulman RJ, Redel CA, Stathos TH. Bolus versus continuous feedings stimulate small-intestinal growth and development in the newborn pig. J Pediatr Gastroenterol Nutr 1994;18(3):350–4.

68. Cho YM, Fujita Y, Kieffer TJ. Glucagon-like peptide-1: glucose homeostasis and beyond. Annu Rev Physiol 2014;76(1):535–59.

69. Jawaheer G, Shaw NJ, Pierro A. Continuous enteral feeding impairs gallbladder emptying in infants. J Pediatr 2001;138(6):822–5.

70. MacLeod JB, Lefton J, Houghton D, et al. Prospective randomized control trial of intermittent versus continuous gastric feeds for critically ill trauma patients. J Trauma 2007;63(1):57–61.

71. Serpa LF, Kimura M, Faintuch J, et al. Effects of continuous versus bolus infusion of enteral nutrition in critical patients. Rev Hosp Clin Fac Med Sao Paulo 2003;58(1):9–14.

72. Maurya I, Pawar M, Garg R, et al. Comparison of respiratory quotient and resting energy expenditure in two regimens of enteral feeding: continuous vs. intermittent in head-injured critically ill patients. Saudi J Anaesth 2011;5(2):195–201.

73. Smith GI, Atherton P, Reeds DN, et al. Dietary omega-3 fatty acid supplementation increases the rate of muscle protein synthesis in older adults: a randomized controlled trial. Am J Clin Nutr 2011; 93(2):402–12.

74. Eaton SB, Konner M. Paleolithic nutrition. A consideration of its nature and current implications. N Engl J Med 1985;312(5):283–9.

75. Leung Yinko SS, Stark KD, Thanassoulis G, et al. Fish consumption and acute coronary syndrome: a meta-analysis. Am J Med 2014;127(9):848–57.e2.

76. Pontes-Arruda A, Demichele S, Seth A, et al. The use of an inflammation-modulating diet in patients with acute lung injury or acute respiratory distress syndrome: a meta-analysis of outcome data. JPEN J Parenter Enteral Nutr 2008;32(6):596–605.

77. Rice TW, Wheeler AP, Thompson BT, et al. Enteral omega-3 fatty acid, gamma-linolenic acid, and antioxidant supplementation in acute lung injury. JAMA 2011;306(14):1574–81.

78. Zhu D, Zhang Y, Li S, et al. Enteral omega-3 fatty acid supplementation in adult patients with acute respiratory distress syndrome: a systematic review of randomized controlled trials with meta-analysis and trial sequential analysis. Intensive Care Med 2014;40(4):504–12.

79. Myers SR, McGuinness OP, Neal DW, et al. Intraportal glucose delivery alters the relationship between net hepatic glucose uptake and the insulin concentration. J Clin Invest 1991;87(3):930–9.

80. Adkins BA, Myers SR, Hendrick GK, et al. Importance of the route of intravenous glucose delivery to hepatic glucose balance in the conscious dog. J Clin Invest 1987;79(2):557–65.

81. Wildhaber BE, Lynn KN, Yang H, et al. Total parenteral nutrition-induced apoptosis in mouse intestinal epithelium: regulation by the Bcl-2 protein family. Pediatr Surg Int 2002;18(7):570–5.

82. Sun X, Spencer AU, Yang H, et al. Impact of caloric intake on parenteral nutrition-associated intestinal morphology and mucosal barrier function. JPEN J Parenter Enteral Nutr 2006;30(6):474–9.

83. Grau T, Bonet A, Rubio M, et al. Liver dysfunction associated with artificial nutrition in critically ill patients. Crit Care 2007;11(1):R10.

84. Li J, Kudsk KA, Gocinski B, et al. Effects of parenteral and enteral nutrition on gut-associated lymphoid tissue. J Trauma 1995;39(1):44–51 [discussion: 51–2].

85. Zheng YJ, Tam YK, Coutts RT. Endotoxin and cytokine released during parenteral nutrition. JPEN J Parenter Enteral Nutr 2004;28(3):163–8.

86. MacFie J, Reddy BS, Gatt M, et al. Bacterial translocation studied in 927 patients over 13 years. Br J Surg 2006;93(1):87–93.

87. Yang H, Kiristioglu I, Fan Y, et al. Interferon-gamma expression by intraepithelial lymphocytes results in a loss of epithelial barrier function in a mouse model of total parenteral nutrition. Ann Surg 2002;236(2):226–34.

88. Gogos CA, Kalfarentzos FE, Zoumbos NC. Effect of different types of total parenteral nutrition on T-lymphocyte subpopulations and NK cells. Am J Clin Nutr 1990;51(1):119–22.

89. Gogos CA, Kalfarentzos F. Total parenteral nutrition and immune system activity: a review. Nutrition 1995;11(4):339–44.

90. Alverdy JC, Burke D. Total parenteral nutrition: iatrogenic immunosuppression. Nutrition 1992;8(5):359–65.

91. Walmsley RS. Refeeding syndrome: screening, incidence, and treatment during parenteral nutrition. J Gastroenterol Hepatol 2013;28(Suppl 4):113–7.

92. Pitkänen O, Hallman M, Andersson S. Generation of free radicals in lipid emulsion used in parenteral nutrition. Pediatr Res 1991;29(1):56–9.

Sleep Loss and Circadian Rhythm Disruption in the Intensive Care Unit

Melissa P. Knauert, MD, PhD[a],*, Jeffrey A. Haspel, MD, PhD[b],
Margaret A. Pisani, MD, MPH[a]

KEYWORDS

- Sleep deprivation • Sleep loss • Circadian rhythm • Circadian misalignment • Delirium
- Intensive care unit • Critical illness

KEY POINTS

- Patients in the intensive care unit (ICU) present on admission with sleep disruption due to acute and chronic medical conditions.
- Sleep disruption includes sleep loss, decrements in N3 sleep, decrements in rapid eye movement (REM) sleep, and circadian misalignment.
- ICU admission reinforces and perpetuates sleep disruption because of environmental, patient, and illness-related factors.
- Clustered care initiatives show promise in improving patient outcomes; this includes decreases in delirium rates.
- Inclusion of other ICU care protocols such as daily sedative interruption and early mobilization may support sleep prolongation, normalization of sleep architecture, and circadian reentrainment.

INTRODUCTION

Critical illness leading to ICU admission creates and propagates a syndrome of sleep loss, poor sleep quality, and circadian misalignment. This syndromic entity is summarized with the term sleep disruption in the context of this review article. Causality is diverse and includes physiologic, psychological, and environmental factors (**Fig. 1**). This syndrome affects virtually all critically ill patients, including mechanically ventilated, nonventilated, septic, nonseptic, and less and more severely ill patients, as well as healthy volunteers exposed to recordings of the ICU environment.[1]

Sleep is a periodic, reversible state of cognitive and sensory disengagement from the external environment. Normal adult sleep occurs overnight and lasts 7 to 9 hours; the sleep period consists of four to six 90- to 100-minute periods during which non-REM (NREM) and REM sleep alternate in a cyclical fashion. NREM sleep includes sequential progression through stages N1, N2, and N3, which grossly correlate to the depth of sleep. In general, N1 comprises 2% to 5% of overnight sleep, N2 comprises 45% to 55% of overnight sleep, and N3 comprises 15% to 20% of overnight sleep. N3 is otherwise known as slow wave sleep (SWS) and is considered necessary for anabolic

The authors have no conflicts of interest to disclose.

[a] Section of Pulmonary, Critical Care and Sleep Medicine, Department of Internal Medicine, Yale University School of Medicine, 300 Cedar Street, TAC-441 South, PO Box 208057, New Haven, CT 06520-8057, USA;
[b] Division of Pulmonary, Critical Care and Sleep Medicine, Department of Internal Medicine, Washington University School of Medicine, 660 South Euclid Avenue, St Louis, MO 63110, USA
* Corresponding author.
E-mail address: melissa.knauert@yale.edu

Clin Chest Med 36 (2015) 419–429
http://dx.doi.org/10.1016/j.ccm.2015.05.008

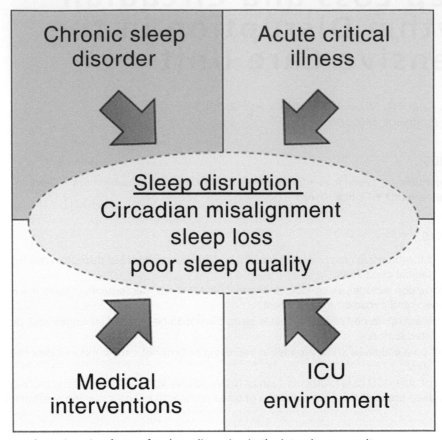

Chronic sleep disorder

Acute critical illness

Sleep disruption
Circadian misalignment
sleep loss
poor sleep quality

Medical interventions

ICU environment

Fig. 1. Causes and perpetuating factors for sleep disruption in the intensive care unit.

cellular recovery. REM sleep occupies 20% to 25% of the total sleep period and is considered to have a critical role in cognition and memory formation.[2,3]

Circadian rhythms are oscillations in biological function that follow a 24-hour cycle and are endogenously generated.[4] These rhythms influence an array of behaviors and physiologic parameters and arise from a genetically based chronometer called the molecular clock that is present in most nucleated cells.[5] This molecular clock is composed of a group of transcription factors and transcription factor regulators that have a feedback effect on one another to produce circadian oscillations in their own transcription. Molecular clock proteins have wide effects on transcriptional activity and metabolism, directly or indirectly causing up to 50% of genes to oscillate body-wide.[6–9] The complement of genes that oscillate in any given organ are largely unique to that organ (outside of the core molecular clock genes themselves),[7,10] indicating that circadian rhythms are heavily embedded in organ physiology. The clocks within individual cells are synchronized at the organ level through incompletely understood mechanisms.

Systemic cues including body temperature, autonomic tone, and circulating hormones such as cortisol are thought to play a role.[11,12] These global cues in turn are under control of a master circadian clock that resides in the neurons of the suprachiasmatic nucleus (SCN).[13] The SCN receives innervation directly from the retina, and its clock is thereby directly pegged to the day-night cycle. The SCN projects to multiple central nervous system regions, including areas of the hypothalamus that regulate arousal, metabolism, and hormone release from the pituitary and pineal glands.[13]

The amount (total sleep time), quality (N3 and REM fractions), and timing (circadian alignment) of sleep are important to human health; all 3 elements are disrupted in the ICU. Studies using 24-hour polysomnography (PSG) in mechanically ventilated and nonventilated patients in the medical ICU (MICU) demonstrate severely reduced overall sleep time, decreased N3, limited REM sleep, frequent arousals, and increased sleep during daytime hours.[1,14–17] Similar findings have been observed in patients in the surgical ICU[18] and in healthy subjects exposed to recordings of the ICU.[19]

CONSEQUENCES OF INTENSIVE CARE UNIT SLEEP DISRUPTION

Acute and chronic sleep disruptions precipitate severe physiologic perturbations and thus contribute to adverse short- and long-term outcomes.[20] Cognitively, acute sleep deprivation diminishes psychomotor performance and short-term memory and impairs executive functioning.[21] Mood disturbances such as fatigue, irritability, difficulty concentrating, disorientation, anxiety, depression, and paranoia also occur.[22] In the context of end-of-life and goals-of-care discussions, clinicians should be particularly alert to sleep disruption and subsequent alterations in patient mood or cognition, which may affect decision making. Similarities between sleep deprivation symptoms and delirium have prompted many experts to draw links between the 2 and question the role of sleep deprivation in causing ICU delirium. Delirium portends worsened ICU outcomes, including higher mortality and increased functional and cognitive impairments.[23–25]

Regarding pulmonary function, sleep deprivation diminishes the respiratory response to hypoxemia and hypercapnea.[26] Forced expiratory volume in 1 second and forced vital capacity have been shown to decrease in sleep-deprived patients with preexisting pulmonary disease.[27] Poor sleep quality or atypical sleep patterns may also predict late failure of noninvasive ventilation in cases of acute hypercarbic respiratory failure.[28]

Normal endocrine function, including anabolic/catabolic balance, is influenced by sleep and disrupted during sleep disturbance. Growth hormone and prolactin, anabolic hormones necessary for cell differentiation and proliferation, follow the sleep-wake cycle and are suppressed during sleep restriction.[29] Similarly, cortisol, the level of which increases in the early morning and peaks in the late morning, loses its periodicity during sleep loss and reentrains during sleep recovery.[30,31] The level of thyroid-stimulating hormone peaks before sleep onset and declines during sleep; thyroid-stimulating hormone is inhibited during N3, and the level increases with sleep deprivation.[30]

The clinical significance of circadian disruption in inpatients is difficult to quantify in isolation. Circadian misalignment is severe in the ICU where normal rhythms, nutritional intake, and arousal clash with circadian synchrony. Although the molecular clocks in various peripheral organs share the same basic genetic makeup, they differ in terms of their sensitivity to particular synchronizers (eg, feeding and light)[11] and as a result can be disassociated from one another.[32] The misalignment of the SCN and peripheral organ clocks is often referred to as internal desynchronization and seems to be interpreted by the body as a form of stress that is additive to, but independent from, sleep deprivation.[33] This internal desynchronization in part explains why long-term night-shift workers have increased incidence of cardiovascular disease, metabolic syndrome, elevated inflammatory markers, and, in women, elevated cancer risk.[34–37] Thus, it follows that circadian disruptions and related molecular changes have an important bearing on the patient's ICU experience and outcomes.

SOURCES OF INTENSIVE CARE UNIT SLEEP DISRUPTION
Chronic Sleep Disorder

Chronic sleep disorders contribute significantly to ICU sleep disruption. Sleep-disordered breathing (SDB) is moderately prevalent in the general population[38] and highly prevalent in patient populations with coronary artery disease,[39,40] diabetes,[41] and stroke[42,43] and therefore likely to be highly prevalent in the critically ill population. Treatment of SDB is often hampered by underrecognition and lack of treatment, and the presence of SDB in an inpatient carries increased risk for complications and poor outcomes during hospitalization.[44] Furthermore, patients with SDB present with chronic sleep disruption most commonly in the form of sleep loss and diminished N3 and REM sleep fractions; this sleep disruption is exacerbated during ICU admission. In addition, patients with chronic obstructive pulmonary disease frequently experience poor sleep quality, including increased sleep latency, decreased total sleep time, and increased arousals[45]; thus these patients present at ICU admission with chronic sleep deprivation. Self-report of poor sleep at home before ICU admission, not surprisingly, predicts worse sleep in the ICU versus patients without preexisting sleep disruption.[46]

Acute Illness–Related Factors

Acute illness is believed to inherently disrupt sleep. The directionality of the relationship between delirium, brain dysfunction, sleep loss, circadian misalignment, and critical illness is not known. Circadian misalignment has been well demonstrated in patients in the ICU (**Table 1**); however, most patients are studied several days postadmission and data are lacking regarding circadian orientation on ICU admission. Circadian abnormalities seem to be grossly proportional to severity of illness. Precise causality is difficult to assign, as circadian misalignment contributes to and is

Table 1
Summary of observational literature on circadian rhythms in patients in the ICU

Parameter	Results	Comments
Vital signs		
Temperature[105–112]	All papers detected circadian temperature rhythms in most patients. Abnormalities included significant patient-to-patient variation in acrophase (5 of 8 papers) and decreased amplitude (4 of 8 papers)	Most articles are based on at least 2 d of serial measurements
BP and HR[113,124]	Loss of BP circadian rhythms in 2 of 2 articles; normal dipping of BP at night was absent. Decreased amplitude or absence of HR circadian rhythm	Papers limited by short duration of observation (24 h). Loss of the dipping pattern in BP is associated with increased mortality
Ventilatory equivalents[114]	Vo_2 and Vco_2 retained circadian rhythms, but amplitudes were low compared with normal historical controls. RQ was arrhythmic	Unknown if the decrease in amplitude was due to patient immobility or masking of the intrinsic circadian clock
Hormones		
Melatonin[73,110,112,115–120]	Circadian variation in melatonin observed in most patients in 3 of 9 studies and in a significant minority in 3 of 9 studies. A common rhythm abnormality was a shifted acrophase into the daylight hours	Studies showing absence of circadian melatonin variation tended to have shorter periods of sampling (48 h or less). Higher-acuity patients seemed less likely to exhibit circadian rhythms in melatonin
Cortisol[110,112,115,121–123]	Loss of circadian variations in cortisol observed in 2 of 6 papers. In 4 of 6 papers a minority of patients were reported to exhibit cortisol rhythms	Patients in the ICU exhibiting cortisol rhythms tended to be in surgical and neurologic ICU settings and less acutely ill
ACTH and leptin[121]	Loss of circadian rhythm	—
Cytokines		
TNF[116,123]	1 of 2 papers reported rhythms in TNF	TNF rhythms reported for patients with sepsis but not with SIRS. Studies with short observation period (24 h)
IL-6[116]	Circadian rhythms in IL-6 noted in patients with sepsis	Short observation period (24 h)
IL-13[123]	Rhythms in IL-13 noted in patients with and without SIRS	IL-13 rhythms in patients with SIRS were in antiphase to rhythms of non-SIRS patients
Other		
RRT calls (clinical deterioration)[124,125]	RRT calls were more common during the day than in the night on the general wards but not in the ICU setting	Results ascribed to circadian variations in the process of care (ie, staffing) rather than intrinsic biology
Glucose[126]	Morning nadirs in blood glucose preserved in diverse populations of patients in the ICU	The amplitude of glucose rhythms is blunted in higher-acuity patients
Clock gene expression[116]	Arrhythmic circadian clock gene expression in peripheral leukocytes of patients with sepsis and ICU controls	No cohort of healthy controls; without this positive control, a lack of observed circadian clock gene expression is difficult to interpret

Abbreviations: ACTH, adrenocorticotropic hormone; BP, blood pressure; HR, heart rate; IL, interleukin; RQ, respiratory quotient; RRT, rapid response team; SIRS, systemic inflammatory response; TNF, tumor necrosis factor; Vco_2, rate of elimination of carbon dioxide; Vo_2, oxygen consumption.

perpetuated by sleep loss and poor sleep quality in the ICU. In addition, the severity of a patient's illness influences the degree of disturbance and clinical intervention required and thus affects the availability of rest periods. Illness severity also relates to the degree of pain and/or anxiety patients are experiencing; pain and anxiety have been linked to poor sleep in the critically ill patient population.[47,48]

Environment Factors

From the earliest days of critical care, excessive noise has been considered a significant source of stress, anxiety, and negative psychological outcomes in hospitalized patients.[49–51] Multiple studies demonstrate high noise levels in ICUs, with average and peak levels of 43 to 80 A-weighted decibels (dBA) and 80 to 90 dBA,[52–56] respectively, despite recommendations for hospital noise maximums of 35 to 45 dBA. Noise has been directly implicated as a disruptor of sleep in the ICU. PSG studies of critically ill patients have demonstrated a correlation between sound peaks greater than 80 dBA and arousals from sleep,[57] with as many as 17% of nighttime arousals occurring because of noise.[15] Moreover, healthy volunteers exposed to simulated ICU sounds experienced decreased REM sleep[19] and reported prolonged sleep latency, increased number of arousals, and poorer sleep quality.[58]

Data on ambient light levels and sleep in the hospital are limited. There are, however, strong theoretic reasons to support that increasing daytime and decreasing nighttime light exposure would benefit critically ill patients. Day-night light cycles are the most important determinant in the entrainment of circadian rhythms via SCN pathways, with the natural decrease in light during evening hours causing a release of melatonin inhibition; the subsequent increase in melatonin promotes sleep. The geriatrics literature suggests that mimicry of normal light cycles improves sleep in institutionalized patients.[59–62]

Medical Interventions

Medical interventions may cause sleep disruption because they are associated with noise, light, pain, anxiety, or movement of the patient. Alternatively, they may fundamentally alter sleep as is the case with many medications and mechanical ventilation (MV). Patients in the ICU experience a tremendous burden of in-room activity. Retrospective chart reviews of 147 patient-nights across 4 ICUs and 180 patient-nights in a surgical ICU demonstrated averages of 42.6 and 51 nocturnal care interactions per room per 12-hour night

shift.[63,64] Moreover, the surgical ICU investigation noted that bathing and mouth, eye, and wound care occurred most frequently between midnight and 5:00 AM.[64] Another observational study of 1831 nighttime patient interactions across 200 patients in 5 ICUs estimated that 13.9% of nocturnal interactions were not time critical.[65]

Medications prescribed during hospitalization can adversely affect sleep quality; medications perceived to promote sleep are often prescribed off-label, may inhibit sleep, and carry untoward side effects.[66,67] Benzodiazepines, γ-aminobutyric acid A (GABA$_A$) benzodiazepine receptor complex agonists, are known to diminish total sleep time and profoundly suppress REM and N3 sleep.[68,69] Sedating antihistamines such as diphenhydramine reversibly antagonize histamine H$_1$ receptors and inhibit histamine-induced wakefulness but do not improve sleep quality on PSG.[70] Trazodone, a tetracyclic antidepressant that inhibits serotonin reuptake and antagonizes the H$_1$ histamine and 5-hydroxytryptamine 1A, 1C, 2 receptors, has been shown to subjectively improve sleep and sleep efficiency; however, PSG data are limited on this drug. In addition, this medication is profoundly sedating and associated with life-threatening arrhythmias and drug-drug interactions.[71] Narcotics, although not considered traditional hypnotics, are frequently prescribed in the inpatient ICU setting and are known to provoke nocturnal awakenings, suppress N3 and REM sleep, and cause central apneas.[72]

Sedative use associated with MV also affects sleep in critically ill patients. A study of 21 sedated mechanically ventilated patients undergoing continuous PSG demonstrated sleep architecture abnormalities and loss of day-night sleep periodicity; only 2 of 21 subjects experienced REM in this study.[73] An observational study of 18 patients comparing intermittent sedation, continuous sedation, and continuous sedation with paralytic use showed abnormal sleep architecture and decreased or no REM sleep on PSG in all 3 study arms; decrements in REM sleep are believed to severely affect cognitive function.[74] Patients experiencing daily interruption of sedating benzodiazepine infusions demonstrated increased SWS and REM as compared with patients on continuous sedation.[75] Newer sedating agents have been investigated for their influence on sleep in the ICU. Neither dexmedetomidine nor propofol demonstrated improvements in REM or SWS in critically ill patients.[76,77]

MV is a well-known cause of severe sleep disruption. In addition to causing pain and anxiety, MV is believed to disrupt sleep via patient-ventilator asynchrony, overventilation leading to apneas and subsequent arousals, and inadequate ventilatory support leading to increased respiratory effort and subsequent arousals.[78] Although extensively studied, there is no strong evidence to support improved patient sleep with one ventilator mode over another.[79] A PSG study of 11 patients comparing assist control (AC) and pressure support ventilation (PSV) demonstrated less sleep fragmentation during PSV; this difference was attributed to diminished patient control of Pco_2 in the AC mode.[80] However, a similar comparison of AC, PSV, and clinician-adjusted PSV revealed poor sleep across all modes.[16] Investigation with alternative ventilator modes, such as proportional assist ventilation with load-adjustable gain and neurally adjusted ventilator assist mode, demonstrates further mixed results.[81–83]

MANAGEMENT GOALS

Goals for ICU sleep promotion include prolonging total sleep time, decreasing the number of arousals, promoting N3 and REM sleep, increasing sleep during night periods, decreasing daytime sleep, and promoting daytime sleep at circadian times. Strategies to achieve these goals are diverse and include recognition and treatment of preexisting sleep disorders (primarily SDB), clustering of care, medication adjustment, pain management, anxiolysis, environmental alterations, and education of patients and clinical staff regarding the importance of sleep and circadian health (**Table 2**).

PHARMACOLOGIC STRATEGIES

Minimization of antihistamine, benzodiazepine, and narcotic medication would likely benefit sleep (despite perceptions of patients and clinical staff that these agents promote sleep). Decreasing use of these medications aligns with the growing body of ICU literature, which supports limitations of sedative agents; these efforts must be carefully balanced with pain management and anxiolysis efforts. Daily sedative interruption is the only known pharmacologic strategy that improves PSG sleep parameters in the ICU.[75] Trazodone should be avoided, as it does not increase restorative sleep. Newer agents such as propofol and dexmedetomidine also do not promote sleep and should not be considered as part of sleep-improvement strategies.

Zolpidem and other members of the nonbenzodiazepine sedative hypnotic family have been shown to improve sleep via agonism of the $GABA_A$ receptor. One ICU study recommended zolpidem for patients without delirium (and haloperidol or an atypical antipsychotic for patients with delirium) as part of a multidisciplinary sleep promotion bundle. Although there was overall benefit in delirium rates for this bundle, the effect of zolpidem on ICU sleep was not established.[84] Zolpidem should be used with caution in the ICU as there is no evidence for overall benefit in critically ill patients, and there is concern for unintentional falls, carryover to outpatient use, and associations between long-term use and increased mortality.[85,86] Melatonin has been considered for patients in the ICU for both its antioxidant and sleep-promoting properties.[87] One small trial suggested sleep extension; however, sleep monitoring in this trial was carried out via Bispectral Index (BIS, Covidien, Mansfield, MA, USA), which is an unreliable method to measure sleep.[88] Further trials are underway.[89]

Table 2
Management goals and strategy summary

	Goals	Strategies
Sleep goals	Increased total sleep time	Recognition/treatment of sleep disorders
	Decreased arousals	Clustering of care activities
	Increased N3 fraction	Strategic medication usage
	Increased REM sleep fractions	Pain management and anxiolysis
Circadian goals	Increasing night sleep	Pharmacologic strategies
	Decreasing daytime sleep	Nonpharmacologic strategies
	Promoting daytime sleep at circadian times	Environmental modification
		Decrease noise and noise peaks
		Increase daytime light
		Decrease nighttime light
		Provision of patient-controlled devices
		Patient and family education
		Clinical staff education
		Promotion of daily sedative interruption, early mobilization, and daytime feeding

NONPHARMACOLOGIC STRATEGIES

Current sleep improvement recommendations emphasize the use of a multidisciplinary, bundled approach aimed at addressing modifiable disruptors of sleep in the ICU setting. These interventions commonly include environmental noise and light reduction via quiet time protocols[90–93] and clustering of patient care activities.[94] Arrangement of patient care activities in strategic clusters allows for periods of nondisturbance during which sleep may more readily occur. Clustering of care creates extensive workflow challenges and cannot be achieved without broad support from the many persons and/or teams that potentially enter and disturb patients in their rooms (**Box 1**); all MICU stakeholders should be included in protocol development.

Additional small studies support the use of nonpharmacologic therapies, such as music therapy,[95] back massage,[96] and aromatherapy,[97] as safe options for sleep promotion. These alternative modalities likely benefit patients via promotion of anxiolysis and pain control. Provision of a signal to sleep and patient education regarding sleep may also be helpful.

Nonpharmacologic circadian entrainment can also be undertaken; use of the key zeitgebers, light, feeding, and exercise, may play an important role in the promotion of ICU circadian health. Maximization of light during the day, including natural light, is an important addition to the sleep promotion bundles, which currently emphasize restriction of light during overnight periods. Adjunctive circadian entrainment with bolus feeding during daytime hours and daytime exercise is safe[98] and may promote resynchronization. Decrements

in delirium duration seen following early mobilization protocols may be attributed, at least in part, to promotion of circadian realignment.[99]

SELF-MANAGEMENT STRATEGIES

Patients frequently report that lack of control over their environment while in the ICU is a major source of stress. Although patient control over much of the ICU environment is difficult, minimization of the impact of noise and light is possible via devices such as earplugs and eye masks. Earplugs and/or eye masks should be offered to patients in the ICU (many patients decline) and have been demonstrated to improve subjective sleep in ICU settings[100,101] and sleep recorded via PSG in simulated ICU settings.[102,103] Patient-directed music therapy is an effective strategy for anxiolysis in ventilated patients[104] and should also be considered. Unrestricted visitation in ICUs has become more popular and likely conveys benefits to patients who experience greater support from loved ones during their admission; however, patient and family education regarding the benefits of overnight sleep coupled with the suggestion to allow rest during overnight hours is reasonable.

SUMMARY/DISCUSSION

ICU sleep disruption, defined by sleep loss, N3 and REM decrements, and circadian misalignment, is a profound physiologic insult resulting from and contributing to acute critical illness. Cognitive and physical critical care outcomes are likely highly affected by the intertwined processes of sleep loss, circadian misalignment and delirium. There exists a panel of low-risk, novel protocols that require ICU workflow alterations and culture change but have tremendous potential to promote sleep and circadian orientation. Challenges in measuring sleep, unpredictable clinical demands, frequent emergencies, and lack of knowledge about sleep and circadian promotion pose some of the largest barriers to implementation of sleep-promoting strategies. However, the critical care field has a rich history of developing and implementing highly successful care bundles. Sleep promotion represents another such opportunity. With the appropriate recruitment and involvement of diverse ICU stakeholders, effective strategies could be created, implemented, and maintained.

Box 1
MICU stakeholders
Patients
Visitors
Physicians
Midlevel providers
Nurses
Care assistants
Respiratory therapists
Pharmacists
Diagnostic imaging
Laboratory medicine
Hospital administration
Facilities/environmental services

REFERENCES

1. Knauert MP, Malik V, Kamdar BB. Sleep and sleep disordered breathing in hospitalized patients. Semin Respir Crit Care Med 2014;35:582–92.

2. Carskadon MA, Dement WC. Normal human sleep. In: Kryger MH, Roth T, Dement WC, editors. Principles and practice of sleep medicine. 5th edition. Philadelphia: Saunders/Elsevier; 2011. p. 16–26.

3. Iber C, Ancoli-Israel S, Chesson AL Jr, et al. The AASM manual for the scoring of sleep and associated events: rules, terminology and technical specifications. Westchester (IL): American Acadmeny of Sleep Medicine; 2007.

4. Refinetti R, Lissen GC, Halberg F. Procedures for numerical analysis of circadian rhythms. Biol Rhythm Res 2007;38:275–325.

5. Green CB, Takahashi JS, Bass J. The meter of metabolism. Cell 2008;134:728–42.

6. Ptitsyn AA, Zvonic S, Conrad SA, et al. Circadian clocks are resounding in peripheral tissues. PLoS Comput Biol 2006;2:e16.

7. Zhang R, Lahens NF, Ballance HI, et al. A circadian gene expression atlas in mammals: implications for biology and medicine. Proc Natl Acad Sci U S A 2014;111:16219–24.

8. Dallmann R, Viola AU, Tarokh L, et al. The human circadian metabolome. Proc Natl Acad Sci U S A 2012;109:2625–9.

9. Eckel-Mahan KL, Patel VR, Mohney RP, et al. Coordination of the transcriptome and metabolome by the circadian clock. Proc Natl Acad Sci U S A 2012;109:5541–6.

10. Storch KF, Lipan O, Leykin I, et al. Extensive and divergent circadian gene expression in liver and heart. Nature 2002;417:78–83.

11. Sujino M, Furukawa K, Koinuma S, et al. Differential entrainment of peripheral clocks in the rat by glucocorticoid and feeding. Endocrinology 2012; 153:2277–86.

12. Buhr ED, Yoo SH, Takahashi JS. Temperature as a universal resetting cue for mammalian circadian oscillators. Science 2010;330:379–85.

13. Kalsbeek A, Yi CX, Cailotto C, et al. Mammalian clock output mechanisms. Essays Biochem 2011; 49:137–51.

14. Cooper AB, Thornley KS, Young GB, et al. Sleep in critically ill patients requiring mechanical ventilation. Chest 2000;117:809–18.

15. Freedman NS, Gazendam J, Levan L, et al. Abnormal sleep/wake cycles and the effect of environmental noise on sleep disruption in the intensive care unit. Am J Respir Crit Care Med 2001;163:451–7.

16. Cabello B, Thille AW, Drouot X, et al. Sleep quality in mechanically ventilated patients: comparison of three ventilatory modes. Crit Care Med 2008;36:1749–55.

17. Elliott R, McKinley S, Cistulli P, et al. Characterisation of sleep in intensive care using 24-hour polysomnography: an observational study. Crit Care 2013;17:R46.

18. Trompeo AC, Vidi Y, Locane MD, et al. Sleep disturbances in the critically ill patients: role of delirium and sedative agents. Minerva Anestesiol 2011;77:604–12.

19. Topf M, Davis JE. Critical care unit noise and rapid eye movement (REM) sleep. Heart Lung 1993;22:252–8.

20. Bonnet MH. Acute sleep deprivation. In: Kryger MH, Roth T, Dement WC, editors. Principles and practice of sleep medicine. 5th edition. Philadelphia: Saunders/Elsevier; 2011. p. 54–66.

21. Pilcher JJ, Huffcutt AI. Effects of sleep deprivation on performance: a meta-analysis. Sleep 1996;19:318–26.

22. Kahn-Greene ET, Killgore DB, Kamimori GH, et al. The effects of sleep deprivation on symptoms of psychopathology in healthy adults. Sleep Med 2007;8:215–21.

23. Pisani MA, Kong SY, Kasl SV, et al. Days of delirium are associated with 1-year mortality in an older intensive care unit population. Am J Respir Crit Care Med 2009;180:1092–7.

24. Ely EW, Gautam S, Margolin R, et al. The impact of delirium in the intensive care unit on hospital length of stay. Intensive Care Med 2001;27:1892–900.

25. Ely EW, Shintani A, Truman B, et al. Delirium as a predictor of mortality in mechanically ventilated patients in the intensive care unit. JAMA 2004;291:1753–62.

26. White DP, Douglas NJ, Pickett CK, et al. Sleep deprivation and the control of ventilation. Am Rev Respir Dis 1983;128:984–6.

27. Phillips BA, Cooper KR, Burke TV. The effect of sleep loss on breathing in chronic obstructive pulmonary disease. Chest 1987;91:29–32.

28. Roche Campo F, Drouot X, Thille AW, et al. Poor sleep quality is associated with late noninvasive ventilation failure in patients with acute hypercapnic respiratory failure. Crit Care Med 2010;38:477–85.

29. Griffin JE, Ojeda SR. Textbook of endocrine physiology. 5th edition. Oxford (United Kingdom); New York: Oxford University Press; 2004.

30. Lee-Chiong TL. Sleep medicine: essentials and review. Oxford (United Kingdom); New York: Oxford University Press; 2008.

31. Schussler P, Uhr M, Ising M, et al. Nocturnal ghrelin, ACTH, GH and cortisol secretion after sleep deprivation in humans. Psychoneuroendocrinology 2006;31:915–23.

32. Yoo SH, Yamazaki S, Lowrey PL, et al. PERIOD2::LUCIFERASE real-time reporting of circadian dynamics reveals persistent circadian oscillations in mouse peripheral tissues. Proc Natl Acad Sci U S A 2004;101:5339–46.

33. Archer SN, Laing EE, Moller-Levet CS, et al. Mistimed sleep disrupts circadian regulation of the

human transcriptome. Proc Natl Acad Sci U S A 2014;111:E682–91.

34. Puttonen S, Viitasalo K, Harma M. Effect of shift work on systemic markers of inflammation. Chronobiol Int 2011;28:528–35.

35. Natti J, Anttila T, Oinas T, et al. Night work and mortality: prospective study among Finnish employees over the time span 1984 to 2008. Chronobiol Int 2012;29:601–9.

36. Vyas MV, Garg AX, Iansavichus AV, et al. Shift work and vascular events: systematic review and meta-analysis. BMJ 2012;345:e4800.

37. Wang F, Zhang L, Zhang Y, et al. Meta-analysis on night shift work and risk of metabolic syndrome. Obes Rev 2014;15:709–20.

38. Peppard PE, Young T, Barnet JH, et al. Increased prevalence of sleep-disordered breathing in adults. Am J Epidemiol 2013;177(9):1006–14.

39. Sanner BM, Konermann M, Doberauer C, et al. Sleep-disordered breathing in patients referred for angina evaluation – association with left ventricular dysfunction. Clin Cardiol 2001;24:146–50.

40. Hetzenecker A, Buchner S, Greimel T, et al. Cardiac workload in patients with sleep-disordered breathing early after acute myocardial infarction. Chest 2013;143:1294–301.

41. Schober AK, Neurath MF, Harsch IA. Prevalence of sleep apnoea in diabetic patients. Clin Respir J 2011;5:165–72.

42. Dyken ME, Somers VK, Yamada T, et al. Investigating the relationship between stroke and obstructive sleep apnea. Stroke 1996;27:401–7.

43. Shahar E, Whitney CW, Redline S, et al. Sleep-disordered breathing and cardiovascular disease: cross-sectional results of the Sleep Heart Health Study. Am J Respir Crit Care Med 2001;163:19–25.

44. Lindenauer PK, Stefan MS, Johnson KG, et al. Prevalence, treatment and outcomes associated with obstructive sleep apnea among patients hospitalized with pneumonia. Chest 2014;145:1032–8.

45. Cormick W, Olson LG, Hensley MJ, et al. Nocturnal hypoxaemia and quality of sleep in patients with chronic obstructive lung disease. Thorax 1986;41:846–54.

46. Bihari S, Doug McEvoy R, Matheson E, et al. Factors affecting sleep quality of patients in intensive care unit. J Clin Sleep Med 2012;8:301–7.

47. Novaes MA, Aronovich A, Ferraz MB, et al. Stressors in ICU: patients' evaluation. Intensive Care Med 1997;23:1282–5.

48. Little A, Ethier C, Ayas N, et al. A patient survey of sleep quality in the intensive care unit. Minerva Anestesiol 2012;78:406–14.

49. Kornfeld DS. Psychiatric view of the intensive care unit. Br Med J 1969;1:108–10.

50. Gabor JY, Cooper AB, Crombach SA, et al. Contribution of the intensive care unit environment to sleep disruption in mechanically ventilated patients and healthy subjects. Am J Respir Crit Care Med 2003;167:708–15.

51. Spence J, Murray T, Tang AS, et al. Nighttime noise issues that interrupt sleep after cardiac surgery. J Nurs Care Qual 2010;26:88–95.

52. Balogh D, Kittinger E, Benzer A, et al. Noise in the ICU. Intensive Care Med 1993;19:343–6.

53. Meyer TJ, Eveloff SE, Bauer MS, et al. Adverse environmental conditions in the respiratory and medical ICU settings. Chest 1994;105:1211–6.

54. Akansel N, Kaymakci S. Effects of intensive care unit noise on patients: a study on coronary artery bypass graft surgery patients. J Clin Nurs 2008;17:1581–90.

55. Lawson N, Thompson K, Saunders G, et al. Sound intensity and noise evaluation in a critical care unit. Am J Crit Care 2010;19:e88–98 [quiz: e99].

56. Cordova AC, Logishetty K, Fauerbach J, et al. Noise levels in a burn intensive care unit. Burns 2013;39(1):44–8.

57. Aaron JN, Carlisle CC, Carskadon MA, et al. Environmental noise as a cause of sleep disruption in an intermediate respiratory care unit. Sleep 1996;19:707–10.

58. Topf M, Bookman M, Arand D. Effects of critical care unit noise on the subjective quality of sleep. J Adv Nurs 1996;24:545–51.

59. Campbell SS, Dawson D, Anderson MW. Alleviation of sleep maintenance insomnia with timed exposure to bright light. J Am Geriatr Soc 1993;41:829–36.

60. Shochat T, Martin J, Marler M, et al. Illumination levels in nursing home patients: effects on sleep and activity rhythms. J Sleep Res 2000;9:373–9.

61. Wakamura T, Tokura H. Influence of bright light during daytime on sleep parameters in hospitalized elderly patients. J Physiol Anthropol Appl Human Sci 2001;20:345–51.

62. Riemersma-van der Lek RF, Swaab DF, Twisk J, et al. Effect of bright light and melatonin on cognitive and noncognitive function in elderly residents of group care facilities: a randomized controlled trial. JAMA 2008;299:2642–55.

63. Tamburri LM, DiBrienza R, Zozula R, et al. Nocturnal care interactions with patients in critical care units. Am J Crit Care 2004;13:102–12 [quiz: 114–5].

64. Celik S, Oztekin D, Akyolcu N, et al. Sleep disturbance: the patient care activities applied at the night shift in the intensive care unit. J Clin Nurs 2005;14:102–6.

65. Le A, Friese RS, Hsu CH, et al. Sleep disruptions and nocturnal nursing interactions in the intensive care unit. J Surg Res 2012;177:310–4.

66. Bourne RS, Mills GH. Sleep disruption in critically ill patients – pharmacological considerations. Anaesthesia 2004;59:374–84.

67. Schweitzer PK. Drugs that disturb sleep and wakefulness. In: Kryger MH, Roth T, Dement WC, editors. Principles and practice of sleep medicine. 5th edition. Philadelphia: Saunders/Elsevier; 2011. p. 542–60.

68. Achermann P, Borbely AA. Dynamics of EEG slow wave activity during physiological sleep and after administration of benzodiazepine hypnotics. Hum Neurobiol 1987;6:203–10.

69. Borbely AA, Mattmann P, Loepfe M, et al. Effect of benzodiazepine hypnotics on all-night sleep EEG spectra. Hum Neurobiol 1985;4:189–94.

70. Morin CM, Koetter U, Bastien C, et al. Valerian-hops combination and diphenhydramine for treating insomnia: a randomized placebo-controlled clinical trial. Sleep 2005;28:1465–71.

71. Buysse D. Clinical pharmacology of other drugs used as hypnotics. In: Kryger MH, Roth T, Dement WC, editors. Principles and practice of sleep medicine. 5th edition. Philadelphia: Saunders/Elsevier; 2011. p. 492–509.

72. Dimsdale JE, Norman D, DeJardin D, et al. The effect of opioids on sleep architecture. J Clin Sleep Med 2007;3:33–6.

73. Gehlbach BK, Chapotot F, Leproult R, et al. Temporal disorganization of circadian rhythmicity and sleep-wake regulation in mechanically ventilated patients receiving continuous intravenous sedation. Sleep 2012;35:1105–14.

74. Hardin KA, Seyal M, Stewart T, et al. Sleep in critically ill chemically paralyzed patients requiring mechanical ventilation. Chest 2006;129:1468–77.

75. Oto J, Yamamoto K, Koike S, et al. Effect of daily sedative interruption on sleep stages of mechanically ventilated patients receiving midazolam by infusion. Anaesth Intensive Care 2011;39:392–400.

76. Oto J, Yamamoto K, Koike S, et al. Sleep quality of mechanically ventilated patients sedated with dexmedetomidine. Intensive Care Med 2012;38:1982–9.

77. Kondili E, Alexopoulou C, Xirouchaki N, et al. Effects of propofol on sleep quality in mechanically ventilated critically ill patients: a physiological study. Intensive Care Med 2012;38:1640–6.

78. Roussos M, Parthasarathy S, Ayas NT. Can we improve sleep quality by changing the way we ventilate patients? Lung 2010;188:1–3.

79. Parthasarathy S. Effects of sleep on patient-ventilator interaction. Respir Care Clin N Am 2005;11:295–305.

80. Parthasarathy S, Tobin MJ. Effect of ventilator mode on sleep quality in critically ill patients. Am J Respir Crit Care Med 2002;166:1423–9.

81. Bosma K, Ferreyra G, Ambrogio C, et al. Patient-ventilator interaction and sleep in mechanically ventilated patients: pressure support versus proportional assist ventilation. Crit Care Med 2007; 35:1048–54.

82. Alexopoulou C, Kondili E, Plataki M, et al. Patient-ventilator synchrony and sleep quality with proportional assist and pressure support ventilation. Intensive Care Med 2013;39:1040–7.

83. Delisle S, Ouellet P, Bellemare P, et al. Sleep quality in mechanically ventilated patients: comparison between NAVA and PSV modes. Ann Intensive Care 2011;1:42.

84. Kamdar BB, King LM, Collop NA, et al. The effect of a quality improvement intervention on perceived sleep quality and cognition in a medical ICU. Crit Care Med 2013;41:800–9.

85. Belleville G. Mortality hazard associated with anxiolytic and hypnotic drug use in the National Population Health Survey. Can J Psychiatry 2010;55: 558–67.

86. Kripke DF, Langer RD, Kline LE. Hypnotics' association with mortality or cancer: a matched cohort study. BMJ Open 2012;2:e000850.

87. Bourne RS, Mills GH. Melatonin: possible implications for the postoperative and critically ill patient. Intensive Care Med 2006;32:371–9.

88. Bourne RS, Mills GH, Minelli C. Melatonin therapy to improve nocturnal sleep in critically ill patients: encouraging results from a small randomised controlled trial. Crit Care 2008;12:R52.

89. Huang H, Jiang L, Shen L, et al. Impact of oral melatonin on critically ill adult patients with ICU sleep deprivation: study protocol for a randomized controlled trial. Trials 2014;15:327.

90. Dennis CM, Lee R, Woodard EK, et al. Benefits of quiet time for neuro-intensive care patients. J Neurosci Nurs 2010;42:217–24.

91. Maidl CA, Leske JS, Garcia AE. The influence of "quiet time" for patients in critical care. Clin Nurs Res 2014;23(5):544–59.

92. Olson DM, Borel CO, Laskowitz DT, et al. Quiet time: a nursing intervention to promote sleep in neurocritical care units. Am J Crit Care 2001;10: 74–8.

93. Faraklas I, Holt B, Tran S, et al. Impact of a nursing-driven sleep hygiene protocol on sleep quality. J Burn Care Res 2013;34:249–54.

94. Barr J, Fraser GL, Puntillo K, et al. Clinical practice guidelines for the management of pain, agitation, and delirium in adult patients in the intensive care unit. Crit Care Med 2013;41:278–80.

95. de Niet G, Tiemens B, Lendemeijer B, et al. Music-assisted relaxation to improve sleep quality: meta-analysis. J Adv Nurs 2009;65:1356–64.

96. Richards KC. Effect of a back massage and relaxation intervention on sleep in critically ill patients. Am J Crit Care 1998;7:288–99.

97. Moeini M, Khadibi M, Bekhradi R, et al. Effect of aromatherapy on the quality of sleep in ischemic heart disease patients hospitalized in intensive care units of heart hospitals of the Isfahan

University of Medical Sciences. Iran J Nurs Midwifery Res 2010;15:234–9.

98. MacLeod JB, Lefton J, Houghton D, et al. Prospective randomized control trial of intermittent versus continuous gastric feeds for critically ill trauma patients. J Trauma 2007;63:57–61.

99. Schweickert WD, Pohlman MC, Pohlman AS, et al. Early physical and occupational therapy in mechanically ventilated, critically ill patients: a randomised controlled trial. Lancet 2009;373:1874–82.

100. Scotto CJ, McClusky C, Spillan S, et al. Earplugs improve patients' subjective experience of sleep in critical care. Nurs Crit Care 2009;14:180–4.

101. Van Rompaey B, Elseviers MM, Van Drom W, et al. The effect of earplugs during the night on the onset of delirium and sleep perception: a randomized controlled trial in intensive care patients. Crit Care 2012;16:R73.

102. Wallace CJ, Robins J, Alvord LS, et al. The effect of earplugs on sleep measures during exposure to simulated intensive care unit noise. Am J Crit Care 1999;8:210–9.

103. Hu RF, Jiang XY, Zeng YM, et al. Effects of earplugs and eye masks on nocturnal sleep, melatonin and cortisol in a simulated intensive care unit environment. Crit Care 2010;14:R66.

104. Chlan LL, Weinert CR, Heiderscheit A, et al. Effects of patient-directed music intervention on anxiety and sedative exposure in critically ill patients receiving mechanical ventilatory support: a randomized clinical trial. JAMA 2013;309:2335–44.

105. Bienert A, Kusza K, Wawrzyniak K, et al. Assessing circadian rhythms in propofol PK and PD during prolonged infusion in ICU patients. J Pharmacokinet Pharmacodyn 2010;37:289–304.

106. Dauch WA, Bauer S. Circadian rhythms in the body temperatures of intensive care patients with brain lesions. J Neurol Neurosurg Psychiatry 1990;53:345–7.

107. Gazendam JA, Van Dongen HP, Grant DA, et al. Altered circadian rhythmicity in patients in the ICU. Chest 2013;144:483–9.

108. Kirkness CJ, Burr RL, Thompson HJ, et al. Temperature rhythm in aneurysmal subarachnoid hemorrhage. Neurocrit Care 2008;8:380–90.

109. Nuttall GA, Kumar M, Murray MJ. No difference exists in the alteration of circadian rhythm between patients with and without intensive care unit psychosis. Crit Care Med 1998;26:1351–5.

110. Pina G, Brun J, Tissot S, et al. Long-term alteration of daily melatonin, 6-sulfatoxymelatonin, cortisol, and temperature profiles in burn patients: a preliminary report. Chronobiol Int 2010;27:378–92.

111. Tweedie IE, Bell CF, Clegg A, et al. Retrospective study of temperature rhythms of intensive care patients. Crit Care Med 1989;17:1159–65.

112. Paul T, Lemmer B. Disturbance of circadian rhythms in analgosedated intensive care unit patients with and without craniocerebral injury. Chronobiol Int 2007;24:45–61.

113. Sturrock ND, George E, Pound N, et al. Non-dipping circadian blood pressure and renal impairment are associated with increased mortality in diabetes mellitus. Diabet Med 2000;17:360–4.

114. van Lanschot JJ, Feenstra BW, Vermeij CG, et al. Accuracy of intermittent metabolic gas exchange recordings extrapolated for diurnal variation. Crit Care Med 1988;16:737–42.

115. Frisk U, Olsson J, Nylen P, et al. Low melatonin excretion during mechanical ventilation in the intensive care unit. Clin Sci (Lond) 2004;107:47–53.

116. Li CX, Liang DD, Xie GH, et al. Altered melatonin secretion and circadian gene expression with increased proinflammatory cytokine expression in early-stage sepsis patients. Mol Med Rep 2013;7:1117–22.

117. Mundigler G, Delle-Karth G, Koreny M, et al. Impaired circadian rhythm of melatonin secretion in sedated critically ill patients with severe sepsis. Crit Care Med 2002;30:536–40.

118. Olofsson K, Alling C, Lundberg D, et al. Abolished circadian rhythm of melatonin secretion in sedated and artificially ventilated intensive care patients. Acta Anaesthesiol Scand 2004;48:679–84.

119. Shilo L, Dagan Y, Smorjik Y, et al. Patients in the intensive care unit suffer from severe lack of sleep associated with loss of normal melatonin secretion pattern. Am J Med Sci 1999;317:278–81.

120. Verceles AC, Silhan L, Terrin M, et al. Circadian rhythm disruption in severe sepsis: the effect of ambient light on urinary 6-sulfatoxymelatonin secretion. Intensive Care Med 2012;38:804–10.

121. Bornstein SR, Licinio J, Tauchnitz R, et al. Plasma leptin levels are increased in survivors of acute sepsis: associated loss of diurnal rhythm, in cortisol and leptin secretion. J Clin Endocrinol Metab 1998;83:280–3.

122. Riutta A, Ylitalo P, Kaukinen S. Diurnal variation of melatonin and cortisol is maintained in non-septic intensive care patients. Intensive Care Med 2009;35:1720–7.

123. Socha LA, Gowardman J, Silva D, et al. Elevation in interleukin 13 levels in patients diagnosed with systemic inflammatory response syndrome. Intensive Care Med 2006;32:244–50.

124. Galhotra S, DeVita MA, Simmons RL, et al. Impact of patient monitoring on the diurnal pattern of medical emergency team activation. Crit Care Med 2006;34:1700–6.

125. Jones D, Bates S, Warrillow S, et al. Circadian pattern of activation of the medical emergency team in a teaching hospital. Crit Care 2005;9:R303–6.

126. Egi M, Bellomo R, Stachowski E, et al. Circadian rhythm of blood glucose values in critically ill patients. Crit Care Med 2007;35:416–21.

Barriers and Challenges to the Successful Implementation of an Intensive Care Unit Mobility Program

Understanding Systems and Human Factors in Search for Practical Solutions

Shyoko Honiden, MSc, MD*, Geoffrey R. Connors, MD

KEYWORDS

- ICU mobility • Quality improvement • Intensive care unit • Critical illness

KEY POINTS

- All change is difficult. Focusing on the environment in which people work, taking an inventory of beliefs held by workers, and assessing the degree of understanding about the change proposed can make facilitating change a more concrete and understandable process.
- Identifying waste, overburden, and inconsistencies is key to improving an environment in order to implement new practices or procedures successfully.
- Appreciating the regulative, normative, and cultural forces at work within an organizational structure is important. In facilitating change, it is vital to address each of these factors.
- The people within an organization need to be accounted for at each step in change implementation, including the leaders of the organization, the champions of the innovation in question, and the end users of that change; in medicine, these include hospital staff, physicians, and patients they care for.

INTRODUCTION

Recent advances in intensive care medicine, combined with an aging population, have led to an increase in the number of survivors following a period of critical illness. However, many of these patients are left with significant sequelae of disease despite surviving the acute phase of their illness. Often patients return home with an inability to function or live as fully as before. Others leave the intensive care unit (ICU) setting but experience prolonged physical disability, permanent loss of function, or the need for repeated hospitalization and ongoing supportive care. The most ill of these critical illness survivors become hospital dependent or chronically critically ill (**Table 1**).[1,2] There is a significant increase in 1-year morbidity for this cohort of patients, despite their having recovered from their critical illnesses.

Although there are many factors that contribute to debility and decline following a period of critical care, one that has a large negative impact on recovery is the development of ICU-acquired weakness.[3,4] Patients who have ICU-acquired

Conflicts of Interest: The authors have no conflicts of interest to disclose.
Section of Pulmonary, Critical Care and Sleep Medicine, Department of Medicine, Yale University School of Medicine, 300 Cedar Street, PO Box 208057, New Haven, CT 06520-8057, USA
* Corresponding author.
E-mail address: shyoko.honiden@yale.edu

Clin Chest Med 36 (2015) 431–440
http://dx.doi.org/10.1016/j.ccm.2015.05.006
0272-5231/15/$ – see front matter © 2015 Elsevier Inc. All rights reserved.

Table 1
Hospital dependency and chronic critical illness

Hospital-dependent Patients	Chronically Critically Ill Patients[a]
Multiple chronic conditions	Continuous need for life-sustaining equipment
Precipitous flares of their disease	Cognitive dysfunction
Decreased physiologic reserve	Neuromuscular weakness
Need for intensive monitoring	Endocrinopathy
Need for immediate medical response	Malnutrition/anasarca
—	Skin breakdown
—	Symptom distress

[a] A chronically critically ill patient has 1 or more of the characteristics of hospital-dependent patients plus at least 1 of the conditions in the right-hand column.

Data from Nelson JE, Cox CE, Hope AA, et al. Chronic critical illness. Am J Respir Crit Care Med 2010;182(4):446–54; and Reuben DB, Tinetti ME. The hospital-dependent patient. N Engl J Med 2014;370(8):694–7.

weakness have higher rates of muscle wasting and weakness,[5] prolonged dependency on mechanical ventilation,[6] and even an increase in complications during their ICU stays, up to and including an increase in mortality.[7] ICU-acquired weakness also has several key elements making it a ready target for intervention: it has a known cause (severe inflammatory illness combined with immobility and possible adverse effects from some medications) and a known intervention (early and aggressive physical therapy and mobility during the period of acute illness) that mitigates its effects.[8,9] In addition, this proven intervention is not cost prohibitive[10] and does not carry significant risk to the patient.[11] However, despite clinicians having identified a problem with significant consequences as well as a potential solution, implementation of early physical therapy and mobility lags behind the evidence for doing so. The questions are therefore these: why are early mobility programs not up and running in all medical and surgical ICUs in this country? What are the barriers to implementing an early mobility program? How can the barriers be overcome?

THE CHALLENGE OF EARLY INTENSIVE CARE UNIT MOBILIZATION AS A CHANGE INITIATIVE

Instituting a new initiative is challenging. The barriers to change in the health care setting are ever more present and intimidating and may contribute to the nihilistic perception that there is an eternal and unbridgeable gap between what is considered best practice and what happens in the real world. There are many pertinent examples in the ICU of practices that are demonstrably good for patients but difficult to get physicians and staff to fully and readily adopt, ranging from hand hygiene to

sedation practices. The issue related to early mobilization of ICU patients is another salient example of expert panels and guideline development seemingly disconnected from bedside adoption of new recommendations. Within the 2013 clinical practice guideline recommendations from the American College of Critical Care Medicine Taskforce, early mobilization of adult ICU patients was strongly endorsed as a way to reduce incidence and duration of delirium.[12] As outlined earlier, studies have shown early mobilization to be safe, feasible, and beneficial by improving delirium days and discharge functional status. Although there is a paucity of data pertaining to true practice patterns surrounding ICU mobilization in the United States, point prevalence studies from other countries show that widespread adoption has been painstakingly slow. For example, in Germany, only 24% of the 783 mechanically ventilated patients among 116 participating ICUs were mobilized out of the bed (defined as sitting on the edge of the bed or higher level of mobilization) on a single survey date.[13] A similar single-day survey study in Australia and New Zealand among 38 participating ICUs reported that none of the 222 mechanically ventilated patients were mobilized out of bed (ie, sat out of bed, stood up, or ambulated), although lesser intensities of mobilization, such as sitting at the edge of the bed or in-bed exercises, occurred with variable frequency over the course of the day.[14]

How can evidence-based change best be cultivated, adopted, and promoted in the health care environment? Although addressing knowledge deficits is a key determinant, focusing on education alone is insufficient to achieve behavioral change.[15] Understanding concepts related to systems and institutional behavior, as well as behavioral psychology, that help to elucidate barriers and motivations at an individual level can be helpful when planning a unit-wide (or hospital-wide) quality improvement initiative, such as that related to ICU mobility. Concrete steps that can be taken to foster a culture of ICU mobilization are outlined later in the article and help to highlight relevant key concepts within organizational and behavioral theories.

START BY LETTING GO OF THE IDEA OF CHANGING CULTURE

What is culture? What does it mean that a hospital or a specific unit within the hospital has a particular culture associated with it? The difficulty in defining a thing such as culture, especially as it applies to a diverse set of workplaces within a hospital system, is immense. More helpful than trying to change something that is difficult to define is to try to define the simple things that need to be changed. When people refer to culture what they mean pertains to how people in a particular environment act based on their beliefs and understandings. Too often when people talk about the culture of a unit they are referring to actions taken by a specific set of people in a specific environment who hold a specific set of beliefs. Thus, using the term culture is both inexact and confusing. Careful observation reveals that culture, a nebulous and elusive concept, is the sum of a few simple and definable parts. Most importantly, each of these parts can be influenced if they are understood and addressed individually.

At its core the definition of culture can be considered as a particular environment and systems of beliefs that lead people to act. The environment to be changed might refer to something as concrete as the physical plant all the way to the daily workflow of the nurses, therapists, and physicians. Changing beliefs and understandings means addressing 2 things: knowledge gaps and real or perceived concerns surrounding the action to be implemented. Focusing on these 2 factors provides a tangible, defined, and finite set of targets at which the efforts could be directed. We think that this frame shift is critically important: the goal is not to change culture but rather to establish an environment and an understanding in which the intervention to be adopted (eg, early ICU mobilization) becomes a daily reality.

Planning for Change at a Systems/Organizational Level: Tackling the Environment by Recognizing Muda (Waste), Muri (Overburden), and Mura (Inconsistency)

One of the prerequisites to improving compliance to any best-practice recommendation is to pay attention to system design. In that regard, the Lean continuous quality improvement (CQI) management system developed by the car manufacturer, Toyota, can be applied within health care as well. The Lean concept hinges on 2 principles. The first is to have a commitment to a systematic approach that works to remove waste and increase value. The second is to have a commitment to respect, challenge, and develop people to create a culture of CQI.

Lean CQI starts by understanding end user needs, defining the current state, and then redesigning processes to minimize the 3 Ms in Japanese: muda, muri, and mura, which translates to waste, overburden, and inconsistency, respectively.

Applying the Toyota Model to an Intensive Care Unit Mobility Project: First Take Inventory of the Current State

In considering an ICU mobility project, identifying end user needs is a useful starting point. Users for this purpose include patients and providers. A baseline survey of the existing mobility users over a discrete period of time (eg, 1 month) can capture the patient experience as well as provider (eg, ICU nurses) perceptions. This survey helps to provide critical information pertaining to existing ICU mobilization. Metrics that can be followed over time should be quantified, such as number of patients mobilized per unit day, number of patients with activity orders that specify bed rest, number of patients with physical therapy orders, and the time lag between the order and certified physical therapist (PT) assessment. This process helps to identify muda or waste within the system that might be remediated, such as the use of scarce skilled resources (eg, PTs) to mobilize patients who could be safely and effectively moved by existing staff (eg, nurses and patient care associates). From a leadership perspective, the initial survey can raise awareness about barriers and misconceptions that need to be strategically addressed, and can help identify champions and leaders who could be recruited later within the CQI process.

One natural concern raised by staff when faced with the start of a new initiative revolves around the perception of additional workload. In keeping with the Lean CQI model, it is critical to ensure a process that has some flexibility, and limits undue stress or unreasonable expectations that could lead to muri or overburden for staff members. Perception of burden or personal experience of overburden (even if isolated to a small number of people) could jeopardize the change initiative. In order to right-size staffing needs during the planning phase, the baseline survey should capture patient-specific parameters such as level of baseline mobility before ICU admission (eg, independent, assisted mobility vs bed bound), as well as prevalence of ongoing advanced ICU interventions (such as noninvasive positive pressure ventilation, mechanical ventilation, vasopressor support, dialysis), and duration of medical ICU length of stay. These metrics help to project how many patients will need to be mobilized and the likely distribution of support intensity, ranging from those capable of getting out of bed with minimal assist versus those who need specialized assessment and support from trained physical therapy staff. In turn, these data points can then be used to create a business plan to advocate for additional dedicated medical ICU PT staffing.

In addition, the baseline assessment may also reveal areas of inconsistencies in a practice, thereby addressing the third M, or help in minimizing mura. Lack of activity orders or infrequent PT consultation requests can be addressed in the era of electronic medical records, through creation of ICU mobility-specific order sets and might help ensure timely and appropriate referral to PT. By generating data pertaining to delays in placement of activity order, PT order, or to time to consultation, additional areas of improvement may be found. Protocol compliance has been shown to improve in other ICU-specific interventions, such as use of a low tidal volume lung protective ventilation strategy when on-screen prompts were embedded into order entry.[16] Additional examples of muda, muri, and mura as they apply to ICU mobility projects are shown in **Box 1**.

Recognizing and fostering an open discussion about the need for additional resources and willingness to start with a limited subset of patients (eg, targeting those deemed to have the highest need and biggest potential gains) helps overcome initial hesitation from staff. Lean CQI seeks to help people work smarter, not harder. Once waste, inappropriate process variation, and staff overburden are identified, simulating various scenarios before project launch is critical to preidentify

---

Box 1
Taking inventory of the status quo: identifying waste, overburden, and inconsistency. An example of system design assessment for an ICU mobility project

Waste (muda)

- Complications caused by inactivity/immobility such as:
  - Delirium
  - Skin breakdown and ulceration
  - Longer time spent in the ICU
  - Longer time spent on the ventilator
  - Longer time spent in the hospital
- Attempting to mobilize patients with limited baseline functioning who will not derive benefit
- Asking specialists (eg, PTs) to perform activities a nurse or care associate could perform safely and effectively (eg, getting a patient who can ambulate with minimal assist out of bed)

Overburden (muri)

- Physician and staff burnout caused by overwork/understaffing
- Asking nonspecialized staff to perform specialized (physical therapy, occupational therapy) activities
- Recognition of other change initiatives occurring in the unit at the same time that will take their own focus and effort
- Recognition of any staff safety concerns regarding mobilization of critically ill patients, even if the perception is greater than the real risk

Inconsistency (mura)

- Missed activity orders for patients
- Missed PT orders, when appropriate
- Missed occupational therapist orders, when appropriate
- Delay in the time from activity or mobility order until the time the patient is mobilized
- Relying on physicians for orders that could be automated using an electronic medical record

potential areas of difficulty. In addition, in this pre-planning phase brainstorming about and creating a mobility screening tool with key stakeholders can be a useful exercise (**Box 2**). Such a tool can be leveraged to help ensure that scarce resources are efficiently allocated, to standardize work flow, to facilitate discussions surrounding mobility action plans during work rounds on a daily basis, and to help identify those who are safe to mobilize and aid in determining how that should be accomplished.

Understanding How Institutions Change: Organizational Sociology

Institutions are social structures that are highly resilient by nature, and therefore resistant to change. To have the highest likelihood of enacting change in this environment and making it permanent, it is important to understand what forces influence its behavior. The first force is regulative, being laws and rules that define what must happen. The second is normative, being a composite of assumptions and expectations that define what should happen. The third is cultural, and relates to mental models about what generally does happen in real life. Each of these forces influences institutions by providing legal sanctions (eg, a penalty for preventable harm, such as pressure ulcers), moral authorization, and cultural support to regulate behavior.[17] As a corollary, institutional change can emerge out of 3 non–mutually exclusive mechanisms. The first is coercive, or top down, such as that related to a change in regulation, exemplified by reporting practices that are now mandated for preventable harm (eg, central line–associated catheter infections). The second pertains to normative expectations, and relates to changing perceptions of what is considered right or reasonable. The third is mimetic, such as when a hospital copies what it considers to be best practice from a sister or competitor institution. In reality, complex change in a complex system is unpredictable, particularly because the human players are unique

---

Box 2
Example of a mobility screening tool for the ICU used at Yale New Haven Hospital

1. Does this patient have a baseline condition that would limit the benefit from out-of-bed mobility?
   - ☐ Comfort measures only or actively dying
   - ☐ Bedbound at baseline
   - ☐ No limiting baseline contraindication: please go on to question #2

2. Is this patient too neurologically impaired to participate in mobility?
   - ☐ Richmond Agitation Sedation Scale less than or equal to −2 or greater than or equal to +3
   - ☐ No neurologic contraindication: please go on to question #3

3. Is this patient not safe from a respiratory standpoint to participate in mobility?
   - ☐ Fraction of inspired oxygen on mechanical ventilation greater than or equal to 60%
   - ☐ Positive end-expiratory pressure on mechanical ventilation greater than or equal to 10
   - ☐ No respiratory contraindications: please go on to question #4

4. Is this patient not safe from a hemodynamic standpoint to participate in mobility?
   - ☐ On more than 1 vasopressor agent
   - ☐ On greater than 50% of the maximum dose of a single vasopressor (vasopressin excluded)
   - ☐ Vasopressor uptitrated within the past 2 hours
   - ☐ Active myocardial ischemia with electrocardiogram changes or rapidly increasing troponin levels
   - ☐ Unstable arrhythmias or persistent sinus tachycardia greater than 120 beats per minute
   - ☐ Ongoing, uncontrolled blood loss or no active bleeding but platelet count less than 20,000/μL
   - ☐ Extracorporeal membrane oxygenation, intracranial pressure monitoring, femoral triple-lumen catheter or hemodialysis catheter in place
   - ☐ No hemodynamic contraindication: please develop a safe mobility plan for the patient

This tool is used to determine whether a patient will benefit from mobility, and also to address staff safety concerns and whether a need for a specialized mobility consult exists based on patient complexity.
Courtesy of YNHH Medical ICU Mobility Screening Tool (draft March 2015), New Haven, CT.

and may behave in an idiosyncratic fashion. Thus, there is no single standardized path that could (or should) be taken to overcome barriers at an institutional level to promote change. However, normative and mimetic forces for change can be powerful, and can be used effectively by deliberate language use and storytelling. This approach may entail a patient story told at the leadership level as a motivation and awareness-raising tool, or it may emerge at a grass roots level as narratives from the bedside to sustain change behavior. These patient success stories can be used as focal points when advocating for additional resources for the ICU with system administrators and managers. In addition, narratives from patients and providers can help maintain momentum once the project has launched.

PLANNING FOR CHANGE AT A LEADERSHIP LEVEL

Once organizational behavior and forces are accounted for, appointing system-level facilitators and leaders becomes critical. A leadership team can formulate a mission statement, plan for resource allocation, and help transform the work climate. It is intuitive that having a management position does not equate to effective leadership. However, being in management may provide an individual with certain kinds of powers that are directly linked to their administrative role, and cannot be dismissed. Positional power and resource power (eg, control over staff and funds) are examples. In contrast, expert power (related to specific skill sets and unique knowledge base) and personal power (eg, charisma) are derived by the unique characteristics of an individual. Individuals who have expert or personal power, with or without positional power, are often referred to as champions in the change initiative. In creating a leadership team, pulling individuals who are able to bring in different power dimensions and matching their strengths to particular tasks is helpful. An optimal team should have leadership representation at a systems level, leaders with expert power and with technical expertise, and day–to-day leadership (ideally, individuals with personal power) that can coach, motivate, and problem solve in real time so that issues can be fixed as they arise (**Fig. 1**).

In group dynamic theory, taking inventory of the various drivers and barriers to change is considered pivotal.[18] In general, a leadership strategy to reduce forces that are resistant to change is thought to be more effective than strengthening driving forces but to some extent attention needs to be paid to both. In addition, leaders need to be aware of the varying responses that individuals

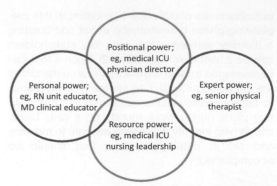

Fig. 1. Sources of power: creating a balanced leadership team. Circles in blue denote power linked to administrative roles. Circles in red denote power linked to personal characteristics. MD, Doctor of Medicine; RN, registered nurse.

could have to change and recognize the different tempos of change adoption that simultaneously exist within a workforce (**Fig. 2**). According to the seminal book by Everett Rogers,[19] first published in 1962, change adoption can be seen early among innovators and later by the late majority and laggards. At some point, innovation reaches a critical mass and the process accelerates. On the whole, the likelihood of change adoption varies depending on individuals' perceptions about benefits and obstacles, as well as their personal motivations. Creating simple processes that fit well within the existing mental model and highlighting observable goals with clear advantages can help transition slower change adopters.

In addition to assessing organizational capacity and developing resources (eg, educational videos for ICU mobility showing how to safely get an intubated patient out of bed), an effective leadership team needs to plan on (1) how the change initiative would be benchmarked, evaluated, and measured; (2) how progress would be demonstrated to stakeholders as part of transparent accountability (eg, weekly, monthly, semiannual feedback); and (3) identifying opportunities for scholarship and research to increase visibility. Evaluation and benchmarking may be important parts of the business plan to bring back to system leadership, especially to justify the need for additional resources if these are sought. Annual progress evaluation can generate data that inform future planning, and may help in deepening the penetration of the program (eg, adoption of innovation at another ICU within the institution). Periodic informal and formal surveys that capture input from leadership, staff competence and knowledge, patient/family-centered satisfaction and outcomes, as well as quality and safety metrics (eg, falls, staff injury, delirium days that would

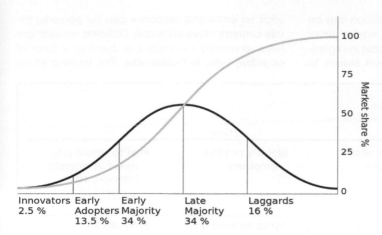

Fig. 2. How ideas and innovations diffuse. The purple line shows the bell curve of innovation adoption. The yellow line shows the cumulative total. With more people adopting the innovation (in purple), the cumulative total (or market share, in yellow) eventually reaches 100%. (*Adapted from* Rogers E. Diffusion of innovations. London; New York: Free Press; 1962.)

be relevant for an ICU mobility project) are vital to fuel an iterative innovation process.

UNDERSTANDING THE PSYCHOLOGY OF CHANGE AND MOTIVATION AT AN INDIVIDUAL LEVEL

Although taking inventory of organizational and leadership qualities is vital, it is difficult to appreciate the science of change without simultaneously accounting for behavioral responses at an individual level. Success ultimately depends on personal motivations that are complicated and poorly understood. Many clinicians are familiar with the transtheoretic model that describes readiness to change.[20] This model is often discussed in the context of smoking cessation and categorizes individuals into 5 stages:

precontemplators, contemplators, in preparation, engaged in action, or maintaining behavior. This model can be applied to any change initiative that is being contemplated in the health care setting. For example, precontemplators are those who, at the moment, have no intention or plans to change. Nonthreatening strategies that focus on raising awareness and consciousness by providing information and asking patients to participate in surveys about ICU mobility may help engage precontemplators. Linking these materials to tangible ideas (eg, highlighting early ICU mobilization benefits measured by reductions in ICU length of stay as opposed to the functional outcome at hospital discharge, which many ICU staff members may not witness and/or appreciate) and infusing messaging with a sense of personal responsibility may help engage this group (**Fig. 3**).

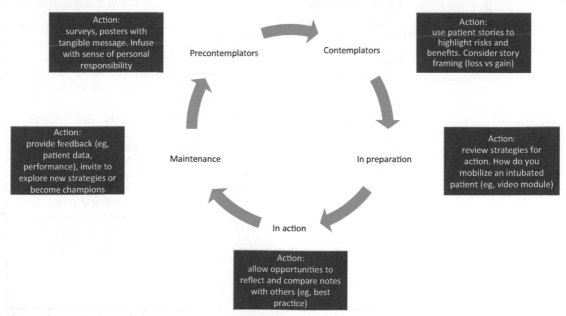

Fig. 3. The psychology of change. Applying the transtheoretic model to ICU mobility adoption.

In contrast, individuals in contemplation may be ready to hear the detailed risks and benefits about early ICU mobilization. As was the case in organizational sociology, the use of patient stories to elicit an emotional response can be powerful for this contemplative audience. Different researchers have examined the impact of framing, a form of cognitive bias, in health care. The framing effect

Table 2
Step-by-step guide to project launch

Steps	Actions		
Prework: assessing emotions	Identify negative emotions	Identify positive emotions	Plan to reevaluate mood at discrete intervals after project launch
Creating a Climate for Change			
Step 1: increase urgency	Create a thought-provoking story bolstered by facts	Avoid reliance on structured presentations	Promote an environment that allows feeling and seeing
Step 2: building teams	Identify problem solvers	Promote credibility/include expert power formal authority	Horizontal and vertical representation over institutional hierarchy
Step 3: getting the vision right	Clear and concise	Asks questions keeping in mind the implications for key stakeholders	Refine until picture of future is clear
Engage and Enable the Whole Organization			
Step 4: communicate for buy-in	Share your vision (can use patient story to make tangible)	Enable open dialogue (eg, FAQ, Q&A sessions)	Enroll the group into effort and secure commitment
Step 5: empower action	Identify barriers and categorize into personnel-related, system-related, or mental barriers, or barriers caused by lack of information	Create practical solutions	For personnel barriers, avoid inundation with facts and figures. Provide opportunities for first-hand experience
Step 6: create short-term wins	Achieve visible, meaningful, unambiguous progress quickly	Create short-term, achievable targets to help build urgency and momentum (eg, targeted patient selection; report on numbers walked)	—
Implement and Sustain Change			
Step 7: do not let up	Even after adoption by most, anticipate problems	Create an automatic cycle of reevaluation to help solve problems quickly	Force the team to self-evaluate compared with best-practice guidelines (or a competitor; eg, another institution, another ICU in the same hospital)
Step 8: make changes permanent	Have a postlive process in place. Recognize that culture change comes last	Strive for dynamic enhancements using performance data and feedback	—

Abbreviations: FAQ, frequently asked questions, Q&A, questions and answers.

talks about how people react to choices in different ways depending on whether this is presented as a loss or a gain. For example, in smoking cessation, some have shown that loss framing is more powerful, whereas in other studies (eg, hand hygiene) gain framing was shown to have more impact.[21,22] Ultimately, the response to gain or loss framing may be variable depending on the target audience and their state of mind. For example, when exploring resource commitments at an organizational level, loss framing might be used strategically knowing that mimetic and normative forces (ie, not embracing best practices accepted at other institutions, financial losses related to prolonged ICU days) are powerful motivators, as described earlier. Moving along the readiness spectrum, individuals in preparation may be eager to learn about different strategies for action (eg, demonstration or video of getting an intubated patient out of bed), whereas those already in action may benefit from opportunities to reflect and compare with others to maintain motivation. In addition, providing feedback to those in the maintenance phase and inviting them to explore new strategies (and thus be engaged in the change process/team itself) may be appropriate. As a group, periodic incentives such as unit recognition for success are helpful. In the end, the key is to accept that the target audience is in different stages of readiness.

Change initiatives need to foster an understanding and commitment that promotes and sustains motivation. The ARCS model for motivational design described by John Keller[23] outlines 4 steps: attention, relevance, confidence, and satisfaction. First, attention can be fostered by developing a varied learning experience, exploring perceptions, and promoting inquiry. Promoting inquiry may be accomplished by encouraging questions (eg, a presentation that incorporates a segment on frequently asked questions), and posing dilemmas and puzzles (eg, how ICU mobilization will be accomplished in a busy day if a patient has to travel for imaging and undergo a bedside procedure). Relevance increases motivation by highlighting how the intervention affects individuals at a personal level. These steps may be particularly relevant for the precontemplators and contemplators described earlier. Maintenance of motivation can be fueled by measures that enhance confidence (eg, providing data about the number of patients mobilized in the unit and providing frequent feedback). Meanwhile, rewards and a sense of achievement provide satisfaction. For some individuals, this is internally generated by self-directed attitudes and beliefs, whereas for others reward is extrinsically generated; for this latter group, social norms (from patients, families, colleagues), audits, and praise (at fixed and variable intervals) may become great motivators. In any case, although gentle peer pressure may be helpful in certain scenarios, forcing change only leads to antagonistic behavior that is best avoided. Prior studies pertaining to nursing hand-washing practices have shown that a combination of factors fuel motivation. Nursing belief about the benefits, a degree of peer pressure from doctors and administrators, and successful role modeling were equally important.[24]

BRINGING IT ALL TOGETHER: A STEP-BY-STEP PRESCRIPTION FOR ENACTING CHANGE IN THE HEALTH CARE ENVIRONMENT

Armed with an understanding and appreciation for systems design and organizational psychology, leadership qualities, as well as individual psychology pertaining to change and motivation, how could this information be distilled into concrete steps that lead to change?

Kotter and Cohen[25] developed a dynamic, nonlinear, 8-step process to characterize management steps relevant to organizational change. Their formulation helps outline the otherwise daunting process in useful, conveniently sized pieces.[25] The first 3 steps (increasing urgency, building guiding teams, and getting the vision right) focus on creating a climate for change. The next 3 steps (communicating for buy-in, enabling action, and creating short-term wins) work to engage and enable the whole organization. The last 2 steps (not letting up, and making it permanent) serve to implement and sustain change. As a preparatory step to all of this, assessing the emotions of key stakeholders is a useful exercise. The goal is to turn negatives such as complacency, anger, pessimism, cynicism, panic, insecurity, anxiety, arrogance, and exhaustion into positives such as faith, trust, optimism, urgency, passion, excitement, hope, and enthusiasm over the course of a change initiative (**Table 2**).

SUMMARY

This article uses the adoption of early mobility and rehabilitation as an example of a common challenge in the ICU. Fostering change, in particular implementing new and innovative programs to cure disease, lessen its incidence, or alleviate suffering, is at the heart of what intensive care leaders do. To do this they must focus on the environment in which they work and have a deeper understanding about the forces that affect people who work there. All change to an environment begins by understanding the system as it exists currently. Remembering the concepts of muda, muri, and mura can help restructure workflow and process to eliminate waste, relieve burden to providers, and reduce inconsistencies. Understanding the impact of the 3 organizational forces (regulative, normative, and cultural) is also critical to implementing change at an organizational level. In terms of managing people and shaping the understandings and beliefs held by a workforce, buy-in from leaders and process champions are key. Once leadership is established, individual learning and behavior change can begin. The 8-step process described by Kotter and Cohen[25] and the ARCS model provide a concrete framework in which individual change can be fostered and the maintenance of change over time can be promoted.

The medical community has worked tirelessly to discover new interventions and to rigorously study risks and benefits for such interventions to provide the best evidence to guide practice. However, this is but only one aspect of the mission we face as critical care physicians. Getting those interventions established and firmly rooted within the hospital environment and creating a shared understanding in an ICU regarding their implementation is entirely another, and is potentially just as challenging.

REFERENCES

1. Nelson JE, Cox CE, Hope AA, et al. Chronic critical illness. Am J Respir Crit Care Med 2010;182(4):446–54.
2. Reuben DB, Tinetti ME. The hospital-dependent patient. N Engl J Med 2014;370(8):694–7.
3. Herridge MS. Legacy of intensive care unit-acquired weakness. Crit Care Med 2009;37(10 Suppl):S457–61.
4. Desai SV, Law TJ, Needham DM. Long-term complications of critical care. Crit Care Med 2011;39(2):371–9.
5. Herridge MS, Cheung AM, Tansey CM, et al. One-year outcomes in survivors of the acute respiratory distress syndrome. N Engl J Med 2003;348(8):683–93.
6. Garnacho-Montero J, Amaya-Villar R, García-Garmendía JL, et al. Effect of critical illness polyneuropathy on the withdrawal from mechanical ventilation and the length of stay in septic patients. Crit Care Med 2005;33(2):349–54.
7. Leijten FS, Harinck-de Weerd JE, Poortvliet DC, et al. The role of polyneuropathy in motor convalescence after prolonged mechanical ventilation. JAMA 1995;274(15):1221–5.
8. Schweickert WD, Pohlman MC, Pohlman AS, et al. Early physical and occupational therapy in mechanically ventilated, critically ill patients: a randomised controlled trial. Lancet 2009;373(9678):1874–82.
9. Morris PE, Griffin L, Berry M, et al. Receiving early mobility during an intensive care unit admission is a predictor of improved outcomes in acute respiratory failure. Am J Med Sci 2011;341(5):373–7.
10. Morris PE, Goad A, Thompson C, et al. Early intensive care unit mobility therapy in the treatment of acute respiratory failure. Crit Care Med 2008;36(8):2238–43.
11. Bailey P, Thomsen GE, Spuhler VJ, et al. Early activity is feasible and safe in respiratory failure patients. Crit Care Med 2007;35(1):139–45.
12. Barr J, Fraser GL, Puntillo K, et al. Clinical practice guidelines for the management of pain, agitation, and delirium in adult patients in the intensive care unit. Crit Care Med 2013;41(1):263–306.
13. Nydahl P, Ruhl AP, Bartoszek G, et al. Early mobilization of mechanically ventilated patients: a 1-day point-prevalence study in Germany. Crit Care Med 2014;42(5):1178–86.
14. Berney SC, Harrold M, Webb SA, et al. Intensive care unit mobility practices in Australia and New Zealand: a point prevalence study. Crit Care Resusc 2013;15(4):260–5.
15. O'Boyle CA, Henly SJ, Larson E. Understanding adherence to hand hygiene recommendations: the theory of planned behavior. Am J Infect Control 2001;29(6):352–60.
16. Bagga S, Paluzzi DE, Chen CY, et al. Better ventilator settings using a computerized clinical tool. Respir Care 2014;59(8):1172–7.
17. Macfarlane F, Barton-Sweeney C, Woodard F, et al. Achieving and sustaining profound institutional change in healthcare: case study using neo-institutional theory. Soc Sci Med 2013;80:10–8.
18. Lewin K. Frontiers in group dynamics: concept, method, and reality in social science; social equilibria and social change. Hum Relat 1947;1(1):5–41.
19. Rogers EM. Diffusion of innovations. 4th edition. New York: The Free Press; 2004.
20. Prochaska JO, DiClemente CC. Stages of change in the modification of problem behaviors. Prog Behav Modif 1992;28:183–218.
21. Wong NC, Harvell LA, Harrison KJ. The unintended target: assessing nonsmokers' reactions to gain- and loss-framed antismoking public service announcements. J Health Commun 2013;18(12):1402–21.
22. Jenner EA, Jones F, Fletcher BC, et al. Hand hygiene posters: selling the message. J Hosp Infect 2005;59(2):77–82.
23. Keller JM. Development and use of the ARCS model of motivational design. J Instr Dev 1987;10(3):2–10.
24. Whitby M, McLaws ML, Ross MW. Why healthcare workers don't wash their hands: a behavioral explanation. Infect Control Hosp Epidemiol 2006;27(5):484–92.
25. Kotter J, Cohen D. The heart of change: real life stories of how people change their organization. Boston: Harvard Business School Press; 2002.

Integration of Palliative Care Services in the Intensive Care Unit
A Roadmap for Overcoming Barriers

Mary Baker, MD[a,b], Jim Luce, MSW[c],
Gabriel T. Bosslet, MD, MA[a,b],*

KEYWORDS

- Palliative care • End-of-life care • Process bundle • Process implementation • ICU integration

KEY POINTS

- Current evidence supports the implementation of palliative care in the ICU.
- Barriers to implementation often stem from misunderstanding of what palliative care services can provide patients, providers, and families.
- Implementation is a process requiring a considerate, step-wise approach.

THE IMPORTANCE OF PALLIATIVE CARE

Clinicians working in the intensive care unit (ICU) confront death and dying daily. As such, intensivists have the dual role of healing patients with survivable illness and supporting families of patients with illnesses that cannot be cured. To emphasize the importance of the latter role, the Institute of Medicine (IOM) released "Dying In America: Improving Quality and Honoring Individual Preferences at the End of Life" in September, 2014.[1] ICU care has been shown to often be inconsistent with a patient's values, preferences, and previously expressed goals of care in many situations.[2,3] The IOM report emphasizes the importance of identifying and honoring patient preferences at the end of life. The IOM endorses the development of standards of care at life's end that would enhance quality of life and foster a more sustainable health care system.

Palliative care bridges the gap between comfort and cure. The World Health Organization defines palliative care as "an approach that improves the quality of life of patients and their families facing the problem associated with life-threatening illness, through the prevention and relief of suffering by means of early identification and impeccable assessment and treatment of pain and other problems, physical, psychosocial and spiritual."[4] Palliative care services are growing quickly in the United States.[5] There have been more than 1000 new hospital-based palliative care programs created since 2000.[5] This represents a 148% increase in the number of palliative care teams in US hospitals during the last 14 years.[6]

Key domains of ICU palliative care have been identified by expert consensus and by patients and families (**Table 1**).[7,8] All major societies representing critical care professionals and the World Health Organization have endorsed addressing palliative care needs for patients who are critically ill or at the end of life.[9–13] These recommendations recognize palliative care as an essential component

Disclosures: The authors have no financial conflicts of interest.
[a] Division of Pulmonary and Critical Care Medicine, Department of Internal Medicine, Indiana University, 1120 W Michigan Street, Indianapolis, IN 46202, USA; [b] Charles Warren Fairbanks Center for Medical Ethics, IU Health Methodist Hospital, 1701 North Senate Boulevard, Indianapolis, IN 46202, USA; [c] Palliative Care, Indiana University Health, Indianapolis, IN, USA
* Corresponding author. Division of Pulmonary, Critical Care, Allergy, and Occupational Medicine, Indiana University School of Medicine, 541 Clinical Drive, CL 285, Indianapolis, IN 46202.
E-mail address: gbosslet@iu.edu

Clin Chest Med 36 (2015) 441–448
http://dx.doi.org/10.1016/j.ccm.2015.05.010
0272-5231/15/$ – see front matter © 2015 Elsevier Inc. All rights reserved.

Table 1
Key domains of ICU palliative care

Expert Consensus[7]	Patient and Family Consensus[8]
Symptom management and comfort care	Timely, compassionate, clear communication and by clinicians
Communication within the team and with patients and families	Patient-focused medical decision making
Emotional and practical support for patients and families	Interdisciplinary support of family including bereavement care
Patient- and family-centered decision making	Proximity of families to patients
Continuity of care	Patient care maintaining comfort, dignity, personhood, privacy
Emotional and organizational support for ICU clinicians	
Spiritual support for patients and families	

of comprehensive ICU care. Successful integration of palliative care services in the ICU aims to promote better quality, lower costs, and improved patient and family satisfaction.[5]

BENEFITS OF PALLIATIVE CARE IN THE INTENSIVE CARE UNIT

The use of palliative care services in the ICU has been associated with improved quality of life for patients,[14] better understanding for the patient and families of the clinical situation and prognosis,[15] increased emotional and spiritual support for patients and families,[16,17] improved mental well-being and care at the time of death,[18] and improved family satisfaction.[19–21] Improved family understanding lowers levels of anxiety among providers and family members.[18,20,21] It also allows for more efficient implementation of care plans in accordance with a patient's values. These plans are likely to be more appropriately focused on goals of care instead of nonbeneficial treatments.[14,15,22] These measures promote less conflict in the ICU[23] and reduce provider burnout,[24] thereby reducing the psychological effects of the ICU on patients and providers.

Palliative care services reduce overall health care costs, even when accounting for the cost of adding the services themselves.[25,26] Palliative care has been shown to reduce the overall costs of inpatient hospitalization,[27–29] and it decreases ICU and overall length of stay.[22,30,31] Palliative care services have also been shown to reduce hospital readmissions.[32] One means of cost reduction is cost avoidance, which is achieved by reduction of nonbeneficial treatments and interventions[14,22] and appropriately downgrading patients from high-cost, high-acuity wards to lower-acuity settings.[33] These actions promote increased ICU resources for those in need. Importantly, the use of palliative care in the ICU has not been associated with an increase in mortality.[14,22,31]

The goal of successful ICU–palliative care integration is to achieve the triple aim: better quality, improved access, and lower costs.[5,34] Additionally, successful integration of palliative care services into ICUs functions to improve the experience of patients, families, and providers.

BARRIERS TO IMPLEMENTATION OF PALLIATIVE CARE

Although the benefits to integrating palliative care in the ICU are many, multiple barriers to implementation have been identified. These barriers result in infrequent use of palliative care even when services are available.[35] A US study of ICU directors of adult ICUs reported perceived challenges to use of palliative care collaboration.[2] These included unrealistic expectations regarding patient prognosis and effectiveness of ICU treatment; inability of patients to partake in treatment discussions; poor training in relevant communication skills; and too many demands for clinician's time. The survey respondents essentially identified barriers at all levels, from patients and families to clinicians and systematic barriers within institutions. Similar barriers have been noted among European intensivists.[36]

Poor understanding of what palliative care provides is a barrier to widespread implementation of palliative care services. Many clinicians misperceive palliative care services, and confuse such care with hospice services.[37–39] Some families may perceive involvement of palliative care as "giving up" and fail to understand that palliative care can complement and support aggressive care rather than simply limit it.[40,41] Physicians are often underprepared to provide comprehensive care to dying and critically ill patients without the support of palliative care specialists.[42,43] Misperceptions abound for providers and patients/families, and efforts at initiation of a palliative care program should focus considerable efforts in this area (discussed later).

With many competing demands on a clinician's time, poor reimbursement for essential yet lengthy family meetings may act as a barrier to quality palliative care in the ICU. Both the American Medical Association and the IOM have called on Medicare and Medicaid to reimburse time spent on end-of-life conversations, Physician Orders for Life-Sustaining Treatment (POLST) paperwork, and family and patient education.[1,44] The ICU is one area where reimbursement for such discussions is already in place. Per Centers for Medicare and Medicaid Services directive, CPT codes 99,291 and 99,292 (critical care time) can be applied toward physician-family discussions regarding goals of care, patient preferences, and end-of-life care, provided that the patient is unable to participate in making treatment decisions, and the discussion is necessary for determining treatment decisions.[45]

Barriers to implementation of palliative care services in ICUs are many, but can be focused on two general areas: the perception that successful palliative care services will entail considerably more time on the part of ICU providers, and an imperfect understanding of what palliative care services are able to provide in the ICU. Strategies aimed at overcoming these barriers is addressed next.

SCREENING TOOLS AND BUNDLING

Palliative care screening tools and other quality improvement measures have been trialed to enhance palliative care use. Such projects as the Improving Palliative Care in the ICU[46] program seek to provide multidisciplinary support to clinicians and hospital administrators working to increase their palliative care reach. **Table 2** provides a list of other World Wide Web–based ICU–palliative care resources.

Screening tools have been proposed as a method to identify the unmet palliative care needs of patients, families, and clinicians, and are a means to begin implementation of ICU–palliative care collaboration. One study selected five trigger criteria for palliative care consultation: (1) ICU care 10 days or more after admission, (2) age greater than 80 or two or more life-threatening comorbidities, (3) active metastatic malignancy, (4) status post cardiac arrest, and (5) intracerebral hemorrhage with mechanical ventilation.[31] Palliative care intervention in patients with one of these criteria resulted in decreased ICU length of stay. Another study[22] used two diagnoses to trigger palliative care consultation: global cerebral ischemia post cardiopulmonary resuscitation and multisystem organ failure. Both diagnostic groups had decreased time to clarification of goals of care and decreased lengths of stay. The multisystem organ failure group also had lower costs when palliative care was involved, presumably because of less use of nonbeneficial treatment.

Process bundling has been used as a means to improve palliative care delivery in the ICU setting. The Voluntary Hospital Association developed the "Care and Communication Bundle"[47] as

---

Table 2
Useful World Wide Web–based palliative care resources for palliative care integration

Resource	Web Site
The IPAL project: Improving Palliative Care	http://www.capc.org/ipal/ipal-icu
Center to Advance Palliative Care	www.capc.org/ http://getpalliativecare.org/
Robert Wood Johnson Foundation: Promoting Excellence in End-of-Life Care- Palliative Care Tools	www.promotingexcellence.org/tools/
National Consensus Project for Quality Palliative Care	www.nationalconsensusproject.org
National Hospice and Palliative Care Organization	www.nhpco.org
Respecting Choices	http://www.gundersenhealth.org/respecting-choices
Intensive Talk: Communication Skills for Intensive Care Physicians	http://depts.washington.edu/icutalk/content/improving-communication-icu
End-of-Life Nursing Education Consortium	http://www.aacn.nche.edu/ELNEC/CriticalCare.htm
Harvard Medical School Palliative Care for Hospitalists and Intensivists course	http://www.hms.harvard.edu/pallcare/PCFHI/PCFHI.htm

a performance initiative (**Table 3**). The bundle, which has been tested in a multicenter trial, targets processes that should occur at certain times during the ICU stay. These include (but are not limited to) determination of resuscitation status and surrogate decision maker (Day 1) and an interdisciplinary family meeting (Day 5). One study[48] indicated improved family communication and compliance with protocols after implementation (although success varied depending on the type of ICU).

Screening tools and bundling of processes of care are just two measures currently being studied as means to improve the process and implementation of palliative care delivery in the ICU. With studies ongoing, there is no consensus on the best method of implementation and improving use of palliative care in the ICU.

SPECIFIC STEPS FOR IMPLEMENTATION AND INTEGRATION OF A PALLIATIVE CARE PROGRAM INTO THE INTENSIVE CARE UNIT

Outlined next are suggested specific steps in the initiation and growth of palliative care services within an ICU culture (**Table 4**). Because culture change is often slow, many of these steps happen in parallel, rather than in series. We provide an evidence base for the areas supported by the literature, but many of these steps are based on the authors' experience with establishment of a local palliative care program and are unsupported by specific empiric data (for reasons the reader will appreciate with the substance of the steps).

Goal 1: Garnering Local Support from Thought Leaders

Integration of palliative care services into ICU workflow is increasingly seen as essential to providing high-quality, comprehensive critical care. Because of the barriers to implementation outlined previously, integration of palliative care services into the ICU should be done in a careful, stepwise fashion that first gathers stakeholders and is attentive to local needs. To address a broad range of ICUs and the needs of various models of care, implementation should begin with "political efforts" of education and solicitation of support from local thought leaders. Without these champions among the leadership of the institution, efforts to obtain resources for palliative care services are often wasted.

The already established key domains of palliative care (see **Table 1**) should be used in initial discussions to educate stakeholders about the goals of palliative care services. These conversations are best initiated by defining local problems that may be ameliorated with improved palliative care services. Examples of such issues include improving patient and family satisfaction surveys, ICU lengths of stay, ICU mortality, and clinician turnover associated with ICU burnout.

As such, data that are often already collected at most institutions (length of stay, patient satisfaction surveys, mortality, cost data) may be helpful to analyze the "initial state" and set tangible goals and benchmarks. Attitude surveys and the development of an understanding of how nurses and clinicians feel about the current delivery of end-of-life care in the ICU may also be helpful. The established key domains of palliative care (see **Table 1**) may serve as a foundation for the attitude surveys to compare local needs and current local behaviors in a specific ICU setting. From this, measurable outcomes of palliative care services can be identified as implementation of end-of-life care improvement measures are used. These outcomes help in education efforts and to tailor interventions to reduce steps that do not achieve improvements in measurable and meaningful outcomes.

An example of this process is to focus on family satisfaction survey results as an outcome measure. An institution that notes a low rating on a scale of quality of patient pain control in their ICU may decide to implement any number of interventions to improve this outcome. Some options may be implementation of a symptom assessment score protocol, an ICU protocol for withdrawal of care and symptom management during the time of the dying process, or mandatory palliative care consultation for dying patients. Observing the effect of one of these palliative care interventions over time either helps to bolster support of the intervention or encourages shifting focus to a different intervention.

The overarching goal of these initial steps is to provide ICU providers and hospital administrators

Table 3 The Voluntary Hospital Association care and communication bundle	
By ICU Day 1	Identify a decision maker Address advance directive status Address cardiopulmonary resuscitation status Distribute family information leaflet Assess pain regularly Manage pain optimally
By ICU Day 3	Offer social work support Offer spiritual support
By ICU Day 5	Interdisciplinary family meeting

Data from Ref.[47]

Table 4
Initiation, integration, and measurable outcomes for integration of palliative care services in the ICU

Goal	Steps	Measurable Outcomes
Garner support from local thought leaders for the need for palliative care	Presentation to institutional leadership regarding needs/benefits/cost	Number of leaders reached Attitude surveys Length of stay Patient satisfaction Mortality
Recruitment and development of a hospital palliative care team	Define and hire needed team members Outline daily workflow data collection for program evaluation and improvement Institutional education efforts and development of local culture "champions"	Number of institution palliative care consultations Satisfaction of providers
Initiation of palliative care services into the ICU culture	Needs assessment Educational initiatives Pilot consultation service Pilot screening tool variables	Number of palliative care consultations from the ICU Staff attitude surveys (before-after) Patient satisfaction surveys Staff satisfaction surveys
Full integration of palliative care services with ICU daily workflow	Develop collaborative leadership relationships with ICU champions Development/pilot of screening tools Develop collaborative rounding structure	Number of palliative care consultations from the ICU Patient satisfaction surveys Staff satisfaction surveys

with end-of-life care quality metrics to be monitored, measured, analyzed, and continuously improved so as to continuously improve end-of-life care in the ICU.[7] Such metric monitoring often achieves provider-level education regarding the utility of such services. Secondarily, demonstrating improvement in tangible outcomes often helps to garner buy-in from skeptical administrators and providers who may otherwise be hesitant to provide resources and time for improved palliative care skills and processes.

Goal 2: Recruitment of a Palliative Care Team and Definition of Roles

Once the case is made for palliative care services using concrete metrics, a palliative care team should be put in place. This may be easier said than done, because a considerable palliative medicine physician shortage is predicted in the coming years.[49] Ideally this interdisciplinary team includes clinicians, case management, social work, and chaplaincy. These are the key people who foster collaboration and ultimately champion the (often slow) change in culture as the shift is made toward ICU–palliative care collaboration. In

some instances, a needs-assessment conducted before recruitment efforts can help further define the roles most needed within the specific institution. Once this team is in place, they can spearhead continued institution-wide education efforts and can help to inculcate palliative care services into local culture.

How the palliative care team functions will likely be dynamic; collaborative agility is of utmost importance for those who are involved in any initial palliative care services. A determination should be made whether the palliative care team will function in a consultative or integrative manner; it is often the case that consultative services are more helpful for ICU cultures that are less open to palliative care assistance, because it allows for more intensivist determination of the frequency and dose of palliative care. Once palliative care consultation is firmly established, screening tools and bundles may be instituted to trigger palliative care consultations in certain situations or patient groups (as discussed previously).

Initiation of palliative care services into an ICU culture requires considerable nimbleness and a willingness to change course and adapt to differing levels of acceptance and integration depending on the cultural milieu into which it is being adopted. Institutional patience and appreciation of small victories in the process becomes extremely important as palliative care services blend into the local culture.

Goals 3 and 4: Initiation of Palliative Care into the Intensive Care Unit and Full Integration into Daily Workflow

Once an ICU is ready for integrative model of palliative care where the palliative care team is "embedded" in the ICU team, designation of a time for daily rounds and goals of the partnership should be negotiated among the team leaders before initiation of services. An effectively integrated palliative care team ideally shares common goals and has a willingness to collaborate within the group structure[50] and devise protocols for the best-practice palliative care approach.[51] Similar to effective ICU teams, the strongest integrated palliative care teams consist of strong communicators who focus on teamwork and function in a nonhierarchical environment.[52]

As services are incorporated into daily workflow, institutional education at all levels should continue and adjust as barriers or successes arise. Quality outcomes previously outlined should be monitored closely, with attention to redesign if indicated and a celebration of outcome improvement shared with all stakeholders. Follow-up surveys and performance measure monitoring should be performed at assigned intervals during the implementation period, and then long-term to ensure continued quality improvement and sustained benefit of ICU–palliative care integration.

SUMMARY

Despite considerable barriers, evidence demonstrates the benefits and improved outcomes from integration of palliative care in the ICU. A rigorous and structured implementation process that focuses on assessment and improvement should be undertaken to overcome the difficulties of education and time constraints that often thwart palliative care initiation and integration. The process of implementing a palliative care program mirrors the content of palliative care services: both are best viewed as a process rather than as a singular event. Success in this process promises to foster better quality care, decreased costs, and improved patient and family satisfaction.

REFERENCES

1. Dying in America: improving quality and honoring individual preferences near the end of life. Washington, DC: The National Academies Press; 2015.

2. Nelson JE. Identifying and overcoming the barriers to high quality palliative care in the intensive care unit. Crit Care Med 2006;34:S324–31.

3. Angus DC, Barnato AE, Linde-Zwirble WT, et al. Use of intensive care at the end of life in the United States: an epidemiologic study. Crit Care Med 2004;32:638–43.

4. World Health Organization definition of palliative care. Available at: www.who.int/cancer/palliative/definition/en. Accessed November 3, 2014.

5. Hughs MT, Smith TJ. The growth of palliative care in the United States. Annu Rev Public Health 2014;35:459–75.

6. CAPC growth analysis. Available at: www.capc.org/capc-growth-analyses-snapshot-2011.pdf. Accessed November 24, 2014.

7. Clarke EB, Curtis JR, Luce JM, et al, Robert Wood Johnson Foundation Critical Care End-of-Life Peer Group. Quality indicators for end-of-life care in the intensive care unit. Crit Care Med 2003;31:2255–62.

8. Nelson JE, Puntillo KA, Pronovost PJ, et al. In their own words: patients and families define high-quality palliative care in the intensive care unit. Crit Care Med 2010;38:808–18.

9. Selecky PA, Eliasson CA, Hall RI, et al, American College of Chest Physicians. Palliative and end-of-life care for patients with cardiopulmonary diseases: American College of Chest Physicians position statement. Chest 2005;128:3599–610.

10. Lanken PN, Terry PB, Delisser HM, et al, ATS End-of-Life Care Task Force. An official American Thoracic Society clinical policy statement: palliative care for patients with respiratory diseases and critical illnesses. Am J Respir Crit Care Med 2008;177:912–27.

11. Truog RD, Campbell ML, Curtis JR, et al, American Academy of Critical Care Medicine. Recommendations for end-of-life care in the intensive care unit: a consensus statement by the American College [corrected] of Critical Care Medicine. Crit Care Med 2008;36:953–63.

12. Carlet J, Thijs LG, Antonelli M, et al. Challenges in end-of-life care in the ICU. Statement of the 5th international Consensus Conference in Critical Care: Brussels, Belgium, April 2003. Intensive Care Med 2004;30:770–84.

13. World Health Organization. Palliative care is an essential part of cancer control. Available at: http://www.who.int/cancer/palliative/en/. Accessed September 26, 2014.

14. O'Mahony S, McHenry J, Blank AE, et al. Preliminary report of the integration of a palliative care team into an intensive care unit. Palliat Med 2010;24:154–65.

15. Azoulay E, Pochard F, Chevret S, et al. Impact of family information leaflet on effectiveness of information provided to family members of intensive care unit patients: a multicenter prospective randomized controlled trial. Am J Respir Crit Care Med 2002;165:438–42.

16. Erdek MA, Pronovost PJ. Improving assessment and treatment of pain in the critically ill. Int J Qual Health Care 2004;16:59–64.

17. Chanques G, Jaber S. Impact of systematic evaluation of pain and agitation in the intensive care unit. Crit Care Med 2006;34:1691–9.

18. Lautrette A, Darmon M, Megarbane B, et al. A communication strategy and brochure for relatives of patients dying in the ICU. N Engl J Med 2007;356:469–78.

19. Hinkle LJ, Bosslet GT, Torke AM. Factors associated with family satisfaction with end-of-life care in the ICU: a systematic review. Chest 2015;147(1):82–93.

20. Stapleton RD, Engleberg RA, Wenrich MD, et al. Clinician statements and family satisfaction with conferences in the intensive care unit. Crit Care Med 2006;34:1679–85.

21. McDonagh JR, Elliott TB, Engelberg RA, et al. Family satisfaction with family conferences about end-of-life care in the intensive care unit: increased proportion of family speech is associated with increased satisfaction. Crit Care Med 2004;32:1484–8.

22. Campbell ML, Guzman JA. Impact of a proactive approach to improve end-of-life care in a medical ICU. Chest 2003;123:266–71.

23. Lilly CM, De Meo DL, Sonna LA, et al. An intensive communication intervention for the critically ill. Am J Med 2000;109:469–75.

24. Quenot JP, Riguad JP, Prin S, et al. Suffering among carers working in critical care can be reduced by an intensive communication strategy on end-of-life practices. Intensive Care Med 2012;38:55–61.

25. Cassel JB, Hager MA, Clark RR, et al. Concentrating hospital-wide deaths in a palliative care unit: the effect on place of death and system-wide mortality. J Palliat Med 2010;13:371–4.

26. Cent. Adv. Palliat. Care 2005 CAPC Impact Calculator. New York: Cent. Adv. Palliat. Care. Available at: http://www.capc.org/impact_calculator_basic/. Accessed November 24, 2014.

27. Morrison RS, Dietrick J, Ladwig S, et al. Palliative care consultation teams cut hospital costs for Medicaid beneficiaries. Health Aff 2011;30:454–63.

28. Morrison RS, Cassel JB, Penrod JD, et al. Cost savings associated with US hospital palliative care consultation programs. Arch Intern Med 2008;168:1783–90.

29. Smith TJ, Coyne P, Cassel JB, et al. A high-volume specialist palliative care unit and team may reduce in-hospital end-of-life care costs. J Palliat Med 2003;6:699–705.

30. Campbell ML, Guzman JA. A proactive approach to improve end-of-life care in a medical intensive care unit for patients with terminal dementia. Crit Care Med 2004;32:1839–43.

31. Norton SA, Hogan LA, Holloway RG, et al. Proactive palliative care in the medical intensive care unit: effects on length of stay for selected high-risk patients. Crit Care Med 2007;35:1530–5.

32. Nelson C, Chand P, Sortais J, et al. Inpatient palliative care consults and the probability of hospital readmissions. Perm J 2011;15:48–51.

33. Smith TJ, Cassel JB. Cost and non-clinical outcomes of palliative care. J Pain Symptom Manage 2009;38:32–44.

34. Peikes D, Zutshi A, Genevro JL, et al. Early evaluations of the medical home: building on a promising start. Am J Manag Care 2012;18:105–16.

35. Penrod JD, Pronovost PJ, Livote EE, et al. Meeting standards of high-quality intensive care unit palliative care: clinical performance and predictors. Crit Care Med 2012;40:1105–12.

36. Alaskan RA, Curtis JM, Nelson JE. The changing role of palliative care in the ICU. Crit Care Med 2014;42:2418–28.

37. Maciasz RM, Arnold RM, Chu E, et al. Does it matter what you call it? A randomized trial of language used to describe palliative care services. Support Care Cancer 2013;21:3411–9.

38. Kavalieratos D, Mitchell M, Carey TS, et al. "Not the 'grim reaper service:'" an assessment of provider knowledge, attitudes, and perceptions regarding palliative care referral barriers in heart failure. J Am Heart Assoc 2014;3:e000544.

39. Matsuyama RK, Balliet WP, Ingram K, et al. Will patients want hospice or palliative care if they do not know what it is? J Hosp Palliat Nurs 2011;13:41–6.

40. Metzger M, Norton SA, Quinn JR, et al. Patient and family members perceptions of palliative care in heart failure. Heart Lung 2013;42:112–9.

41. CAPC 2011 Public Opinion Research on Palliative Care. Available at: http://www.capc.org/tools-for-palliative-care-programs/marketing/public-opinion-research/2011-public-opinion-research-on-palliative-care.pdf. Accessed September 27, 2014.

42. Tulsky JA, Chesney MA, Lo B. How do medical residents discuss resuscitation with patients? J Gen Intern Med 1995;10:436–42.

43. Plauth WH, Pantilat SZ, Wachter RM, et al. Hospitalists perceptions of their residency training needs: results of a national survey. AM J Med 2001;111:247–54.

44. Belluck P. Coverage for end-of-life talks gaining ground. New York Times 2014. Available at: http://www.nytimes.com/2014/08/31/health/end-of-life-talks-may-finally-overcome-politics.html?_r=0. Accessed August 31, 2014.

45. Lustbader DR, Nelson JE, Weissman DE, et al, The IPAL-ICU Project. Physician reimbursement for critical care services integrating palliative care for patients who are critically ill. Chest 2012;141:787–92.

46. The IPAL project: improving palliative care. Available at: http://www.capc.org/ipal/ipal-icu. Accessed August 29, 2014.

47. Nelson JE, Mulkerin CM, Adams LL, et al. Improving comfort and communication in the ICU: a practical new tool for palliative care performance measurement and feedback. Qual Saf Health Care 2006; 15(4):264–71.

48. Black MD, Vigorito MC, Curtis JR, et al. A multifaceted intervention to improve compliance with process measures for ICU clinician communication with ICU patients and families. Crit Care Med 2013;41:2275–83.

49. Lupu D, American Academy of Hospice and Palliative Medicine Workforce Task Force. Estimate of current hospice and palliative medicine physician workforce shortage. J Pain Symptom Manage 2010;40:899–911.

50. Larson CE, LeFasto FM. Teamwork: what must go right; what can go wrong. Newbury Park (CA): Sage; 1989.

51. Flacker JM, Won A, Kiely DK, et al. Differing perceptions of end-of-life care in long-term care. J Palliat Med 2001;4:9–13.

52. Vachon M. Recent research into staff stress in palliative care. Eur J Palliat Care 1997;4:99–110.

Clinical Reasoning and Risk in the Intensive Care Unit

Geoffrey R. Connors, MD*, Jonathan M. Siner, MD

KEYWORDS

- Clinical reasoning • Risk assessment • Bayesian analysis • Risk benefit • Intensive care

KEY POINTS

- Clinical reasoning, the process by which clinicians make diagnostic and treatment decisions in medicine, is particularly challenging in the ICU because clinicians often work with incomplete information and in an evolving physiologic context.
- Novices and experts, both of whom practice in an academic intensive care environment, think and reason differently from one another. Understanding and appreciating these differences is important for educators and learners in the ICU.
- Understanding the risk related to the disease and the medical treatment is the critical final piece to the clinical reasoning and decision-making process because risk and benefit determine the treatment threshold.
- We propose a modified bayesian reasoning approach to clinical reasoning, which is replicable, works for experts and novices, and incorporates not just diagnostic algorithms but also accounts for treatment thresholds, leading to a standard approach to risk assessment and intervention.

INTRODUCTION

"Clinical reasoning" is a commonly used phrase in medicine, although one that can be difficult to define and means different things to different people. A reasonably succinct definition of clinical reasoning is "the ability to sort through a cluster of features presented by a patient and accurately assign a diagnostic label, with the development of an appropriate treatment as the end goal."[1] This definition captures the diagnostic component of reasoning without forgetting the larger picture, namely the patient requiring treatment or intervention.

Clinical reasoning and decision-making face particular challenges in an intensive care unit (ICU) environment. ICU medicine is practiced at a fast pace. Patients are unstable from a hemodynamic or respiratory perspective, therefore decision-making occurs under greater stress, making accurate diagnostic reasoning more difficult.[2] In addition to the pressure of needing to act quickly, the reduced time to make a clinical decision also means that the information ICU physicians work with is often incomplete, leading to an increase in biased reasoning.[3] The ICU is a continuously evolving environment. The correct intervention one moment (fluids for septic shock) can become incorrect the next (when the stress of sepsis induces an acute cardiomyopathy and markedly reduced ejection fraction) meaning practitioners cannot rely on a single course of action to remain the correct course of action. Finally, in a standard academic ICU, there are decision-makers at many

The authors have no conflicts of interest to disclose.
Section of Pulmonary, Critical Care and Sleep Medicine, Department of Internal Medicine, Yale University School of Medicine, 300 Cedar Street, TAC-441 South, PO Box 208057, New Haven, CT 06520-8057, USA
* Corresponding author.
E-mail address: geoffrey.connors@yale.edu

Clin Chest Med 36 (2015) 449–459
http://dx.doi.org/10.1016/j.ccm.2015.05.016

different levels of training: students, subinterns, junior and senior residents, junior and senior fellows, all the way up to attending physicians. Each of these practitioners has their own breadth of experience, which affects how they see the case in front of them.[4] Each of these practitioners brings different reasoning skills to the bedside and approaches problems with a unique style and ability.[5,6]

Thus, it is important to think about reasoning and risk in a structured manner. The use of a methodology provides structure, reliability, and reproducibility to a process that is rooted in uncertainty and dynamism. The methodology we propose is a modified bayesian reasoning method that can be adapted to the practitioner or learner. A goal of this article is to help define a method of clinical reasoning and show how it can work in an ICU environment. We also demonstrate the differences between novice and expert reasoning and shed light on how this affects the education and oversight of these practitioners. Finally, we define the term "treatment threshold" and make clear the relationship between reasoning and risk in the ICU.

ANALYSIS, INTUITION, AND METHOD

There are many methods that have been proposed to achieve the goal of correctly reasoning through a diagnostic challenge. Despite this variability, the core elements of good reasoning remain the same. The first step in any diagnostic challenge is to frame the question or identification of the chief concern (complaint, historically). The physician then gathers information about the patient including information on the historical state of the patient (past medical history, past surgical history, social history, family history, any medications they were taking when the concern started) and the current state of the patient (history of present illness, vital signs, physical examination, and any available test results). The doctor then moves through six core critical thinking skills to assess

this trove of information: (1) interpretation, (2) analysis, (3) evaluation, (4) inference, (5) explanation, and (6) self-regulation; the last refers to looking back on one's performance in the first five.[7] Finally, the physician must then decide if the evidence at hand is consistent with a known diagnosis and institute therapy if the benefit is greater than the risk. Together this is the art of clinical reasoning.

Clinical reasoning has traditionally been performed via several different methodologies, each with proponents and critics, advantages and disadvantages.[8] The largest camps align themselves similar to the Five Subscale Critical Thinking Processes proposed by Facione and Facione[9] where reasoning was broken into inductive and deductive styles and analytical and intuitive thinking. Deductive reasoning starts with a firm hypothesis followed by a search for facts to support or refute that belief. Inductive reasoning values the open-minded search for clues that can, once gathered and assessed, add up to a conclusion or hypothesis. Intuitive thinking looks for key elements of the story to draw reasonable conclusions regarding already-formed hypotheses, whereas analytical thinking values facts, clues, and evidence that is used to generate a conclusion. According to their methods, the intuitive thinkers tend toward deductive reasoning and the analytical thinkers tend toward a more inductive reasoning process. Each of these approaches has its strengths and weaknesses that have to be recognized or the practitioner risks adding significant error into the reasoning process (**Table 1**).

EXPERTS AND NOVICES: NOT ALL REASONING IS DONE THE SAME WAY

Although all physicians and trainees use pieces of each of these reasoning and thinking methods in their actual practice, reliance on one versus the other changes over time. This is important to understand when using reasoning on one's own

---

Table 1
Relative strengths and weaknesses of intuitive and analytical reasoning

Intuitive/Deductive		Analytical/Inductive	
Strengths	Weaknesses	Strengths	Weaknesses
Hypothesis-based	Open to early closure, confirmation, and choice-support biases	Thorough/rigorous	Susceptible to availability, anchoring, and framing biases
Relies on prior experience	Can be "too fast"	Does not require much prior experience	Slow
Fast	Requires experience	Methodical	Laborious
			"Paralysis by analysis"

or when teaching others how to clinically reason: experts and novices are not the same (**Fig. 1**).[1,10] Experts, by definition, have experience and tend to rely on it. They use their prior experience to intuit a quick hypothesis and then use deductive reasoning to determine what condition is present in their patient. They may find an analytical/inductive approach to a problem slow, boring, unnecessary, and rote. And although this does open them up to various reasoning errors, often their experience can make up for the lack of rigor and even exceed it. Novices, however, do not have this advantage. Their efforts tend to focus on overwhelming their lack of experience with facts and attempting to join those facts into a coherent conclusion.[11] This does not mean that both groups do not use the methods of the other; in fact, they do.[12] It is just that they tend not to perform as well when operating outside their comfort zone. This sets up an obvious difficulty in teaching clinical reasoning in the ICU, where the difference between expert and novice can be large. Communication between expert and novice can be difficult because they are (unwittingly) working through the same problem but using different methods. It also means that trainees on the path from one to the other group (senior residents, fellows, and junior attendings) are at greatest risk of not having a firm footing in either domain.

A METHOD OF CLINICAL REASONING: THE MODIFIED BAYESIAN APPROACH FOR THE INTENSIVE CARE UNIT

For all these reasons, we propose a method of clinical reasoning that deliberately combines intuitive with analytical methods, inductive with deductive critical thinking, and places great value on moving forward and backward, offering large doses of self-reflection.[13] It is also bayesian at its core, meaning that all new evidence is evaluated in the context of prior impressions and folded into the deliberation going forward, changing pretest probabilities into posttest (or posterior) probabilities.[14] At the end of a bayesian process one is left with a probability of disease, not necessarily a "right" answer. It focuses equally on hypothesis generation and testing, and gathering new information as it becomes available, viewing all evidence (physical examination, testing, and radiography) against pretest probability of disease. This is in contrast to nonbayesian approaches where accounting of all hypotheses and tests occurs until a correct answer emerges. The bayesian approach allows for more uncertainty in diagnosis and, as demonstrated in this article, allows one to evaluate a diagnosis versus its treatment and help determine the risk-benefit ratio and how it relates to treatment decisions.

This method of clinical reasoning has several advantages and is built specifically to counter some of the difficulties noted previously. To be successful in the ICU, a clinical reasoning approach must be (1) methodical, to account for the need for quick action and to help absorb some of the stress of the situation; (2) flexible, to account for the different levels of learner and the ever-changing nature of an ICU patient; (3) dynamic, to allow for the acute treatment and stabilization of a patient during the reasoning process and to take the effect of those treatments into account in the formation of a differential; (4) reproducible, so that a student or resident can be evaluated in their ability to complete each of the tasks; and (5) consistent, to account for heuristic errors or common reasoning mistakes made by novices and experts alike.

The classic, six-step, expert-level approach to patient care and clinical reasoning is demonstrated in **Fig. 2**. The steps involved are familiar

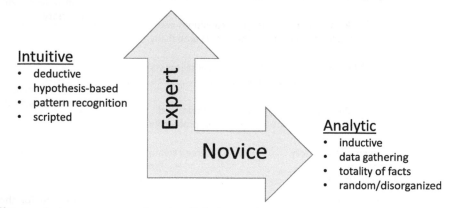

Fig. 1. Differences between expert and novice clinical reasoning.

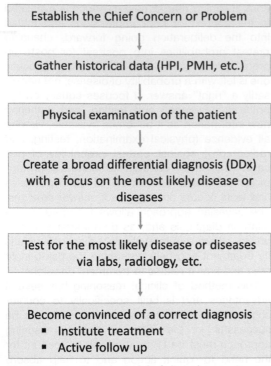

Fig. 2. Classic, six-step model of clinical reasoning and treatment. HPI, history of present illness; PMH, past medical history.

and start with establishing the patient baseline (who they are historically), move to things that can be known about their current condition including the physical examination, vital signs, and testing (who they are currently), and then assimilate that information to create an argument that the person is suffering from a particular condition requiring a particular treatment. Looking at **Fig. 3**, one sees a much more complex process. This is the modified bayesian approach to clinical reasoning. It accounts for the intermittent need for immediate, life-sustaining intervention during diagnosis, that these complex patients need simplification of their condition at various steps in the reasoning process to not become mentally overwhelming, and the reality that information may change during (and because of) the work-up, necessitating going backward through the process to revisit the patient's history or physical examination in addition to additional testing. The steps in this model (as enumerated in **Fig. 3** and **Fig. 4**) are as follows:

1. Establish the chief concern or problem
   - Important first step in any reasoning paradigm, knowing the nature of the problem to be addressed

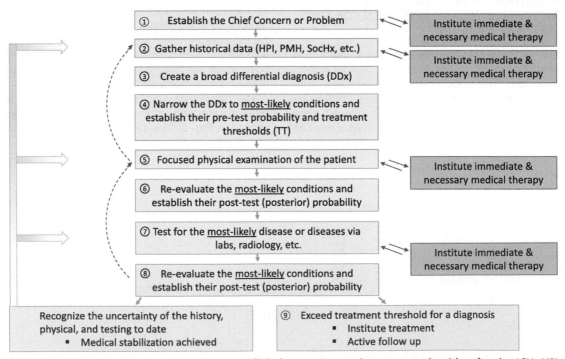

Fig. 3. Modified bayesian reasoning, nine-step clinical reasoning, and treatment algorithm for the ICU. HPI, history of present illness; PMH, past medical history; SocHx, social history.

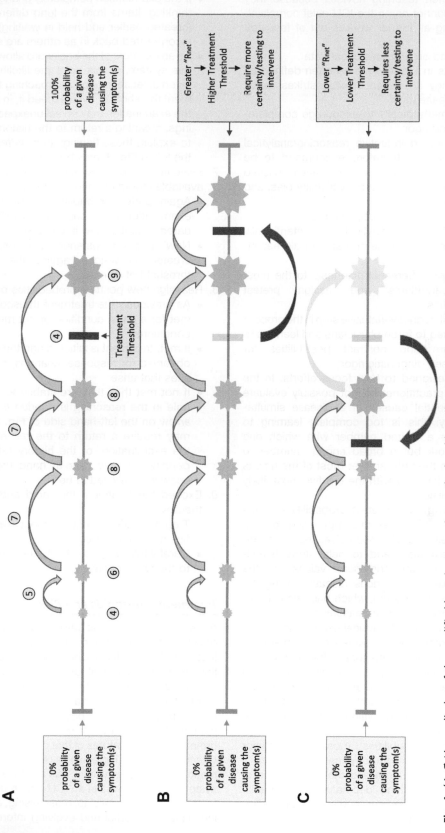

Fig. 4. (A–C) Linear display of the modified bayesian reasoning method and how the treatment threshold affects the decision to treat or to stop/continue evaluation.

- Key when teaching novices because they often cannot name the ICU chief complaint, meaning all further work is out of focus/off track

2. Gather and organize historical data
   - Patients in the ICU are as often defined by who they are when disease strikes as by the disease itself
   - Done methodically to encourage completeness and rigor
   - Grounded in inductive reasoning/analytical thinking, and therefore encouraged to be expansive so no important fact is missed (avoiding early closure, availability bias, and so forth)
3. Create a broad differential diagnosis
   - Also inductive/analytical and intentionally broad to encourage inclusion of all reasonable possibilities
4. Narrow the differential diagnosis to the most likely candidates and assign pretest probabilities
   - The first deductive/intuitive step in the process
   - Designed to force physicians and learners to compare and contrast possibilities for increased diagnostic rigor
   - Also designed to help focus efforts. In the ICU a practitioner cannot possibly evaluate all potential causes of a disease simultaneously, this is too complex; learning to choose a limited number with which one can work but a broad enough number to contain the right answer most of the time is critical (starting with the top five most likely possibilities).
   - Assigning strict pretest probabilities serves two main purposes: to compare and contrast the likelihood of various diseases as a clarifying exercise; and to help students/residents assign numerical values to the possibilities of various diseases being the disease in question, which has been shown to improve bayesian reasoning
5. Perform a focused physical examination
   - Encourage all organ systems to be examined in a broad way with special focus on the organ systems that should show or could show abnormality based on the narrowed differential diagnosis and pretest probabilities
   - Demonstrates the value of the physical in modern medicine
6. Reassign probabilities (posttest, posterior probabilities) after the physical examination
   - The physical increases the probabilities of certain conditions, decreases the probabilities of other diseases, and some can be eliminated entirely

- If the examination completely changes one's thinking, items from the long differential list (created earlier and held in waiting) may be incorporated back in as others are excluded
- As an example of the backward allowances in this system, at this point the likelihood of a given disease may be approaching the treatment threshold or even exceed it; in contrast, the examination may reveal unexpected findings, meaning a return to the history looking to explain those findings (the *dotted line* on the left in **Fig. 3**) may be required

7. Evaluate the posttest differential against the available laboratory and radiographic studies
   - Again, pretest probabilities (or post physical examination, in this case) are critically reevaluated in light of new information
   - New posttest/posterior probabilities are created and weighed against the treatment threshold of disease
8. Reassign new posttest probabilities of disease
   - As previously the treatment threshold will be met for a given condition or not met for any conditions
   - If met, treatment is initiated and the patient is observed for response, changes, or new issues that arise
   - If not met then they are stabilized while the hole in the reasoning is queried (*large blue arrow* on the left-hand side of **Fig. 3**), which may require a return to the testing phase, the examination, or the history taking, depending on how near at hand the correct answer is believed to be
9. Exceed the treatment threshold and institute therapy
   - Treatment of the identified most likely causative disease can begin
   - Careful follow-up for effect, need for change to the plan continues

Treatment Thresholds and Risk

A key component of this bayesian process comes down to a simple question: what do I do with a posttest probability of disease once I have created it? In this way, the classical diagnostic approach is simpler: work up the patient and decide, at some point, does the patient have disease X. But in a bayesian or modified bayesian structure, the patient often does not clearly have disease X but rather has many features of that disease with a picture that becomes increasingly clear as more information becomes available. This is why a bayesian system works so well in an ICU where one needs to be constantly assessing, reassessing, and treating based on partial and evolving information. It allows for flexibility and adaptation while still moving forward to a final diagnosis. Once a posttest probability has been created, it can now be compared with the treatment threshold (see **Fig. 4**) to decide whether or not to institute therapy.

Fig. 4A demonstrates a linear model of how a pretest probability (generated from steps 1–3) of the reasoning process can, through examination of the patient and testing (steps 5–8), turn into a posttest probability. (In this figure the result of repeated positive testing increasing the possibility of disease is shown, although it could go in the other direction if a negative test or examination maneuver made the proposed diagnosis less likely.) **Fig. 4**B and C demonstrate what happens when the treatment threshold increases or decreases. The treatment threshold itself (indicated by the *red bar* in **Fig. 4**) is determined by a combination of factors including the following:

- Severity of illness (the more acutely ill a patient is, the less sure one needs to be to attempt an intervention because the less the patient has to lose)
- Frailty of the patient (the more robust the patient, the more relative harm or side effect they can tolerate)
- Risk of intervention (the greater the risk of intervening, the more sure one needs to be about the diagnosis; an example of this is the difference between initiating heparin vs a thrombolytic vs sending a patient to cardiothoracic surgery for a thrombectomy for suspected pulmonary embolus; one needs to have a much higher treatment threshold for cardiothoracic surgery than for tissue plasminogen activator than for initiating heparin, something clinicians often do before confirmatory testing is completed)
- Risk of not intervening (relates to the known outcome of the disease if left untreated)
- Patient tolerance for risk
- Physician tolerance for decision-making in uncertainty

For these reasons, any clinical reasoning algorithm is intricately tied to the decision to treat. The decision to treat is tied to the treatment threshold, which is grounded in the next topic: risk, benefit, and the balance of those two considerations.

INTERVENTION IN THE CRITICALLY ILL: RISK VERSUS BENEFIT

Although clinicians commonly use the word "risk" to describe the potential of a poor outcome from an intervention, the topic is not frequently discussed during a practitioner's medical education and training. A reasonable definition of risk is a description of the probability and magnitude of future harm. We introduce the topic of risk here as it pertains to clinical reasoning because it highlights key elements of the reasoning process specifically as it relates to the concept of treatment thresholds.

A reasonable way to approach a risk in a clinical setting is to distinguish the clinician's estimate of risk in a given scenario from the patient's perception of risk. Assessing risks with regards to an intervention is a process that ICU clinicians do frequently, albeit implicitly rather than explicitly, as part of their decision-making. Less attention is paid to the perception of risk, which can bias the clinician and certainly the patient or surrogate decision-maker. Clinicians do address risk frequently in regards to benefits of individual therapies, particularly with procedures requiring informed consent, yet one of the predominant paradigms in medicine obscures the particulars of risk. This obscuring of risk results from a focus on specific outcomes that are typical of large randomized controlled trials. Although adverse events are often addressed or acknowledged they are frequently discounted if there is a mortality benefit (a net benefit) as a result of the intervention. Although that is appropriate when considering the intervention from a population perspective, the appropriate interpretation for an individual patient is the one where the incremental benefit outweighs the incremental risk. The relative benefits and risks may vary substantially between individual patients. An example of this is the initial publication on Early Goal Directed Therapy in which there is an extensive discussion of the improved outcomes but little to suggest an increase in risk, despite the intervention arm receiving substantially more red blood cell transfusions (which has known risks) than the control group.[15] Many clinicians do not pursue the red blood cell transfusion component of the Early Goal Directed Therapy protocol likely, in part, because they did indeed make a calculus about the risks of the individual component interventions as they apply to the benefits for individual patients. With large clinical trials there may be percentage or point estimates of risk surrounding a specific disease state known as "historical risk" (eg, risk of a pneumothorax during insertion of a subclavian triple lumen catheter or the risk of certain infections from a red blood cell transfusion). This type of risk is distinguished from risks that are new, meaning that there is presumed risk but little data to quantify the incidence or magnitude of harm. Another important element when defining risk is distinguishing absolute risk (the number of people who will be harmed divided by all those who receive the intervention) from incremental risk defined as the increased risk of one intervention relative to the alternative therapeutic options, which is the most common scenario in clinical situations.

By definition, the assessment of risk is an inherently uncertain process. This uncertainty can be caused by a stochastic process meaning whether a specific risk is encountered (whether a patient is placed in a room that was previously occupied by a patient with a resistant bacteria). Systematic uncertainty describes risks that are not unique to that situation but would apply to another individual in the same situation. An example of systematic risk is how well a room is cleaned between patients in a particular hospital or unit when the prior occupant of a room is known to have a highly resistant bacterial infection. One final important element frequently forgotten in risk assessment is the role of time. Any estimate of risk must have boundaries defined as the duration the patient was exposed to some risk. Therefore a clinician must aggregate historical information and adjust for stochastic and systematic risk and impose a time period to arrive at an estimate of risk.

PERCEPTION VERSUS REALITY OR PERCEPTION AS REALITY?

Risk perception is a complex field that often focuses on population risks (nuclear power plants) or economic risk but the findings are highly applicable to medical decision-making. In general, risk perception is affected by people's beliefs before the scenario, their dispositions, and how information is presented to them. Early work by Starr[16] suggested that individuals may accept greater risks if they believe they have greater control over a particular situation, although this effect may not be as significant as initially thought. Tversky and Kahneman[3] developed a list of theories about the heuristics people use to evaluate probabilities. Although a full exploration of these findings is beyond the scope of this article these authors found that several common heuristics affect people's perception of risk including anchoring (being influenced more by initial information than subsequent information), availability (ideas that come to mind have a greater influence on assessment of probability), and representativeness (overreliance on membership in a class to assign characteristics).

Furthermore, Fischhoff's work in 1978 indicated that that a major determinant of risk is the immediacy of effect. Events are viewed as more risky if the adverse outcome occurs immediately rather than in the future.[17] Although the discovery of these heuristics explained many of the apparent illogical decisions individuals make, additional investigation has implicated the role of personal affect in risk perception. Initial work by Slovic[18] suggests that specific elements of emotions that he labels as voluntariness, dread, novelty, and control have substantial influence on risk perception. Additional investigation demonstrated an inverse relationship between perceived risk and benefit, which is modulated by affect meaning that if an individual's feeling toward a given intervention is positive, then risks are perceived as lower and benefits are assessed as higher (as compared with negative feelings toward the intervention). In addition, the more quickly these decisions have to be made, the stronger this effect became.[19] Framing of risk discussions has also been shown to have a substantial impact on perception. In an investigation of particular relevance to medical care, Slovic and coworkers[20] observed that a "20% risk" of death is perceived as describing much lower risk than when a person is told "20 out of 100 of patients undergoing this procedure will die." Another example derived from the medical literature is that when standard therapeutic interventions have been unsuccessful and patients are offered enrollment in clinical trials with a low likelihood of benefit they frequently overestimate the benefits of these experimental interventions.[21] These latter two examples demonstrate how framing of the scenario has substantial impact on risk perception. Although there is no question that basic heuristics contribute to risk perception more recent work demonstrates that affect and how information is presented also make substantial contributions.

To further illustrate the impact of risk assessment and risk perception we next review an example related to the infectious and procedural complications of placement and maintenance of an internal jugular, multilumen central venous catheter. Risks of placement of such a catheter include risk during the insertion procedure (pneumothorax, carotid cannulation, hematoma, infection) and during maintenance of the line (infectious, accidental dislocation). Although there are quoted statistics around the rate of pneumothorax the stochastic risk (whether an experienced operator is the medical provider the day of the procedure) and the systematic risk (whether the institution has good training programs and policies) are major determinants of risk not well accounted for by citing the literature (ie, the historical risk). A patient's affect (whether they believe the intervention is likely to benefit them) is expected to have substantial impact on whether they believe a low pneumothorax rate or infectious risk is significant. Looking at this example further, with regard to the infectious risk, it is known that with good techniques the infectious risk in a population of patients with these devices is low.[22] Thus, a young woman with streptococcal pneumonia who is admitted with septic shock and requires this device has a substantial benefit and essentially a negligible risk. From a risk-benefit perspective the net risk ($Risk_{net}$ or R_{net}) is described by the formula where net risk is proportional to the estimation of risk divided by the estimated benefit: R_{net} α Risk/Benefit. The scenario of a young woman with pneumonia describes a situation with a very low risk of a complication from a central line and substantial benefit and thus has a very low net risk (R_{net}). However, using population estimates from the data of Pronovost and coworkers[22] is not necessarily useful in all scenarios. For example, a middle-aged man with cirrhosis who is still actively drinking alcohol and who is not a candidate for a liver transplant develops septic shock and renal failure with progression over several days to multisystem organ failure. In the setting of cirrhosis, he does not opsonize bacteria well and his infectious risk is therefore increased. Because of coagulopathy, his wound is likely to ooze blood significantly following the insertion, further increasing the infectious risk. Given the nature of his illness and lack of effective therapy for his liver disease, he is not likely to recover quickly and the device may be in for a more extended duration (giving him a long time of exposure and increased risk). Finally, given that he has multisystem organ failure and is not a transplant candidate (the intervention that might save his life) his benefit from these interventions in the face of a 95% or greater 6-month mortality rate is extremely low. In this situation, with a substantially increased risk and very low (close to zero) benefit, one could

describe the situation as "infinite risk" meaning that given minimal benefit the patient can essentially only experience adverse events in aggregate because the risks are so disproportional to the benefits. Although the latter example may seem extreme, similar situations arise routinely in the ICU and a formal approach of attempting to broadly categorize risk and benefit is very useful for the provider and also aids in communication with patients or medical decision-makers. A close inspection of adverse events in an ICU demonstrates this principal and viewing interventions in situations of low benefit and high risk does allow a clearer accounting of the use of interventions.

Clinical reasoning involves assessment of pretest probability and use of test characteristics to determine a posttest probability and make a clinical decision. Importantly, without an accurate assessment of treatment threshold the accuracy of a diagnosis or efficacy of an intervention cannot actually be determined because the previously described net risk (R_{net}) has a dramatic impact on whether the calculated posttest probability is above or below the treatment threshold. As described and shown in **Fig. 5**, the range of risk and benefit in the ICU is often much more significant than standard historical numbers and therefore the treatment threshold can vary from extremely low to high enough that almost no diagnosis or treatment can alter the outcome, thus presenting "infinite risk."

Every disease has a treatment or a set of possible treatments that advance a cure. Each of these interventions comes at a price or a risk to the patient. When a clinician is reasoning and has established a certain posttest probability of disease, the treatment threshold is the degree of certainty that they must possess to say that the risk of the intervention to treat the disease is less than the probability of the disease being present and not being treated. It also takes into account the perceived risk of the patient and doctor and

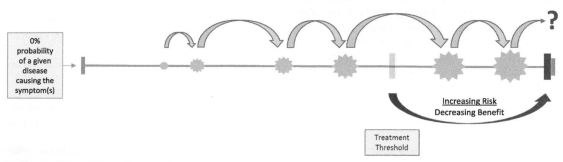

Fig. 5. "Infinite risk" in the very ill patient. Serial diagnostic testing with increased diagnostic certainty does not reach the treatment threshold in a scenario of high risk and low benefit (infinite risk).

their comfort with uncertainty in outcome. It is different for every disease and for every intervention as it is for every person. Thus, our process of reasoning led us to establish a probability of disease, we can compare this probability with the treatment threshold, and we establish this treatment threshold by having a basic understanding of risk and the proportional relationship to the expected benefit.

SUMMARY

Clinical reasoning is a process by which many facts are compiled to generate a hypothesis about why a patient has become ill and what is the cause of their illness. Reasoning and diagnosis is accomplished in many different ways, each with their strengths and weakness, and practitioners of different ability reason differently. Ultimately, the purpose of diagnostic assessment is to make a decision about therapeutic interventions. Whether to intervene or not requires knowing the diagnosis and treatment and assessing the relative risks and benefits of the intervention from the patient and clinician perspective.

The ICU environment requires a structured approach to clinical reasoning because of the pace of decision-making, the high acuity of illness, the need to work with incomplete information, and the iterative nature of data acquisition and intervention. The nine-step modified bayesian reasoning method is a representation of how clinicians approach clinical decision-making and problems in the ICU and is a composite method for experts and novices. It accounts for common reasoning errors, increasing fidelity in the search for a diagnosis. The method also defines and makes explicit a complex process, allowing for active assessment and feedback for ourselves and for our learners. Finally, the use of posttest probabilities and treatment thresholds allow practitioners to consider risk and benefit when deciding for or against an intervention, making the method practical and patient-centered. The modified bayesian reasoning method provides structure and flexibility, assessment and outcome, and frames history taking, examination, and testing in terms of risk and benefit to allow providers to determine whether or not to intervene on the patients for whom they care.

REFERENCES

1. Eva KW. What every teacher needs to know about clinical reasoning. Med Educ 2005;39(1):98–106.

2. Pottier P, Dejoie T, Hardouin JB, et al. Effect of stress on clinical reasoning during simulated ambulatory consultations. Med Teach 2013;35(6): 472–80.

3. Tversky A, Kahneman D. Judgment under uncertainty: heuristics and biases. Science 1974; 185(4157):1124–31.

4. Bowen JL. Educational strategies to promote clinical diagnostic reasoning. N Engl J Med 2006;355(21): 2217–25.

5. Boshuizen HPA, Schmidt HG. On the role of biomedical knowledge in clinical reasoning by experts, intermediates and novices. Cogn Sci 1992;16(2): 153–84.

6. Patel VL, Groen GJ. Knowledge based solution strategies in medical reasoning. Cogn Sci 1986;10(1): 91–116.

7. Facione PA, Facione NC, Giancarlo CAF. California critical thinking disposition inventory: CCTDI. Millbrae, CA: California Academic Press; 2001.

8. Custers EJ, Regehr G, Norman GR. Mental representations of medical diagnostic knowledge: a review. Acad Med 1996;71(10 Suppl):S55–61.

9. Facione PA, Facione NC. Thinking and reasoning in human decision making: the method of argument and heuristic analysis. Millbrae, CA: California Academic Press; 2007.

10. Norman G, Young M, Brooks L. Non-analytical models of clinical reasoning: the role of experience. Med Educ 2007;41(12):1140–5.

11. Norman GR, Eva KW. Diagnostic error and clinical reasoning. Med Educ 2010;44(1):94–100.

12. Norman GR, Brooks LR. The non-analytical basis of clinical reasoning. Adv Health Sci Educ Theory Pract 1997;2(2):173–84.

13. Eva KW, Hatala RM, Leblanc VR, et al. Teaching from the clinical reasoning literature: combined reasoning strategies help novice diagnosticians overcome misleading information. Med Educ 2007; 41(12):1152–8.

14. Brase GL, Hill WT. Good fences make for good neighbors but bad science: a review of what improves bayesian reasoning and why. Front Psychol 2015;6:340.

15. Rivers E, Nguyen B, Havstad S, et al. Early goal-directed therapy in the treatment of severe sepsis and septic shock. N Engl J Med 2001;345(19): 1368–77.

16. Starr C. Social benefit versus technological risk. Science 1969;165(3899):1232–8.

17. Fischhoff B, Slovic P, Lichtenstein S, et al. How safe is safe enough? A psychometric study of attitudes toward technological risks and benefits. Policy Sci 1978;9:25.

18. Slovic P. Perception of risk. Science 1987; 236(4799):280–5.

19. Alhakami AS, Slovic P. A psychological study of the inverse relationship between perceived risk and perceived benefit. Risk Anal 1994;14(6):1085–96.

20. Slovic P, Monahan J, MacGregor DG. Violence risk assessment and risk communication: the effects of using actual cases, providing instruction, and employing probability versus frequency formats. Law I lum Behav 2000;24(3).271–96.

21. Appelbaum PS, Roth LH, Lidz CW, et al. False hopes and best data: consent to research and the therapeutic misconception. Hastings Cent Rep 1987; 17(2):20–4.

22. Pronovost P, Needham D, Berenholtz S, et al. An intervention to decrease catheter-related bloodstream infections in the ICU. N Engl J Med 2006; 355(26):2725–32.

Adverse Event Reporting and Quality Improvement in the Intensive Care Unit

Jason J. Heavner, MD*, Jonathan M. Siner, MD

KEYWORDS

• Safety • Quality • Adverse event • Error • Reporting • Safety culture

KEY POINTS

- Patients in the intensive care unit (ICU) are at increased risk for adverse events and errors.
- Adverse events are associated, directly and indirectly, with poor patient outcomes including increased mortality.
- In multiple studies, most errors are not routinely detected. The unknown frequency of medical errors and adverse events is a major limitation to improvements in quality and safety.
- Adverse events detected by voluntary reporting are important in fostering a culture of safety and are complimentary to other detection strategies.
- Voluntary adverse event reporting is significantly underutilized.

INTRODUCTION

Patients in the ICU are at high-risk for adverse events. The variety of high-acuity health care needs of these vulnerable patients exposes them to numerous medications, procedures, and health care providers. During the past 15 years, health care quality and patient safety have become major focuses in the optimization of health care delivery. However, the origins of the current construct of outcomes measurement and patient safety began in the early twentieth century with Ernest Codman, the first physician in the United States to systematically track patients throughout their hospitalizations and beyond. After receiving significant opposition from other physicians and the hospitals in which he worked for what essentially amounted to outcomes documentation, Codman established his own hospital and published the clinical outcomes in *A Study in Hospital Efficiency*.[1] Later, Dr Codman became an initial founder of the American College of Surgeons along with its Hospital Standardization Program. The latter became, as we know it today, The Joint Commission.

DEFINITIONS OF ADVERSE EVENT AND ERRORS

In the Institute of Medicine's (IOM) report *To Err is Human*, safety is defined as freedom from injury and error.[2] An adverse event is an unanticipated consequence of medical care and is defined by an occurrence that always reaches the patient. Adverse events can occur from the appropriate delivery of health care or from an error. Errors can result from a failure of a planned action to be completed as intended (error of execution) or from use of an incorrect plan to achieve a goal (error of planning).[2] Errors also can occur from inappropriate action (error of commission) or from unintentionally not doing the correct action (error of omission).[2] In addition, errors can be latent as a result of a systems defect or active such as those occurring because of the actions of frontline staff.

The authors have nothing to disclose.

Section of Pulmonary, Critical Care and Sleep Medicine, Department of Internal Medicine, Yale School of Medicine, New Haven, CT, USA

* Corresponding author. 300 Cedar Street, TAC-441 South PO Box 208057, New Haven, CT 06520-8057.

E-mail address: jason.heavner@yale.edu

Clin Chest Med 36 (2015) 461–467

http://dx.doi.org/10.1016/j.ccm.2015.05.005

An error that does not reach the patient or does not cause harm to the patient is a near miss.[2]

RISK FACTORS

There have been many studies demonstrating risk factors for errors, which, for the ICU, include the use of mechanical ventilation, hypoglycemic agents, central venous catheterization, nonelective surgery, and above-target nursing ratios.[3,4] Patients in the medical ICU older than 65 years with more than 2 organ system failures are at increased risk for adverse events.[5] A multicenter European study demonstrated that the risk of adverse events could be predicted based on the presence of organ failure, high workload, and the amount of time the patient is exposed to risk.[6] It is difficult to assess the impact of individual or cumulative adverse events on patient outcomes; however, in one study, the risk of death was increased 3-fold when a patient encountered more than 2 adverse events in the ICU.[3]

HISTORICAL BACKGROUND

In 1991, it was reported that 3.7% of hospitalizations had adverse events.[7] In 1995, it was reported that 1.7 errors occurred per patient per day in the ICU.[8] Despite the availability of this information, there was no national priority for quality improvement during this time. However, in 1999, after the IOM released its report *To Err is Human*, quality and safety became a national health care priority.[2] In this report, the IOM estimated that 44,000 to 98,000 patients die each year as a result of medical errors, with a national cost of $17 billion to $29 billion yearly.[2] These issues were attributed to what was called a cycle of inaction and an acceptance of status quo.[2] It was strongly stated that it would be "irresponsible" to expect anything less than a 50% reduction in errors over 5 years.[2] *To Err is Human* and the subsequent report *Crossing the Quality Chasm* (2001) publicized that medical errors were common and affected the quality of health care received by patients.[2,9]

By 2004, there were not enough available data to assess if the IOM 5-year benchmark of 50% reduction in errors was reached. However, by 5 years, many things had changed, and groundwork for improvement was established.[10] Regulatory changes were initiated, and accrediting and governmental organizations focused on improving safety goals to enhance organizational accountability.[10] There was evidence of an improved reporting culture.[10] The National Quality Forum was established to promote public reporting of quality metrics to improve health care quality and safety. Likewise, states began requiring health care organizations to publicly disclose health care–associated infection rates, which proved to be a powerful motivator both from a reputational perspective as well as in the use of these rates to determine hospital reimbursement for Medicare patients. Medical training regulations also changed. In 2003, the Accreditation Council for Graduate Medical Education (ACGME) limited duty hours.[11] The ACGME also articulated practice-based learning and systems-based practice as 2 of the core professional competencies required in all accredited residency training programs.[11] The Agency for Healthcare Research and Quality (AHRQ) was created and funded as a federal investment. In these 5 years, publications of original research in patient safety nearly doubled and federal funding awards saw a 28-fold increase.[10]

The 2008 National Healthcare Quality Report by the AHRQ noted that patient safety was actually getting worse.[12] A 2008 study revealed that only 55% of adults received the recommended therapies for any particular disease.[12] Similarly, a 2010 study found no significant change over time in the rate of harms identified.[13] This group hypothesized that simple things were not being changed, which prevented more focus on addressing complex issues.[13] For example, in 2008, only 1.5% of hospitals in the United States had implemented a comprehensive electronic medical record, compliance with hand washing remained poor, adverse event reporting was infrequent, and there were difficulties in fostering the necessary organizational change.[13]

EVENT DETECTION

A major limitation to understanding the scope of medical errors and adverse events is the unknown frequency of these events. It is estimated that 50% to 96% of errors are not routinely detected.[14] In 2005, the Critical Care Safety Study attempted to identify and characterize all adverse events and serious medical errors in their teaching hospital ICUs[15]; this included 1 year of direct continuous observation of on-call interns, both voluntary and solicited event reports, computerized adverse drug event detection monitoring, and chart abstraction. The study detected 80 adverse events per 1000 patient-days and 150 serious errors per 1000 patient-days.[15] Only 23% of events were discovered by more than 1 detection method.[15] Nurses were the most frequent reporters. The most frequent physician reports were from physicians reporting an event involving another physician.[15] It was extrapolated that 148,000 life-threatening serious errors occur annually in teaching ICUs.[15] Much of the adverse event review has focused on pharmacy and nursing reported events, and, similarly, this study did not find many diagnostic errors. However, in a large review in 2012, 28% of patients in the ICU who were autopsied had at least 1 misdiagnosis.[16] Of these, 8% were major and potentially lethal.[16] Autopsy rates have declined substantially necessitating alternative methods for identifying these errors.

Since 2007, there has been increased emphasis and available funding for diagnostic error research; however, most methods for detecting adverse events have difficulty detecting these types of errors.[17] Because no institution has the capability to routinely assess for errors as thoroughly and comprehensively as was done in the Critical Care Safety Study or the Harvard Medical Practice Study, there remains a need for an efficient way of identifying harms.[7,15] The Institute for Healthcare Improvement (IHI) developed the Global Trigger Tool using directed chart reviews as a way to measure the overall level of harm in an institution. In an evaluation of the IHI Trigger Tool, more than 12,000 charts were reviewed between 2001 and 2004 from 62 ICUs.[18] The prevalence of adverse events was 11.3 per 100 ICU days.[18] Forty-one percent of the identified adverse events were thought to have contributed directly to death, and 11.4% events required intervention to sustain life.[18] Permanent harm was associated with 2% of the adverse events, and 24.3% of the events caused temporary harm requiring hospitalization or prolonged stay in the hospital.[18] Temporary harm requiring intervention was found in 64.5% events.[18]

Evaluating the frequency of adverse events is difficult because of differences in definitions of events and harm. Medication errors are the most frequently reported adverse events, which exemplifies the difficulties in achieving the goal of attaining the 5 Rights of Medication Management in the ICU: the right patient, the right drug, the right dose, the right route, and the right time.[19] In the Sentinel Events Evaluation study, parenteral medication errors occurred at a rate of 745 per 1000 patient-days.[6,20] Using direct observation, a tool only sustainable for research purposes, 20% of medication doses were found to involve an error.[21] The medications associated with most errors include antimicrobials, vasoactive agents, anticoagulants, sedatives, and insulin.[20,22,23] Many of the adverse events and errors in the ICU are related to procedures or equipment that are unique to this care setting. Mechanical ventilation has been associated with adverse events in 69% of ventilated

patients.[24] Pneumothorax as a consequence of barotrauma or as a complication from a procedure occurs in 1.5% of patients in the ICU and has been associated with an increased risk of death.[25] Likewise, the support devices required in the care of patients in the ICU can be dislodged causing harm. Unplanned endotracheal tube displacements are associated with an increased risk of death.[26]

APPROACHES TO QUALITY EVALUATION

There are 2 general approaches to the understanding and improvement of quality of care. In a continuous improvement process, a problem is identified, a plan is created to correct the problem, and the effectiveness of the plan is evaluated. This approach is also known as the plan-do-study-act cycle (PDSA), which was developed from W. Edwards Deming's iterative cycles of evaluation and improvement.[27] The second approach involves a monitoring system that identifies and characterizes events using valid, sensitive, and specific process, structural, and outcome indicators. These processes are not exclusive of one another. For example, monitoring quality indicators can identify areas needing improvement that can be evaluated and changed using PDSA cycles.

Although there is acknowledgment that the frequency of adverse events and errors must be reduced and quality improved in the ICU, it is not yet apparent how best to measure these events. Arguments have been made to measure errors related to adverse events or to measure errors and extrapolate to potential adverse events.[18] However, most errors do not cause direct harm to patients.[18] These medical errors may be a sign of potential issues, but a causal relationship to most actual adverse events is poor.[18,28,29] Adverse events detected by voluntary reporting are important in creating the culture of safety and are complementary to other measurement strategies, but voluntary reporting significantly underreports the true adverse event rate and changes in event reporting does not correlate with the actual frequency of detected events.[18,30,31]

Direct observation requires an exhaustive amount of personnel resources and is not routinely sustainable. Therefore, the role of direct observation is usually limited to research purposes.[21] Specific chart reviews are also resource intensive and require a high level of diligence to identify actual adverse events and errors.[15,18] Chart reviews that are targeted to specific types of events can be helpful, such as the use of particular medications (eg, naloxone), the use of mechanical ventilation or other life support devices, and mortality reviews. Chart reviews have several difficulties, including the substantial resources needed to perform the task, skilled reviewers for identification and interpretation of events, variability or incorrect terminology, and the presence of typos in the medical record.

Recognizing the limitations of these methods of detecting adverse events, the IHI evaluated an adverse event detection process called the ICU Trigger Tool in an initial group of 13 ICUs within the Idealized Design of the Intensive Care Unit collaboration in 2001.[18] The trigger tool was first used as a method of detecting medication-related adverse events via computerized evaluation of pharmacy records. The concurrent nature of the review allows rapid identification of potential or actual adverse events when the full chart was examined. By focusing the chart review, the rate of identifying adverse events or errors in the reviewed charts was increased. The ICU trigger tool is easy to use and enables ICUs to measure a harm rate and follow the harm rate over time as resources are used for improvement work.[18] In addition, organizations can subsequently prioritize the findings, direct improvement resources, and evaluate the effect of the improvement effort by trending adverse events over time.[18] The ICU trigger tool is intended as a standardized method to detect a rate of events; it is not a comprehensive approach to measure the true frequency of all adverse events in the ICU.[18] Recent reports have emphasized the subjective nature of the IHI trigger tool and its variability when implemented as well as evidence that it may identify fewer events than some historically used tools.[32–34] As mentioned previously, it is reasonable to conclude that the IHI global trigger tool is useful for efficiently identifying many adverse events, but it may not be able to reliably generate data for temporal trends or comparisons between institutions.

ADVERSE EVENT AND ERROR REPORTING

Voluntary reporting is the most frequently used tool to identify adverse events and errors. This reporting method is the most useful for promoting attitude and behavioral changes by allowing individuals to participate in the event recognition process as well as engaging these individuals in process improvement and feedback mechanisms. The implementation of a multidisciplinary quality improvement and safety team augments robust voluntary reporting. Despite this, voluntary reporting is underutilized. It is estimated that 50% to 96% of errors are underreported.[14] Nurses and pharmacists have consistently been shown to report most of the identified adverse events, and most of these events are medication related.[12] These groups rarely report diagnostic errors.[12] Multiple studies have demonstrated that few physicians report at baseline; however, physician reports are unique and, therefore, their reporting should be optimized. During a reporting intervention for internal medicine residents, 6.4% of the reports involved diagnostic error.[35] During their 3-month study period, there were 58 reports in the hospital-wide incident reporting system and 100 resident reports.[35] Of the total 158 events reported, only 1 of the events reported by the residents was reported by someone else in the hospital's anonymous reporting system,[35] which emphasizes the need to have all members of the care team involved in event reporting.[35]

Historically, physician participation in voluntary event reporting has been low for a variety of reasons. It has been shown that there is a fear of litigation, disciplinary action, and fear of loss of reputation.[36] Other reasons for the lack of reporting include the voluntary nature of reporting, lack of agreement on a standardized definition of a reportable event, perceived lack of benefit, apathy, lack of feedback, time constraints, and unfamiliarity with the process.[37,38] In 2002, Leape[37] discussed the reporting of adverse events.[37] He noted 7 characteristics of a successful reporting system: nonpunitive, confidential, independent, expert analysis, timely, systems oriented, and responsive.

In 2004, the Patient Safety Study Group at Washington University and Barnes-Jewish Hospital implemented a SAFE card report system.[39] The SAFE acronym referred to safety, actions, focus, and everyone.[39] The SAFE reporting system was anonymous, simple, and required basic information, which triggered follow-up.[39] These cards were kept in piles near each patient room and in charting rooms.[39] Nurses submitted reports most frequently.[39] SAFE described more events than the hospital-wide computer database, and the system identified a larger number of preventable incidents.[39] However, this process itself did not have a mechanism to address issues in real time, it did not account for the Hawthorne effect, and sustainability was not demonstrated.[39]

In 2011, a prospective, interventional study in 2 ICUs at a Canadian academic center implemented the SAFE card system.[38] There was a significant increase in event reports, including those from physicians, compared with years prior.[38] House staff and attending physicians were educated about the results of the SAFE card reports in a monthly quality improvement meeting, but plans for change or follow-up were not routinely relayed.[38] Subsequently, their SAFE reporting system was phased out to an electronic system. There were no physician reports after this time.[38] During their transition to an electronic system, many physicians reported not knowing that the online system existed, and those that did thought the login was difficult to complete.[38] In addition, the new system was not entirely anonymous.[38]

Peer modeling may be one method of improving physician engagement. At an academic hospital in Boston, a general medicine Fellow met with junior and senior residents during care coordination rounds a few times per week to solicit information about events and errors.[35] Participation in this process was voluntary. During the course of 3 months, there were 28 encounters with the fellow, and 100 events were reported.[35] After the emergency department, house officers were most likely to identify themselves as the responsible party. In this study, the interviewer was a Fellow who knew most of the residents well and was likely viewed as a peer, suggesting that residents may be more likely to report errors or events to a trusted peer.[35] This system did not capture nights and weekends and most weekdays, so there would need to be a fulltime personnel assignment to create a sustainable model.[35] There was no specified mechanism to act on reports.[35]

Errors occurring in the ICU are caused by both human factors and system factors.[40] Human errors are common, ranging from 31% to 63%.[41,42] Human errors are unavoidable, and, as such, interventions to increase education, effort, and focus among health care workers are not effective. Many human errors are related to less-than-ideal human organization, such as staffing models and failure to mitigate factors associated with burnout.[4,43] Interventions should be designed to minimize the opportunity for human error from a systems approach. The goal is to determine how the error occurred not who is at fault for the error. Once the underlying contributory factors leading up to the error are identified, the system can be modified to prevent future occurrences of the error. This methodology prevents the individual provider from receiving the blame, which allows for enhancement of the institution's safety culture.

SAFETY CULTURE

The term safety culture was first used in the International Nuclear Safety Group's 1986 summary report following the Chernobyl nuclear accident. Safety culture was described as "that assembly of characteristics and attitudes in organizations and individuals which establishes that, as an overriding priority, nuclear plant safety issues receive the attention warranted by their significance."[44]

As identified by the AHRQ, a more optimal definition of safety culture has been developed by the Health and Safety Commission of Great Britain: "the safety culture of an organization is the product of individual and group values, attitudes, perceptions, competencies, and patterns of behavior that determine the commitment to, and style and proficiency of, an organization's health and safety management."[45] During the development of the safety attitudes questionnaire, 6 safety attitude domains were identified: teamwork climate, safety climate, perceptions of management, job satisfaction, working conditions, and stress recognition.[46] This questionnaire allows for institutions to be benchmarked so that areas for improvement can be identified and success of interventions can be measured.[46] Although such surveys do convey staff perceptions and attitudes, it remains unclear whether this is a direct correlate of patient safety.[47]

Adverse events and errors are common occurrences in ICUs, and these events are associated with increased risk of harm and death in the most vulnerable patients. It is essential that adverse events and errors are identified and monitored via a complementary set of methods. Trends in event frequency and identification of specific events allow for identification of areas to focus quality improvement efforts as well as to evaluate the impact of these interventions over time. Adverse event reporting is a first step in this process. Although there is a need to report adverse events so that they can be categorized and evaluated, improving safety culture when individuals are more comfortable with reporting also involves real-time adverse event identification, mitigation, and reporting. A robust adverse event reporting system improves the detection of events and is associated with improved safety culture of an organization. Physicians do not routinely report adverse events for the variety of reasons discussed. However, given that diagnostic errors and judgment errors can lead to major adverse events, further understanding these types of adverse events likely requires improved physician reporting. It is unclear, however, which comes first, a good safety culture or a good reporting culture. More research is needed to understand the relationship between lack of physician reporting and safety culture, attitudes, communication skills, reliability, team work, and outcomes.

REFERENCES

1. Codman EA. A study in hospital efficiency: as demonstrated by the case report of the first five years of a private hospital. Boston: Thomas Todd Co; 1918. p. 1–192.

2. Kohn LT, Corrigan JM, Donaldson MS. To err is human: building a safer health system, vol. 627. Washington, DC: National Academies Press; 2000.

3. Garrouste-Orgeas M, Timsit JF, Vesin A, et al. Selected medical errors in the intensive care unit: results of the IATROREF study: parts I and II. Am J Respir Crit Care Med 2010;181(2):134–42.

4. Needleman J, Buerhaus P, Pankratz VS, et al. Nurse staffing and inpatient hospital mortality. N Engl J Med 2011;364(11):1037–45.

5. Giraud T, Dhainaut JF, Vaxelaire JF, et al. Iatrogenic complications in adult intensive care units: a prospective two-center study. Crit Care Med 1993;21(1):40–51.

6. Valentin A, Capuzzo M, Guidet B, et al. Patient safety in intensive care: results from the multinational Sentinel Events Evaluation (SEE) study. Intensive Care Med 2006;32(10):1591–8.

7. Brennan TA, Leape LL, Laird NM, et al. Incidence of adverse events and negligence in hospitalized patients. Results of the Harvard Medical Practice Study I. N Engl J Med 1991;324(6):370–6.

8. Donchin Y, Gopher D, Olin M, et al. A look into the nature and causes of human errors in the intensive-care unit. Crit Care Med 1995;23(2):294–300.

9. Committee on Quality of Health Care in America. Crossing the quality chasm: a new health system for the 21st century. Washington, DC: National Academies Press; 2001.

10. Wachter RM. The end of the beginning: patient safety five years after "To Err Is Human". Health Aff 2004;23(11):534–45.

11. Leape LL, Berwick DM. Five years after To Err is Human: what have we learned? JAMA 2005;293(19):2384–90.

12. Clancy CM. Ten years after To Err is Human. Am J Med Qual 2009;24(6):525–8.

13. Landrigan CP, Parry GJ, Bones CB, et al. Temporal trends in rates of patient harm resulting from medical care. N Engl J Med 2010;363(22):2124–34.

14. Barach P, Small SD. Reporting and preventing medical mishaps: lessons from non-medical near miss reporting systems. BMJ 2000;320(7237):759–63.

15. Rothschild JM, Landrigan CP, Cronin JW, et al. The Critical Care Safety Study: the incidence and nature of adverse events and serious medical errors in intensive care. Crit Care Med 2005;33(8):1694–700.

16. Winters B, Custer J, Galvagno SM Jr, et al. Diagnostic errors in the intensive care unit: a systematic review of autopsy studies. BMJ Qual Saf 2012;21(11):894–902.

17. Newman-Toker DE, Pronovost PJ. Diagnostic errors—the next frontier for patient safety. JAMA 2009;301(10):1060–2.

18. Resar RK, Rozich JD, Simmonds T, et al. A trigger tool to identify adverse events in the intensive care unit. Jt Comm J Qual Patient Saf 2006;32(10):585–90.

19. Little J, Mark S. Pharmacy patient bill of rights: practice advancement from the patient perspective. Hosp Pharm 2013;48(5):351–3.

20. Valentin A, Capuzzo M, Guidet B, et al. Errors in administration of parenteral drugs in intensive care units: multinational prospective study. BMJ 2009;338:b814.

21. Kopp BJ, Erstad BL, Allen ME, et al. Medication errors and adverse drug events in an intensive care unit: direct observation approach for detection. Crit Care Med 2006;34(2):415–25.

22. Buckley MS, LeBlanc JM, Cawley MJ. Electrolyte disturbances associated with commonly prescribed medications in the intensive care unit. Crit Care Med 2010;38:S253–64.

23. Adrogué HJ, Madias NE. Hypernatremia. N Engl J Med 2000;342(20):1493–9.

24. Auriant I, Reignier J, Pibarot M, et al. Critical incidents related to invasive mechanical ventilation in the ICU: preliminary descriptive study. Intensive Care Med 2002;28(4):452–8.

25. de Lassence A, Timsit J-F, Tafflet M, et al. Pneumothorax in the intensive care unit: incidence, risk factors, and outcome. Anesthesiology 2006;104(1):5–13.

26. Thille AW, Harrois A, Schortgen F, et al. Outcomes of extubation failure in medical intensive care unit patients. Crit Care Med 2011;39(12):2612–8.

27. Deming WE. Out of the crisis, 1986. Cambridge (United Kingdom): Mass: Massachusetts Institute of Technology Center for Advanced Engineering Study; 1991. p. 507, xiii.

28. Rozich JD, Haraden CR, Resar RK. Adverse drug event trigger tool: a practical methodology for measuring medication related harm. Qual Saf Health Care 2003;12(3):194–200.

29. Resar RK, Rozich JD, Classen D. Methodology and rationale for the measurement of harm with trigger tools. Qual Saf Health Care 2003;12(Suppl 2):ii39–45.

30. Wu AW, Pronovost P, Morlock L. ICU incident reporting systems. J Crit Care 2002;17(2):86–94.

31. Cullen DJ, Bates DW, Small SD, et al. The incident reporting system does not detect adverse drug events: a problem for quality improvement. Jt Comm J Qual Improv 1995;21(10):541–8.

32. Schildmeijer K, Nilsson L, Årestedt K, et al. Assessment of adverse events in medical care: lack of consistency between experienced teams using the global trigger tool. BMJ Qual Saf 2012;21(4):307–14.

33. Mattsson TO, Knudsen JL, Lauritsen J, et al. Assessment of the global trigger tool to measure, monitor and evaluate patient safety in cancer patients: reliability concerns are raised. BMJ Qual Saf 2013;22(7):571–9.

34. Unbeck M, Schildmeijer K, Henriksson P, et al. Is detection of adverse events affected by record review methodology? An evaluation of the "Harvard

Medical Practice Study" method and the "Global Trigger Tool". Patient Saf Surg 2013;7(1):10.

35. Weingart SN, Ship AN, Aronson MD. Confidential clinician-reported surveillance of adverse events among medical inpatients. J Gen Intern Med 2000; 15(7):470–7.

36. Schuerer DJ, Nast PA, Harris CB, et al. A new safety event reporting system improves physician reporting in the surgical intensive care unit. J Am Coll Surg 2006;202(6):881–7.

37. Leape LL. Reporting of adverse events. N Engl J Med 2002;347(20):1633–8.

38. Ilan R, Squires M, Panopoulos C, et al. Increasing patient safety event reporting in 2 intensive care units: a prospective interventional study. J Crit Care 2011;26(4):431.e11–8.

39. Osmon S, Harris CB, Dunagan WC, et al. Reporting of medical errors: an intensive care unit experience. Crit Care Med 2004;32(3):727–33.

40. Reason J. Human error: models and management. BMJ 2000;320(7237):768–70.

41. Abramson NS, Wald KS, Grenvik AN, et al. Adverse occurrences in intensive care units. JAMA 1980; 244(14):1582–4.

42. Bracco D, Favre J-B, Bissonnette B, et al. Human errors in a multidisciplinary intensive care unit: a 1-year prospective study. Intensive Care Med 2001; 27(1):137–45.

43. Landrigan CP, Rothschild JM, Cronin JW, et al. Effect of reducing interns' work hours on serious medical errors in intensive care units. N Engl J Med 2004; 351(18):1838–48.

44. Summary report on the post-accident review meeting on the Chernobyl accident. Safety Series No. 75-INSAG-1. IAEA, Vienna, Austria: International Atomic Energy Agency; 1986.

45. Health and Safety Commission. Organizing for safety: third report of the Human Factors Study Group of ACSNI. Sudbury (United Kingdom): HSE Books; 1993.

46. Sexton J, Helmreich R, Neilands T, et al. The Safety Attitudes Questionnaire: psychometric properties, benchmarking data, and emerging research. BMC Health Serv Res 2006;6(1):44.

47. Farup PG. Are measurements of patient safety culture and adverse events valid and reliable? Results from a cross-sectional study. BMC Health Serv Res 2015;15(1):186.

Five Questions Critical Care Educators Should Ask About Simulation-Based Medical Education

Dominique Piquette, MD, MSc, MEd, PhD[a],*,
Vicki R. LeBlanc, PhD[b]

KEYWORDS

• Medical education • Simulation • Critical care • Learning outcomes

KEY POINTS

• Simulation-based medical education (SBME) is an instructional medium that refers to the use of multiple simulation modalities.

• SBME presents favorable characteristics for the achievement of educational goals that may not be fully addressed during clinical-based training.

• Numerous studies support the use of SBME for the improvement of knowledge, technical and nontechnical tasks (teamwork, communication skills), and system issues in different clinical domains.

• More research is needed to better understand the most effective use of SBME as part of a broader medical curriculum.

INTRODUCTION

Simulation is rapidly permeating into every sphere of medical education, including teaching, assessment, and research.[1] Publications about SBME have grown exponentially over the past 10 years.[1,2] In addition, the quality of the studies published on SBME has consistently increased, as illustrated by a series of reviews published by Issenberg, McGaghie and colleagues.[3–5] This impressive body of evidence now includes original studies, narrative and systematic reviews, opinion and position papers in different clinical domains, as well as a fewer number of publications specifically related to critical care medicine. These studies combined with the research findings in other clinical areas demonstrate the relevance of SBME for critical care health professionals.[6–11] In the presence of such an extensive literature, it seemed superfluous to undertake another systematic review on the topic of simulation in critical care medicine. However, this abundance of information on SBME can be overwhelming for critical care educators who attempt, in the midst of many other professional responsibilities, to design, implement, and evaluate sound educational innovations or curricula for their trainees. The focus of this review on SBME is therefore to summarize the evidence relevant for frontline educators in critical care medicine. The authors briefly examine 5 practical questions aimed at better understanding the nature of SBME, its theoretic and proven benefits,

Disclosure Statement: None of the authors have any conflict of interest to declare.
[a] Department of Critical Care Medicine, Sunnybrook Health Sciences Centre, 2075 Bayview Avenue, Room D108, Toronto, Ontario M4N 3M5, Canada; [b] Wilson Centre, University of Toronto, 200 Elizabeth Street, 1ES-565, Toronto, Ontario M5G 2C4, Canada
* Corresponding author.
E-mail address: dominique.piquette@sunnybrook.ca

Clin Chest Med 36 (2015) 469–479
http://dx.doi.org/10.1016/j.ccm.2015.05.003
0272-5231/15/$ – see front matter © 2015 Elsevier Inc. All rights reserved.

its delivery, as well as the challenges posed by SBME. The term SBME is used broadly to include education of all health care professionals. Although SBME has traditionally been predominantly focused on physicians, simulation studies are increasingly directed toward other health care professionals, such as nurses, pharmacists, and dieticians.[12–14]

WHAT IS SIMULATION-BASED MEDICAL EDUCATION?

Simulation has been broadly defined as "an instructional medium used for education, assessment, and research, which includes several modalities that have in common the reproduction of certain characteristics of the clinical reality."[15] Simulation modalities typically include part-task trainers (interactions with a physical or virtual model requiring the use of specific psychomotor skills to complete procedures), human simulation (interactions with a simulated or standardized patient), computer-based simulation (interaction with a screen-based interface), and simulated clinical immersion (interaction with a physical or virtual work environment including team members, computer-driven manikin patient, and equipment).[9,10,15–17] More recently, simulation modalities have been combined into hybrid simulations to facilitate the simultaneous and integrative practice of complementary skills (eg, part-task trainer on a simulated patient to practice suturing and communication skills).[18] In addition, simulators have been placed in real clinical environments to create in situ simulations.[19] In the face of such variety of simulation modalities, medical educators need to choose a modality that best aligns with the learning objectives of their training programs and depending upon the benefits and limitations of each modality.[9,15]

WHY SHOULD SIMULATION-BASED MEDICAL EDUCATION BE USED?

If simulation has ever elicited doubts among health care educators about its roles in medical education, many think that we have now moved beyond the need to justify its use.[13,20,21] Based on a growing body of evidence, the use of simulation seems judicious for certain aspects of health care training. The need to better define how to use SBME optimally and cost effectively has been identified as the next question to be answered by the medical education community.[7,13,20]

It is worthwhile to briefly consider the context in which SBME rapidly gained popularity over the recent years, after initial delays in the uptake of a technology developed more than three decades ago.[7,9] As medical education evolved, educators developed a better understanding of the learning processes involved in health care education, such as deliberate practice,[22,23] reflection,[24–26] and feedback.[27–29] Meanwhile, the traditional apprenticeship model, based on the prolonged and repeated interactions between junior and senior health care professionals, was increasingly under threat because of numerous changes in the health care system: increased clinical workload; rapid turnover of patients and health care professionals in a given clinical unit; competing academic roles of faculty as clinicians, educators, and researchers; and so on.[9,30–32] Such changes led to perceived inadequacies of the medical training system: the key processes thought to benefit clinical learning seemed increasingly hard to experience in acute care environments.[7,32] Furthermore, growing concerns about patient safety made the idea of inexperienced trainees practicing their skills on real patients morally inacceptable.[17,31,33] Working hour limitations and increased patient supervision were implemented to increase the quality of care provided in teaching hospitals.[9,17,32–35] The educational shortcomings of this new form of time-limited, autonomy-restricted clinical experience needed to be compensated.[31,36] In addition to individual competencies, human factors and teamwork were identified as a common source of medical errors.[9,37] Specific training for interdisciplinary teams was strongly recommended to further improve the quality of care.[37]

Simulation represented a natural response to these problems for several reasons.[17,38] First, simulation can provide a safe learning environment where mistakes can be made, reviewed, corrected, and reflected upon.[9,17] Second, simulation offers the opportunity to practice clinical skills and to achieve a certain level of proficiency or mastery before caring of real patients.[7] Third, simulation offers greater control and predictability of the learning experience in terms of type, order, number, and length of the sessions; type of feedback provided; number and level of participants; and so on.[17] In theory, SBME therefore presents desirable characteristics to meet the educational needs of health care professionals in training, as well as the moral obligation to prioritize patient safety in real clinical situations.[9,17]

The medical education literature provides clear evidence that SBME can fulfill an important role within health care professional training. At least 3 systematic reviews have now demonstrated that SBME, as an instructional medium, can positively affect learning and can translate into benefits for the patients.[13,14,39] However, the heterogeneity of the literature on SBME justifies taking a closer look at the potential educational benefits of SBME. This topic is the focus of the following section.

WHAT CAN BE TAUGHT AND ASSESSED WITH SIMULATION-BASED MEDICAL EDUCATION?

Simulation-based education has been used to teach and study a broad range of knowledge, skills, and attitudes. Multiple reviews have attempted to summarize the current evidence supporting the use of SBME. Some of these reviews are specific for critical care medicine,[6,9–11,40] whereas others are related to different clinical specialties, such as anesthesia,[1,41] obstetrics,[42] emergency medicine,[17,43] surgery,[44] or pediatrics.[45] Specific modalities or groups of modalities have also been the object of literature reviews, including simulated patients,[46] virtual simulation,[47] technology-enhanced simulation,[13] computer-assisted learning,[48] and in situ simulation.[19] The following conclusions can be derived from the examination of these reviews:

1. Simulation is generally well accepted by learners as a teaching strategy, as illustrated by the positive ratings consistently reported in trainee satisfaction surveys.[9]
2. The types of learning outcomes measured to demonstrate the benefits of SBME are not equally represented in the literature: studies showing short-term gain in knowledge and skills in the simulation environment (levels 1 and 2 of Kirkpatrick's model[49] presented in **Box 1**) are overrepresented when compared with studies

assessing long-term (eg, 6–12 months) gain of knowledge and skills, or changes in behaviors transferred to real clinical environments and benefiting patients (levels 3 and 4 of Kirkpatrick's model).[50]
3. The quality of the evidence on SBME is generally limited, as indicated by small sample sizes, lack of control group or randomization, scarcity of multicenter studies, and poor reporting.[13,51]
4. Improvement of knowledge, technical and nontechnical tasks,[10] teamwork, communication skills, and system issues has been achieved by SBME in certain areas.

SBME has shown promising results in many areas relevant for critical care educators. Specific examples related to technical and nontechnical skills, system issues, and assessment tools are presented in **Box 2**. When appropriate, the Kirkpatrick's level of learning outcomes measured by individual studies is indicated. Simulation is also being increasingly considered in 2 other educational domains: high-stakes assessment and mass casualty training. Simulation-based assessment is not a new phenomenon and has been incorporated in licensure and certification examination at the undergraduate and postgraduate level for many years.[52] More recently, simulation has also been used in regulatory programs for practicing physicians in the fields of anesthesia, internal medicine, and family medicine.[52] In addition to part-task trainers and simulated patients, full-body manikin simulators are now increasingly used for high-stakes assessment.[53] As the caveats of simulation-based assessment are better understood and slowly overcome (eg, psychometric properties and technological limitations),[53] simulation will likely play an important role in high-stakes assessment in critical care. Finally, SBME has been shown to be useful for mass casualty training[54] and may represent a useful tool for health care professional training in response to specific threats, such as the recent Ebola epidemic.[55]

There are also studies in the domains of neonatal resuscitation,[56,57] teamwork during cardiac arrests,[58] airway management,[59] and Advanced Trauma Life Support (ATLS) skills[60] that have failed to demonstrate a clear benefit of SBME. Most of these studies have compared SBME with other types of educational interventions such as video training, case-based or problem-based discussions, and traditional teaching. Limitations in the methodological rigor of many studies supporting the role of SBME, as well as inconsistencies regarding its efficacy

---

Box 1
Kirkpatrick's model

Level 1: Reaction

  Level of satisfaction regarding training

Level 2: Learning

  Knowledge, skills, and attitudes acquired

Level 3: Behavior

  Transfer of learning to workplace

Level 4: Results

  Transfer or impact on society (patients)

Adapted from Kirkpatrick DL. Evaluating Training Programs. 2nd edition. San Francisco (CA): Berrett-Koehler; 1998.

Box 2
Selected evidence supporting a role for SBME in different domains relevant to critical care

Technical skills

Procedures

 Central line insertion (KL 1–4)[46,64–67]

 Airway management and endotracheal intubation (KL 2, 3, 4)[68–71]

 Bronchoscopy (KL 2–3)[72,73]

 Cricothyroidotomy (KL 2)[74]

 Thoracocentesis (KL 2)[75]

 Paracentesis (KL 2)[76]

 Ultrasonography skills, including echocardiography (KL 1, 2)[77,78]

Task-related technical skills

 Neurocritical skills (KL 1)[79]

 ACLS skills (KL 1–4)[14,80–83]

 Task management of critical care crises (KL 1, 2)[84–89]

 Task management of patients with trauma (KL 1, 2)[84,90]

 Knowledge and skills in respiratory mechanics, mechanical ventilation, and circulation (KL 3)[91]

Nontechnical skills/teamwork

Crisis resource management skills (KL 1, 2)[40,92–95]

Team behaviors during ATLS (KL 2)[90,96]

Team crisis responses, including outcomes of simulated patient and communication (KL 2)[97]

Interprofessional team responses of undergraduate students (KL 1)[98]

MET performance (KL 2, 4)[99]

Teamwork during postcardiac surgery pediatric cardiac arrest (KL 1)[100]

System-based processes

Interphysician variability in ICU admission of patients with end-stage cancer[101]

Nursing hand-offs of patients in ICU[102]

Discrepancies between institutional or departmental policies and clinical practice related to obstetric emergencies[103]

Infectious disease challenges during SARS cardiac arrests[104]

Assessment tools: validation studies

Teamwork

 Mayo High Performance Teamwork scale for CRM skills[105]

 Self-assessment tool of teamwork in critical care[106]

 Clinical Teamwork Scale[107]

 Crisis management behavior performance markers[108]

 TEAM[109]

Individual nontechnical skills

 Anesthesia nontechnical skills system[110]

 Ottawa Global Rating Scale for nontechnical skills[111,112]

 Family Conference OSCE for professionalism and communication skills[113]

 Checklist for professionalism during ethical dilemma[114]

Individual technical or mixed skills

    Interdisciplinary management of septic shock[115]

    Integrated Procedural Performance Instrument for technical and communication skills[116]

    Scenario-specific performance checklist for pediatric scenarios,[117] undergraduates,[118] and acute care scenarios[119,120]

    IPETT for emergency technical and nontechnical skills[121]

    Comparison between written examination, simulation-based, and oral viva examinations for procedural skills[122]

Abbreviations: ACLS, Advanced Cardiac Life Support; ATLS, Advanced Trauma Life Support; CRM, crisis resource management; ICU, intensive care unit; IPETT, Imperial Pediatric Emergency Training Toolkit; KL, Kirkpatrick's level; MET, medical emergency team; OSCE, Objective Structured Clinical Examination; SARS, severe acute respiratory syndrome; TEAM, Team Emergency Assessment Measure.

when compared with other learning strategies, call for thoughtful reflection as to when simulation should, or should not, be used for critical care instruction. In this regard, another type of literature on SBME, described in the following section, helps to further inform the judicious use of SBME in critical care medicine.

HOW SHOULD SIMULATION-BASED MEDICAL EDUCATION BE USED?

SBME is a time-consuming, potentially costly enterprise and must therefore be carefully planned to maximize its educational benefits and minimize its resource requirements. Thankfully, the body of literature dedicated to the understanding of the features characterizing effective SBME is slowly growing.[5] **Box 3** summarizes the types of questions that critical care educators should consider when planning a simulation-based curricular activity.[4,5]

Chiniara and colleagues[15] have also nicely summarized many issues related to the instructional design of SBME. The investigators discussed the learning objectives for which simulation may be the most appropriate medium, the choice of a simulation modality, the choice of an instructional method (self-directed or instructor-based method), and the simulation presentation (including feedback, fidelity, type of simulator, scenarios, and team composition).[15]

Studies assessing the best ways to deliver SBME have been increasingly conducted in the critical care setting. For example, Springer and colleagues[61] concluded that multiple 30-min simulation sessions held over 3 consecutive days were more effective than one 90-min session to improve resident knowledge regarding recognition and management of septic shock. Ali and colleagues[62] reported that both students and instructors perceived the use of mechanical simulators and of simulated patients as equally satisfactory for

ATLS training. Such studies can contribute to the improvement of SBME by increasing its efficacy or reducing its costs. However, there are still a large number of unanswered questions regarding the best ways to optimize the use of SBME. This is an area that requires further high-quality research.

Box 3
Important questions to consider when planning a simulation-based educational intervention

How is this intervention integrated with other aspects of the curriculum?

Based on the learning objectives, should this training be interdisciplinary and/or focused on team training?

How will the facilitator/instructor be chosen and trained (clinical, educational, and interpersonal skills)?

How should the right level of simulation fidelity be chosen (physical, psychological, and sociocultural)?

How much and what type of practice will be required of the participants (repetitive, deliberate, massed, or distributed)?

How will the feedback be provided (by whom, when, how often, how)?

How will each practice session differ from the other (progressive difficulty, variety of cases, adapted to individual learners)?

When will the intervention end (achievement of mastery learning)?

How and where will the outcomes of this intervention be measured (in the simulation setting or in real clinical environments)?

How can it be ensured that the knowledge and skills acquired will be maintained?

WHAT ARE THE CHALLENGES RELATED TO SIMULATION-BASED MEDICAL EDUCATION?

As described earlier, the rising popularity of SBME has emerged in a specific context where traditional clinical-based training is increasingly challenging because of complex and interdependent societal and organizational changes. Based on the current evidence, the use of SBME to prevent medical errors and adverse events seems totally legitimate. However, the authors foresee important challenges that critical care educators should carefully consider before engaging in SBME activities.

First, the authors feel the need to address the aspects of health care professional training that SBME will not address. Clinical training is challenging in part because of the lack of availability of dedicated clinical teachers (who struggle to fulfill other professional responsibilities) and motivated trainees (overwhelming workload, working hours limitation, etc.). Health care resources are globally limited. The lack of time and scarcity of human and financial resources identified as

barriers for clinical learning also apply to SBME. Clinically competent, properly trained simulation instructors are a rarity in most institutions. Training faculty to fulfill these responsibilities is time and resource consuming. Furthermore, the authors do not share the enthusiasm of others regarding the potential to add hours of SBME to the working hours of medical trainees. The educational value of any training completed beyond 80 hours of clinical work is questionable. Although the mistakes committed in a simulated environment will not harm any patient, tired trainees are unlikely to efficiently learn and to positively process their simulation experience. Furthermore, the time and energy invested in SBME necessarily redirect part of the energy and resources from clinical-based training toward SBME. Such unilateral shift could potentially represent additional impediments to the improvement of clinical-based learning, still recognized, even among the strongest proponents of SBME, as a core component of health care education. The authors believe that clinical-based learning and SBME can inform and complement each other in many aspects of

---

Box 4
Development and curricular integration of SBME

1. Identification of an educational problem

    Which educational need is not adequately addressed by the current curriculum?

    How is this problem currently addressed?

    Could SBME help address this problem?

2. Targeted need assessment

    Which learners should be targeted for this program/activity?

    What are the learners' specific needs?

    Is a simulated learning environment appropriate to address these needs?

3. Goals and objectives

    What are the general goals of this program/activity?

    What are the measurable objectives that will be achieved?

4. Educational strategies

    Which simulation modality is the most appropriate to achieve these goals?

    Which instructional method will be the most helpful?

    How should the simulation activity/program be presented (timing, duration, feedback, etc.)?

5. Implementation

    Which kind of support/resources will be required?

    Which barriers to implementation can be expected?

6. Evaluation and feedback

    How will feedback be obtained from individual learners?

    How will this activity be assessed at the program level?

training. In their opinion, recent calls for better curricular integration of SBME are an encouraging step in the right direction. SBME is not a panacea that will fix all the medical education problems, and clinical-based training should continue to be a high priority for medical educators and researchers.

The second challenge faced by SBME is the significant gap between the theoretic understanding of how SBME should be delivered and the way it is currently delivered in most institutions. With the exception of a few programs led by groups of committed and trained educators, SBME is frequently delivered in an ad hoc and unsystematic manner, separate from the broader curriculum. **Box 4** suggests an approach to SBME based on general principles of curriculum development.[63] Far from wanting to blame educators, their intention is rather to highlight how difficult it can be for an educational intervention to present most of the features of effective SBME. In an attempt to be pragmatic about the implementation of SBME, educators must often select one of 2 features on which to focus their time and energy. The real benefits of SBME as currently applied may therefore be less than the ones presented in the literature.

SUMMARY

SBME has come a long way since the introduction of the first simulator more than 30 years ago. The authors have many reasons to be optimistic about SBME: the role of SBME is expanding (identification of gaps in clinical training and practice; undergraduate, postgraduate, and continuing education; formative and high-stakes assessment), the quality of evidence to support its use is increasing, and the strategies to implement SBME effectively and efficiently are better understood. There seems to be a consensus in the literature that SBME has an important role to play in the improvement of the safety of the care delivered in health care institutions; patient outcomes can be affected by our educational choices. These conclusions likely apply to the critical care environment in which patient outcomes critically depend on timely, complex, and highly coordinated care. However, significant research is still needed to further explore the advantages and limitations of SBME for specific clinical activities completed in particular clinical contexts. Such efforts should be coordinated with larger educational initiatives aimed at providing the best and most comprehensive educational experience for the critical care trainees.

REFERENCES

1. Ross AJ, Kodate N, Anderson JE, et al. Review of simulation studies in anaesthesia journals, 2001–2010: mapping and content analysis. Br J Anaesth 2012;109(1):99–109.
2. Leblanc VR, Bould MD, McNaughton N, et al. Simulation in postgraduate medical education. Ottawa, Canada: Members of the FMEC PG consortium; 2011.
3. Issenberg SB, McGaghie WC, Hart IR, et al. Simulation technology for health care professional skills training and assessment. JAMA 1999;282(9):861–6.
4. Issenberg SB, McGaghie WC, Petrusa ER, et al. Features and uses of high-fidelity medical simulations that lead to effective learning: a BEME systematic review. Med Teach 2005;27(1):10–28.
5. McGaghie WC, Issenberg SB, Petrusa ER, et al. A critical review of simulation-based medical education research: 2003–2009. Med Educ 2010; 44(1):50–63.
6. Greenberg SB, Tokarczyk A, Small S. Critical care simulation. Dis Mon 2011;57(11):715–22.
7. Ventre KM. Toward a sustainable future for simulation-based critical care training: facing a few "inconvenient truths". Pediatr Crit Care Med 2009;10(2):264–5.
8. Murray D. Clinical skills in acute care: a role for simulation training. Crit Care Med 2006;34(1): 252–3.
9. Lam G, Ayas NT, Griesdale DE, et al. Medical simulation in respiratory and critical care medicine. Lung 2010;188(6):445–57.
10. Lighthall GK, Barr J. The use of clinical simulation systems to train critical care physicians. J Intensive Care Med 2007;22(5):257–69.
11. Hammond J. Simulation in critical care and trauma education and training. Curr Opin Crit Care 2004; 10:325–9.
12. Fox-Robichaud AE, Nimmo GR. Education and simulation techniques for improving reliability of care. Curr Opin Crit Care 2007;13:737–41.
13. Cook DA, Hatala R, Brydges R, et al. Technology-enhanced simulation for health professions education: a systemic review and meta-analysis. JAMA 2011;306(9):978–88.
14. Yuan HB, Williams BA, Fang JB, et al. A systematic review of selected evidence on improving knowledge and skills through high-fidelity simulation. Nurse Educ Today 2012;32(3):294–8.
15. Chiniara G, Cole G, Brisbin K, et al. Simulation in healthcare: a taxonomy and a conceptual framework for instructional design and media selection. Med Teach 2013;35(8):e1380–95.
16. Naik VN, Brien SE. Review article: simulation: a means to address and improve patient safety. Can J Anaesth 2013;60(2):192–200.

17. McLaughlin S, Fitch MT, Goyal DG, et al. Simulation in graduate medical education 2008: a review for emergency medicine. Acad Emerg Med 2008; 15(11):1117–29.

18. Ellaway RH, Kneebone R, Lachapelle K, et al. Practica continua: connecting and combining simulation modalities for integrated teaching, learning and assessment. Med Teach 2009;31(8): 725–31.

19. Rosen MA, Hunt EA, Pronovost PJ, et al. In situ simulation in continuing education for the health care professions: a systematic review. J Contin Educ Health Prof 2012;32(4):243–54.

20. Brindley PG. Medical simulation: no longer "why" but "how". J Crit Care 2009;24(1):153–4.

21. Ziv A, Root Wolpe P, Small SD, et al. Simulation-based medical education: an ethical imperative. Acad Med 2003;78:783–8.

22. Ericsson KA, Krampe RT, Tesh-Romer C. The role of deliberate practice in the acquisition of expert performance. Psychol Rev 1993;100:363–406.

23. Ericsson KA. Deliberate practice and the acquisition and maintenance of expert performance in medicine and related domains. Acad Med 2004; 79(10 Suppl):S70–81.

24. Mann K, Gordon J, MacLeod A. Reflection and reflective practice in health professions education: a systematic review. Adv Health Sci Educ Theory Pract 2009;14(4):595–621.

25. Sandars J. The use of reflection in medical education: AMEE Guide No. 44. Med Teach 2009;31(8): 685–95.

26. Schön D. The reflective practitioner: how professionals think in action. Aldershot (United Kingdom): Ashgate Publishing Limited; 1983.

27. Ende J. Feedback in clinical medical education. JAMA 1983;250(6):777–81.

28. Kluger A, DeNisi A. The effects of feedback interventions on performance: historical review, a meta-analysis and a preliminary feedback intervention theory. Psychol Bull 1996;119:254–84.

29. van de Ridder JM, Stokking KM, McGaghie WC, et al. What is feedback in clinical education? Med Educ 2008;42(2):189–97.

30. Kennedy TJ, Regehr G, Baker GR, et al. Progressive independence in clinical training: a tradition worth defending? Acad Med 2005;80(10 Suppl): S106–11.

31. Cox M, Irby DM. American medical education 100 years after the Flexner report. N Engl J Med 2006; 355:1339–44.

32. Swanwick T. Informal learning in postgraduate medical education: from cognitivism to 'culturism'. Med Educ 2005;39(8):859–65.

33. IOM. To err is human: building a safer health system. Washington, DC: National Academic Press; 2000.

34. IOM. Resident duty hours: enhancing sleep, supervision, and safety. Washington, DC: National Academies Press; 2009.

35. Landrigan CP, Rothschild JM, Cronin JW, et al. Effect of reducing interns' work hours on serious medical errors in intensive care units. N Engl J Med 2004;351(18):1838–48.

36. Woodrow SI, Segouin C, Armbruster J, et al. Duty hours reforms in the United States, France, and Canada: is it time to refocus our attention on education? Acad Med 2006;81(12):1045–51.

37. Kohn L, Corrigan J, Donaldson M. To err is human: building a safer health system. Washington, DC: Institute of Medicine; 1999.

38. Gould DA, Chalmers N, Johnson SJ, et al. Simulation: moving from technology challenge to human factors success. Cardiovasc Intervent Radiol 2012;35(3):445–53.

39. McGaghie WC, Issenberg SB, Cohen ER, et al. Does simulation-based medical education with deliberate practice yield better results than traditional clinical education? A meta-analytic comparative review of the evidence. Acad Med 2011;86(6): 706–11.

40. Cheng A, Donoghue A, Gilfoyle E, et al. Simulation-based crisis resource management training for pediatric critical care medicine: a review for instructors. Pediatr Crit Care Med 2012;13(2): 197–203.

41. Leblanc VR. Review article: simulation in anesthesia: state of the science and looking forward. Can J Anaesth 2012;59(2):193–202.

42. Pratt SD. Recent trends in simulation for obstetric anesthesia. Curr Opin Anaesthesiol 2012;25(3): 271–6.

43. McFetrich J. A structured literature review on the use of high fidelity patient simulators for teaching in emergency medicine. Emerg Med J 2006; 23(7):509–11.

44. Sutherland LM, Middleton PF, Anthony A, et al. Surgical simulation: a systematic review. Ann Surg 2006;243(3):291–300.

45. Mills DM, Williams DC, Dobson JV. Simulation training as a mechanism for procedural and resuscitation education for pediatric residents: a systematic review. Hosp Pediatr 2013;3(2):167–76.

46. Ma IW, Brindle ME, Ronksley PE, et al. Use of simulation-based education to improve outcomes of central venous catheterization: a systematic review and meta-analysis. Acad Med 2011;86(9): 1137–47.

47. Cook DA, Triola MM. Virtual patients: a critical literature review and proposed next steps. Med Educ 2009;43(4):303–11.

48. Tegtmeyer K, Ibsen L, Goldstein B. Computer-assisted learning in critical care: from ENIAC to HAL. Crit Care Med 2001;29(8):N177–82.

49. Kirkpatrick DL. Evaluating training programs. 2nd edition. San Francisco (CA): Berrett-Koehler; 1998.

50. Shear TD, Greenberg SB, Tokarczyk A. Does training with human patient simulation translate to improved patient safety and outcome? Curr Opin Anaesthesiol 2013;26(2):159–63.

51. McGaghie WC, Issenberg SB, Petrusa ER, et al. Effect of practice on standardised learning outcomes in simulation-based medical education. Med Educ 2006;40(8):792–7.

52. Holmboe E, Rizzolo MA, Sachdeva AK, et al. Simulation-based assessment and the regulation of healthcare professionals. Simul Healthc 2011; 6(Suppl):S58–62.

53. Boulet JR. Summative assessment in medicine: the promise of simulation for high-stakes evaluation. Acad Emerg Med 2008;15(11):1017–24.

54. Weinberg ER, Auerbach MA, Shah NB. The use of simulation for pediatric training and assessment. Curr Opin Pediatr 2009;21(3):282–7.

55. Decker BK, Sevransky JE, Barrett K, et al. Preparing for critical care services to patients with Ebola. Ann Intern Med 2014;161(1):831–3.

56. Curran VR, Aziz K, O'Young S, et al. Evaluation of the effect of a computerized training simulator (ANAKIN) on the retention of neonatal resuscitation skills. Teach Learn Med 2004;16(2):157–64.

57. Cavaleiro AP, Guimaraes H, Calheiros F. Training neonatal skills with simulators? Acta Paediatr 2009;98(4):636–9.

58. Frengley RW, Weller JM, Torrie J, et al. The effect of a simulation-based training intervention on the performance of established critical care unit teams. Crit Care Med 2011;39(12):2605–11.

59. Wenk M, Waurick R, Schotes D, et al. Simulation-based medical education is no better than problem-based discussions and induces misjudgment in self-assessment. Adv Health Sci Educ Theory Pract 2009;14(2):159–71.

60. Cherry RA, Williams J, George J, et al. The effectiveness of a human patient simulator in the ATLS shock skills station. J Surg Res 2007; 139(2):229–35.

61. Springer R, Mah J, Shusdock I, et al. Simulation training in critical care: does practice make perfect? Surgery 2013;154(2):345–50.

62. Ali J, Dunn J, Eason M, et al. Comparing the standardized live trauma patient and the mechanical simulator models in the ATLS initial assessment station. J Surg Res 2010;162(1):7–10.

63. Kern DE, Thomas PA, Hughes MT. Curriculum development for medical education: a six-step approach. 2nd edition. Baltimore (MA): JHU Press; 2010.

64. Smith CC, Huang GC, Newman LR, et al. Simulation training and its effect on long-term resident performance in central venous catheterization. Simul Healthc 2010;5(3):146–51.

65. Barsuk JH, McGaghie WC, Cohen ER, et al. Simulation-based mastery learning reduces complications during central venous catheter insertion in a medical intensive care unit. Crit Care Med 2009; 37(10):2697–701.

66. Britt RC, Novosel TJ, Britt LD, et al. The impact of central line simulation before the ICU experience. Am J Surg 2009;197(4):533–6.

67. Barsuk JH, Cohen ER, Potts S, et al. Dissemination of a simulation-based mastery learning intervention reduces central line-associated bloodstream infections. BMJ Qual Saf 2014;23(9):749–56.

68. Mayo PH, Hackney JE, Mueck JT, et al. Achieving house staff competence in emergency airway management: results of a teaching program using a computerized patient simulator*. Crit Care Med 2004;32(12):2422–7.

69. Kuduvalli PM, Jervis A, Tighe SQ, et al. Unanticipated difficult airway management in anaesthetised patients: a prospective study of the effect of mannequin training on management strategies and skill retention. Anaesthesia 2008;63(4): 364–9.

70. Rosenthal ME, Adachi M, Ribaudo V, et al. Achieving housestaff competence in emergency airway management using scenario based simulation training: comparison of attending vs housestaff trainers. Chest 2006;129(6):1453–8.

71. Kory PD, Eisen LA, Adachi M, et al. Initial airway management skills of senior residents: simulation training compared with traditional training. Chest 2007;132(6):1927–31.

72. Ost D, DeRosiers A, Britt EJ, et al. Assessment of a bronchoscopy simulator. Am J Respir Crit Care Med 2001;164(12):2248–55.

73. Wahidi MM, Silvestri GA, Coakley RD, et al. A prospective multicenter study of competency metrics and educational interventions in the learning of bronchoscopy among new pulmonary fellows. Chest 2010;137(5):1040–9.

74. Boet S, Borges BC, Naik VN, et al. Complex procedural skills are retained for a minimum of 1 yr after a single high-fidelity simulation training session. Br J Anaesth 2011;107(4):533–9.

75. Wayne DB, Barsuk JH, O'Leary KJ, et al. Mastery learning of thoracentesis skills by internal medicine residents using simulation technology and deliberate practice. J Hosp Med 2008;3(1):48–54.

76. Barsuk JH, Cohen ER, Vozenilek JA, et al. Simulation-based education with mastery learning improves paracentesis skills. J Grad Med Educ 2012;4(1):23–7.

77. Sekiguchi H, Bhagra A, Gajic O, et al. A general Critical Care Ultrasonography workshop: results of a novel Web-based learning program combined with simulation-based hands-on training. J Crit Care 2013;28(2):217.e7–12.

78. Clau-Terré F, Sharma V, Cholley B, et al. Can simulation help to answer the demand for echography education. Anesthesiology 2014;120:32–41.

79. Musacchio MJ Jr, Smith AP, McNeal CA, et al. Neuro-critical care skills training using a human patient simulator. Neurocrit Care 2010;13(2):169–75.

80. Wayne DB, Didwania A, Feinglass J, et al. Simulation-based education improves quality of care during cardiac arrest team responses at an academic teaching hospital: a case-control study. Chest 2008;133(1):56–61.

81. Wayne DB, Butter J, Siddall VJ, et al. Mastery learning of advanced cardiac life support skills by internal medicine residents using simulation technology and deliberate practice. J Gen Intern Med 2006;21(3):251–6.

82. Wayne DB, Butter J, Siddall VJ, et al. Simulation-based training of internal medicine residents in advanced cardiac life support protocols: a randomized trial. Teach Learn Med 2005;17(3):210–6.

83. Andreatta P, Saxton E, Thompson M, et al. Simulation-based mock codes significantly correlate with improved pediatric patient cardiopulmonary arrest survival rates. Pediatr Crit Care Med 2011;12(1):33–8.

84. Shukla A, Kline D, Cherian A, et al. A simulation course on lifesaving techniques for third-year medical students. Simul Healthc 2007;2:11–5.

85. Hammond J, Bermann M, Chen B, et al. Incorporation of a computerized human patient simulator in critical care training: a preliminary report. J Trauma 2002;53(6):1064–7.

86. Nishisaki A, Hales R, Biagas K, et al. A multi-institutional high-fidelity simulation "boot camp" orientation and training program for first year pediatric critical care fellows. Pediatr Crit Care Med 2009; 10(2):157–62.

87. Freeman J, Dobbie A. Simulation enhances resident confidence in critical care and procedural skills. Fam Med 2008;40(3):165–7.

88. Hedrick TL, Young JS. The use of "war games" to enhance high-risk clinical decision-making in students and residents. Am J Surg 2008;195(6): 843–9.

89. Steadman RH, Coates WC, Huang YM, et al. Simulation-based training is superior to problem-based learning for the acquisition of critical assessment and management skills*. Crit Care Med 2006; 34(1):151–7.

90. Holcomb JB, Dumire RD, Crommett JW, et al. Evaluation of trauma team performance using an advanced human patient simulator for resuscitation training. J Trauma 2002;52(6):1078–85 [discussion: 1085–6].

91. Schroedl CJ, Corbridge TC, Cohen ER, et al. Use of simulation-based education to improve resident learning and patient care in the medical intensive

care unit: a randomized trial. J Crit Care 2012; 27(2):219.e2–13.

92. Jankouskas T, Bush MC, Murray B, et al. Crisis resource management: evaluating outcomes of a multidisciplinary team. Simul Healthc 2007;2(2): 96–101.

93. Lighthall GK, Barr J, Howard SK, et al. Use of a fully simulated intensive care unit environment for critical event management training for internal medicine residents. Crit Care Med 2003;31(10): 2437–43.

94. Reznek M, Smith-Coggins R, Howard S, et al. Emergency medicine crisis resource management (EMCRM): pilot study of a simulation-based crisis management course for emergency medicine. Acad Emerg Med 2003;10(4):386–9.

95. Yee B, Naik VN, Joo HS, et al. Nontechnical skills in anesthesia crisis management with repeated exposure to simulation-based education. Anesthesiology 2005;103(2):241–8.

96. Roberts NK, Williams RG, Schwind CJ, et al. The impact of brief team communication, leadership and team behavior training on ad hoc team performance in trauma care settings. Am J Surg 2014; 207(2):170–8.

97. DeVita MA, Schaefer J, Lutz J, et al. Improving medical crisis team performance. Crit Care Med 2004;32(Supplement):S61–5.

98. Kyrkjebo JM, Brattebo G, Smith-Strom H. Improving patient safety by using interprofessional simulation training in health professional education. J Interprof Care 2006;20(5):507–16.

99. DeVita MA, Schaefer J, Lutz J, et al. Improving medical emergency team (MET) performance using a novel curriculum and a computerized human patient simulator. Qual Saf Health Care 2005;14(5): 326–31.

100. Figueroa MI, Sepanski R, Goldberg SP, et al. Improving teamwork, confidence, and collaboration among members of a pediatric cardiovascular intensive care unit multidisciplinary team using simulation-based team training. Pediatr Cardiol 2013;34(3):612–9.

101. Barnato AE, Hsu HE, Bryce CL, et al. Using simulation to isolate physician variation in intensive care unit admission decision making for critically ill elders with end-stage cancer: a pilot feasibility study. Crit Care Med 2008;36(12):3156–63.

102. Berkenstadt H, Haviv Y, Tuval A, et al. Improving handoff communications in critical care: utilizing simulation-based training toward process improvement in managing patient risk. Chest 2008;134(1): 158–62.

103. Andreatta P, Frankel J, Boblick Smith S, et al. Interdisciplinary team training identifies discrepancies in institutional policies and practices. Am J Obstet Gynecol 2011;205(4):298–301

104. Abrahamson SD, Canzian S, Brunet F. Using simulation for training and to change protocol during the outbreak of severe acute respiratory syndrome. Crit Care 2006;10(1):R3.

105. Malec JF, Torsher LC, Dunn WF, et al. The mayo high performance teamwork scale: reliability and validity for evaluating key crew resource management skills. Simul Healthc 2007;2(1):4–10.

106. Weller J, Shulruf B, Torrie J, et al. Validation of a measurement tool for self-assessment of teamwork in intensive care. Br J Anaesth 2013;111(3):460–7.

107. Guise JM, Deering SH, Kanki BG, et al. Validation of a tool to measure and promote clinical teamwork. Simul Healthc 2008;3(4):217–23.

108. Gaba DM, Howard SK, Flanagan B, et al. Assessment of clinical performance during simulated crises using both technical and behavioral ratings. Anesthesiology 1998;89(1):8–18.

109. Cooper S, Cant R, Porter J, et al. Rating medical emergency teamwork performance: development of the Team Emergency Assessment Measure (TEAM). Resuscitation 2010;81(4):446–52.

110. Fletcher G, Flin R, McGeorge P, et al. Anaesthetists' Non-Technical Skills (ANTS): evaluation of a behavioural marker system. Br J Anaesth 2003; 90(5):580–8.

111. Kim J, Neilipovitz D, Cardinal P, et al. A pilot study using high-fidelity simulation to formally evaluate performance in the resuscitation of critically ill patients: the University of Ottawa Critical Care Medicine, High-Fidelity Simulation, and Crisis Resource Management I Study. Crit Care Med 2006;34(8):2167–74.

112. Kim J, Neilipovitz D, Cardinal P, et al. A comparison of global rating scale and checklist scores in the validation of an evaluation tool to assess performance in the resuscitation of critically ill patients during simulated emergencies (abbreviated as "CRM simulator study IB"). Simul Healthc 2009; 4(1):6–16.

113. Schmitz CC, Chipman JG, Luxenberg MG, et al. Professionalism and communication in the intensive care unit: reliability and validity of a simulated family conference. Simul Healthc 2008;3(4):224–38.

114. Gisondi MA, Smith-Coggins R, Harter PM, et al. Assessment of resident professionalism using high-fidelity simulation of ethical dilemmas. Acad Emerg Med 2004;11(9):931–7.

115. Ottestad E, Boulet JR, Lighthall GK. Evaluating the management of septic shock using patient simulation. Crit Care Med 2007;35(3):769–75.

116. LeBlanc VR, Tabak D, Kneebone R, et al. Psychometric properties of an integrated assessment of technical and communication skills. Am J Surg 2009;197(1):96–101.

117. Adler MD, Trainor JL, Siddall VJ, et al. Development and evaluation of high-fidelity simulation case scenarios for pediatric resident education. Ambul Pediatr 2007;7(2):182–6.

118. Morgan PJ, Cleave-Hogg D, DeSousa S, et al. High-fidelity patient simulation: validation of performance checklists. Br J Anaesth 2004;92(3):388–92.

119. Murray D, Boulet J, Ziv A, et al. An acute care skills evaluation for graduating medical students: a pilot study using clinical simulation. Med Educ 2002;36: 833–41.

120. Boulet JR, Murray D, Kras J, et al. Reliability and validity of a simulation-based acute care skills assessment for medical students and residents. Anesthesiology 2003;99:1270–80.

121. Lambden S, DeMunter C, Dowson A, et al. The Imperial Paediatric Emergency Training Toolkit (IPETT) for use in paediatric emergency training: development and evaluation of feasibility and validity. Resuscitation 2013;84(6):831–6.

122. Nunnink L, Ventkatesh B, Krishnan A, et al. A prospective comparison between written examination and either simulation-based or oral viva examination of intensive care trainees' procedural skills. Anaesth Intensive Care 2010;38:876–82.

Recent Advances in the Management of the Acute Respiratory Distress Syndrome

David N. Hager, MD, PhD

KEYWORDS

- ARDS • ALI • Epidemiology • Advances • Management • PEEP • Driving pressure
- Mechanical ventilation

KEY POINTS

- Low tidal volume ventilation (6 mL/kg predicted body weight) with limits on plateau pressure is the standard of care for patients with acute respiratory distress syndrome.
- A fluid conservative strategy decreases ventilator days and intensive care unit length of stay.
- The best approach to the titration of positive end-expiratory pressure has not been determined, but a strategy that minimizes driving pressure is promising.
- Recent clinical trials strongly support the use of neuromuscular blockers and prone positioning for severe and refractory hypoxemia.
- A focus on acute respiratory distress syndrome risk factor reduction and the development of tools predicting progression to acute respiratory distress syndrome have the potential to further reduce the incidence, morbidity, and mortality of this syndrome.

INTRODUCTION

The acute respiratory distress syndrome (ARDS) has been the subject of intense research efforts since it was first described in 1967.[1] The understanding of ARDS benefitted greatly from the development of a consensus definition in 1994 that allowed investigators to more consistently identify the syndrome.[2] As a result of subsequent study, the understanding and management of ARDS has improved. Standard of care has changed, and outcomes are better. This review highlights the new definition and epidemiology of the syndrome, key advances in management, areas of continued uncertainty, and future directions.

DEFINITIONS AND EPIDEMIOLOGY

The American-European Consensus Conference (AECC) defined ARDS in 1994 as the acute onset of hypoxemia (partial pressure of oxygen, arterial [Pao_2]/fraction of inspired oxygen [Fio_2] $\leq$200 mm Hg) with new bilateral infiltrates in the setting of either a normal pulmonary arterial wedge pressure (PAWP $\leq$18 mm Hg) or the absence of suspected of left atrial hypertension when PAWP was not available.[2] In the setting of less severe hypoxemia (Pao_2/Fio_2 $\leq$300 mm Hg), the term *acute lung injury* (ALI) was applied. Although these definitions have provided an important mechanism to identify patients with ALI and ARDS for both management and research purposes, several limitations have been appreciated. For example, "acute" was not well defined, although most clinical trials of patients with ALI and ARDS have limited enrollment to patients meeting the other criteria for less than 72 hours. Further, in some patients, the magnitude of the Pao_2/Fio_2 ratio (P/F ratio) changes with the application of positive end-expiratory pressure (PEEP).[3] In addition, the presence of new bilateral infiltrates on chest radiographs was not

No Disclosures.
Johns Hopkins University, Sheikh Zayed Tower, 1800 Orleans Street, Suite 9121, Baltimore, MD 21287, USA
E-mail address: dhager1@jhmi.edu

Clin Chest Med 36 (2015) 481–496
http://dx.doi.org/10.1016/j.ccm.2015.05.002
0272-5231/15/$ – see front matter © 2015 Elsevier Inc. All rights reserved.

consistently appreciated by providers (poor inter-observer reliability). Lastly, the distinction of non-hydrostatic versus hydrostatic pulmonary edema was not well appreciated. As a result, the definition of ALI and ARDS was refined in 2012 (**Table 1**).[4]

The extent to which the new definition will improve the identification or study of patients with ARDS is not yet clear. However, it does provide a more precise definition of "acute," gives a more granular description of severity, and provides better guidance in assessing those patients with components of both hydrostatic and nonhydrostatic pulmonary edema. In the remainder of this review, the acronym *ARDS* will include patients with ALI and ARDS unless otherwise stated. This is consistent with the new definition.

Incidence and Outcomes

Because the Berlin Definition is new, there are few epidemiologic data based on its criteria. Estimates of incidence and outcomes are, therefore, predominantly limited to data from studies relying on the AECC criteria, some of which are now 10 years old. In one such study of 1113 ARDS patients undergoing mechanical ventilation in King County, Washington, the overall incidence was estimated at 79 cases per 100,000 person-years. Hospital mortality rate was 38.5% (42.2% among the subgroup of 828 patients with ARDS).[5] Of note, incidence and mortality increased with age. For patients 15 to 19 years old, incidence was 16 per 100,000 person-years, whereas the incidence for

patients 75 to 84 years old 306 per 100,000 person-years. Mortality rates in these age groups increased from 24% to 60%, respectively. Based on these data, it was estimated that there were 190,600 new cases of ARDS in the United States each year with a case fatality rate of 39% (74,500 deaths), and 3.6 million associated hospital days.

In another population-based cohort, the incidence of ARDS based on the AECC definition decreased from 82 to 39 cases per 100,000 person-years between 2001 and 2008 (**Fig. 1**).[6] Of note, this decrease was attributed to ARDS acquired after hospitalization and may be the result of changes in clinical practice intended to decreased ARDS risk factors. These changes included the use of lung protective ventilatory strategies, efforts to limit blood product exposure, and improved protocols for the management of sepsis and pneumonia.

Two studies compared the performance of the AECC and Berlin Definition for ARDS.[7,8] In a 6-month observational study of patients admitted to 10 intensive care units (ICUs) in France undergoing noninvasive ventilation (NIV) or invasive mechanical ventilation, 278 of 3504 patients fulfilled the AECC criteria.[7] Of these, 18 would not have been identified by the Berlin Definition because PEEP was less than 5 cm H_2O, and another 20 would not have fit into a category because the P/F ratio was $\leq$200 while receiving support from NIV (Note: Berlin Definition does not categorize patients on NIV and P/F $\leq$200). Of the 240 patients meeting criteria for ARDS by the Berlin Definition,

---

Table 1
Limitations of AECC criteria for ARDS and solution proposed by the Berlin definition for ARDS

	AECC Limitations	Berlin Solution
Timing of onset	• Acute not defined	• $\leq$7 d of known risk factor or new or worsening symptoms
P/F ratio & pressure	• P/F $\leq$300 • Irrespective of PEEP[a]	• P/F $\leq$300 on PEEP or Continuous positive airway pressure[b] $\geq$of 5 cm H_2O
Severity	• ALI if P/F $\leq$300 • ARDS if P/F $\leq$200	• Mild ARDS: P/F $\leq$300[b] • Moderate ARDS: P/F $\leq$200 • Severe ARDS: P/F $\leq$100
Chest radiograph	• Inconsistent interpretation	• Specific chest radiograph criteria defined[c] • Example chest radiograph produced
PAWP	• PAWP $\leq$18 mm Hg *or* • No suspicion of left atrial hypertension	• PAWP requirement removed • Hydrostatic edema cannot be primary cause of respiratory failure
Risk factor	• None defined	• Risk factor needs to be present • If risk factor not clear, hydrostatic edema must be ruled out

[a] Intubation and mechanical ventilation not required.
[b] Continuous positive airway pressure may be delivered by noninvasive means, but limits severity to mild ARDS.
[c] Criteria may be met on computed tomography as well as chest radiograph.

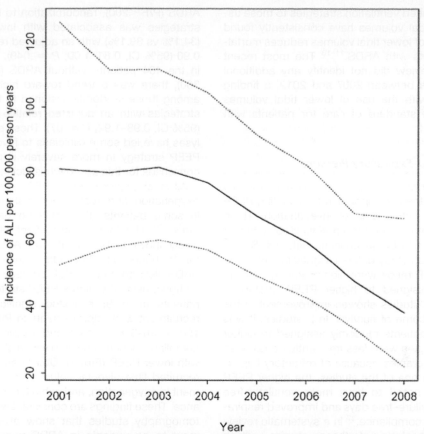

Fig. 1. Trends in age- and sex-specific incidence of acute respiratory distress syndrome from 2001 to 2008 in Olmsted County, Minnesota; dotted lines represent 95% confidence intervals and solid line is the mean incidence of ALI per 100,000 person years. (*From* Li G, Malinchoc M, Cartin-Ceba R, et al. Eight-year trend of acute respiratory distress syndrome: a population-based study in Olmsted County, Minnesota. Am J Respir Crit Care Med 2011;183(1):61; with permission. Copyright © 2015 American Thoracic Society.)

42 (18%) were classified as mild, 123 (51%) as moderate, and 75 (31%) as severe with 28-day mortality rates of 31%, 28%, and 49%, respectively. Based on these numbers, the overall estimated incidence for ARDS was 32 per 100,000 person-years. By severity, the incidence was 5.6, 16.3, and 10 per 100,000 person-years for mild, moderate, and severe ARDS, respectively. In a second study, 130 of 7133 patients admitted to any of 14 hospitals in Brazil during 2006 and 2007 were identified as having ARDS by both AECC criteria and the Berlin Definition.[8] However, patients undergoing NIV and patients in whom left atrial hypertension was evident were not included. As a result, incidence and prevalence data could not be estimated for either definition. Which of the definitions will be used clinically and which will be used to identify patients for research studies in the future remains to be seen. In general, most patients with ARDS seem to be captured by both definitions.

VENTILATOR STRATEGIES
Tidal Volume Reduction

Perhaps the most significant advance in the management ARDS is the use of volume and pressure-limited ventilation as shown in the first trial published by the ARDS Network.[9] In 861 patients randomly assigned to a lung protective strategy consisting of low tidal volume (6 mL/kg predicted body weight [PBW]) and end inspiratory pressure limited to a plateau pressure (P_{plat}) $\leq$30 cm H_2O versus a traditional tidal volume (12 mL/kg PBW) with higher P_{plat} limit ($\leq$50 cm H_2O), mortality rate was 9% lower in patients randomly assigned to the lower tidal volume strategy. This approach was the first to meaningfully decrease mortality in patients with ARDS. In a secondary analysis of this study, it was further determined that tidal volume reduction was of value regardless of plateau pressure.[10] Systematic reviews and a meta-analysis of studies comparing volume and pressure-limited ventilation strategies to those using larger tidal volumes have consistently found that the use of lower tidal volumes reduces mortality in patients with ARDS.[11–13] The most recent Cochrane review did not identify any additional such studies between 2007 and 2012, a finding consistent with the use of lower tidal volumes becoming a standard of care for patients with ARDS.[14]

Positive End-Expiratory Pressure

Although the value of tidal volume reduction seems to be clear, the best approach to adjusting PEEP remains an active area of investigation. Three large, randomized, controlled trials studied higher versus lower PEEP in patients with ARDS.[15–17] Although each study differed slightly in methodology, and P/F ratios were higher among patients randomly assigned to higher PEEP strategies, none of the studies showed improvement in the primary outcome of survival. In 2 studies, it was noted that patients randomly assigned to higher PEEP strategies were less frequently transitioned to rescue therapies because of refractory hypoxemia.[16,17] In one of the studies, the higher PEEP group was noted to have more ventilator-free and organ failure–free days and improved respiratory system compliance.[17] In a systematic review and meta-analysis of these studies, which included a total of 2299 individual patients, mortality rates in the lower versus higher PEEP groups were 35.2% and 32.9%, respectively, with an adjusted relative risk of 0.94 (95% confidence interval [CI], 0.86–1.04; $P = .25$).[18] However, when the analysis was limited to the 1892 patients with

ARDS (P/F $\leq$200), randomization to higher PEEP strategies was associated with lower mortality (34.1% vs 39.1%) with an adjusted relative risk of 0.90 (95% CI, 0.81–1.00; $P = .049$). By contrast, in the 404 patients without ARDS (P/F of 201–300), there was a trend toward higher mortality among those randomly assigned to higher PEEP strategies with an adjusted relative risk of 1.37 (95% CI, 0.98–1.92; $P = .07$). These posthoc analyses have led some clinicians to favor the higher PEEP strategy in more severely ill patients, but consensus for this approach is lacking.

Although higher levels of PEEP clearly improve oxygenation and respiratory system mechanics in some patients, they may be detrimental to others.[19] The inconsistent effect of PEEP was nicely shown in 19 patients with ARDS ventilated for 12 hours with low tidal volumes using the ARDS Network lower PEEP strategy, followed by 12 hours using the higher PEEP strategy.[20] Some patients (n = 9) exhibited significant alveolar recruitment with improvements in P/F ratio (from 150 $\pm$ 36–396 $\pm$ 138) and respiratory system compliance when ventilated with higher compared with lower PEEP (**Fig. 2**). Other patients (n = 10) recruited little alveolar volume, had no improvement in oxygenation, and exhibited worse compliance. These findings are consistent with computer tomography studies that show alveolar recruitment to be variable in ARDS patients.[21,22] For example, in one study, increasing PEEP from 0 to 15 cm H_2O failed to recruit some regions of atelectasis or consolidation in patients with ARDS, whereas aerated portions become hyperinflated.[22] Over time, hyperinflation can cause additional inflammation of the lung.[19] These

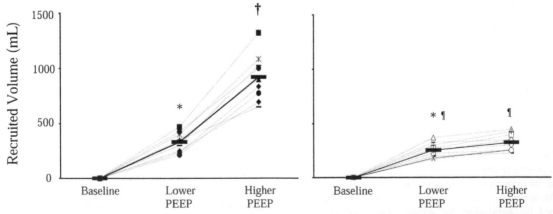

Fig. 2. Alveolar recruitment induced by lower and higher PEEP strategies compared with baseline. Panel on left demonstrates responders. Panel on right demonstrates nonresponders. *Lower PEEP strategy versus baseline in the same group ($P<.05$); †Higher versus lower PEEP strategy in the same group ($P<.05$); ¶Between the two groups in the same experimental condition ($P<.05$). (*From* Grasso S, Fanelli V, Cafarelli A, et al. Effects of high vs low positive end-expiratory pressures in acute respiratory distress syndrome. Am J Respir Crit Care Med 2005;171(9):1004; with permission. Copyright © 2015 American Thoracic Society.)

observations may explain the negative results of the 3 large trials comparing lower and higher PEEP strategies in patients with ARDS. It is likely that both PEEP responders and nonresponders were randomly assigned to both higher and lower PEEP strategies. Responders that received lower PEEP did not have the opportunity to benefit from higher PEEP. By contrast, nonresponders that received higher PEEP may have been harmed. Of note, prescription of PEEP and F_{IO_2} based on a table is reasonable in patients that respond to PEEP. However, in the nonresponder, tables prevent additional oxygen from being administered without a simultaneous increase in PEEP. This may be injurious to some patients.

Approaches that set PEEP according to respiratory mechanics rather than PEEP:F_{IO_2} tables have been proposed. In an early study of lung protective ventilation with lower tidal volumes, pressure volume curves were constructed, and PEEP was set at 2 cm H_2O above the lower inflection point (LIP) on the inspiratory limb of the pressure volume curve.[23] It is thought that the LIP represents the pressure at which a large population of alveoli is recruited. Maintaining PEEP at a slightly higher level is thought to limit overall cyclic recruitment/derecruitment injury. Unfortunately, this approach has not been tested in a randomized trial in which both patient groups receive lower tidal volumes. Further, the approach is limited by the need to deeply sedate and paralyze patients for accurate curve construction. And, even with a relaxed patient, there is significant interobserver and intraobserver variability in identifying the LIP.[24] In some patients, the LIP cannot be accurately identified.[23,25]

Another approach is the use of the stress index.[26–28] With this approach, airway pressure is observed over time during constant flow inflation. The pressure curve generated is described by:

Airway Pressure = a (inspiratory time)^b + c,

where a is the slope of the airway pressure–time relationship, c is the airway pressure at time zero of the maneuver, and b is the stress index, which describes the shape of the curve. If b is less than 1, the curve has a downward concavity consistent with lung recruitment and improving compliance. If b is greater than >1, the curve has an upward concavity and is consistent with overdistention and worsening compliance. When $b = 1$, compliance is constant over the volume shift of the delivered breath. Performing this maneuver serially while increasing PEEP until $b = 1$ would theoretically balance the potentially beneficial effects of limiting cyclic recruitment/derecruitment and cyclic overdistention

with each breath. When this approach was used in patients with ARDS with low potential for alveolar recruitment based on computed tomography appearance (focal consolidation), plasma inflammatory markers and static lung elastance were lower than when the same patients were ventilated using the ARDS Network lower PEEP strategy.[19] Although the protocol allowed for increased sedation during periods of physiologic measurements, no neuromuscular blockers were used. Whether this approach effectively guides PEEP titration in patients with recruitable lung has not been demonstrated.

The use of esophageal pressure (P_{es}) as a surrogate for pleural pressure (P_{pl}) has more recently been considered as a means of guiding PEEP titration. In healthy upright controls, P_{es} can be used to deconstruct the distending pressure of the respiratory system into lung (P_{tp}) and chest wall (P_{cw}) components.[29] The extent to which P_{es} is a fair surrogate of P_{pl} in supine patients with ARDS has been debated.[30,31] However, one small trial using P_{es} to a targeted P_{tp} of 0 to 10 cm H_2O has shown promising results when compared with PEEP managed per the PEEP:F_{IO_2} table of the ARDS Network.[32] In that study of 61 patients, those randomly assigned to P_{es}-guided PEEP titration had higher P/F ratios at 72 hours and better respiratory system compliance. Average PEEP was significantly higher in the P_{es}-guided group at 24, 48, and 72 hours. After adjusting for baseline APACHE II scores, the P_{es}-guided protocol was associated with a significant reduction in mortality relative risk (0.46; 95% CI, 0.19–1.0; $P = .05$). To further explore the value of P_{es}-guided PEEP titration, a multicenter phase 2 trial of 200 ARDS patients is currently underway. Enrollment began in 2012 and is planned to conclude in 2016 (ClinicalTrials.gov NCT01681225).[33]

Recently, using data from 3562 ARDS patients enrolled in 9 different clinical trials, driving pressure (ΔP) was investigated as an independent variable associated with survival.[34]

Driving Pressure = P_{plat} − PEEP

In this analysis, adjustments in tidal volume and PEEP were associated with improved outcomes only when the adjustment resulted in a simultaneous reduction in ΔP. In other words, variables that have historically received much focus, such as P_{plat} and PEEP, should be considered in the context of the associated ΔP. Recall that compliance of the respiratory system is composed of chest wall compliance and lung compliance in series. In the short term, chest wall compliance is often relatively stable. As a result, in the setting of ARDS, changes in respiratory system compliance are more often a function of the volume of aerated lung available for tidal ventilation. The aerated volume, or functional volume, is reduced because of inflammation and atelectasis in ARDS. As PEEP is increased from lower to higher levels, additional volume may be recruited. Using a constant tidal volume, increases in PEEP that improve respiratory system compliance will be indicated by decreases in ΔP. If ΔP increases as PEEP is increased, it indicates increased risk for overdistention injury to the functional lung. Such patients may do better with increases in inspired oxygen concentration than increases in PEEP. Although simple bedside ΔP assessments may turn out to be a better guide for PEEP titration than other approaches (eg, PEEP:F_{IO_2} tables, assessment of the LIP, and P_{tp}), it will require prospective study before it can be integrated fully into clinical practice. However, in patients that do not appear PEEP responsive, it is reasonable to consider adjusting PEEP to minimize ΔP, rather than committing patients to a PEEP:F_{IO_2} table.

ALTERNATE MODES OF VENTILATION
High-Frequency Oscillatory Ventilation

Although the ideal approach to PEEP is still under study, it is accepted that some level of PEEP is necessary to minimize low volume recruitment/derecruitment injury. However, increases in PEEP, even when tidal volumes are not large, are limited by accepted standards of airway pressure.[35] High-frequency oscillatory ventilation (HFOV), which delivers small tidal volumes at high rates (3–15 Hz), has been considered an alternative means of lung protective ventilation. During HFOV, generous mean airway pressures (mean P_{aw}) are applied to limit cyclic end-expiratory alveolar collapse, whereas small tidal volumes limit end-inspiratory overdistention.[36]

Early case series of patients ventilated with HFOV show that most patients exhibit an improvement in oxygenation based on increases in the P/F ratio and decreases in the oxygenation index.[37–40]

$$Oxygenation\ Index = F_{IO_2} * mean\ P_{aw} * 100/P_{aO_2}$$

An early randomized, controlled trial of 148 adults with ARDS comparing HFOV with conventional mechanical ventilation showed a trend toward decreased mortality among patients randomly assigned to HFOV at 30 days (37% vs 52%; $P = .10$).[41] A significant limitation of this study was the use of tidal volumes that are no longer reflective of standard of care (10.6 mL/kg

ideal body weight). However, the trend toward decreased mortality in this study and the successful use of HFOV in animal models resulted in renewed enthusiasm for further development of HFOV techniques and follow-up comparisons with conventional lung protective approaches.

In a roundtable discussion by HFOV expert users, emphasis was placed on maximizing ventilator frequency to minimize tidal volume delivery.[42] HFOV protocols had previously recommended initiating oscillations at 5 Hz with the option to decrease frequency to 3 Hz if ventilation was poor.[43] Although tidal volumes delivered during HFOV at 5 Hz are smaller (~ 2.5 mL/kg PBW) than those delivered by conventional ventilators, in many patients much higher frequencies, and therefore smaller tidal volumes, are feasible.[44,45] For example, at 12 Hz, tidal volume can be as low as 1.1 mL/kg PBW.[45] In addition to emphasizing the importance of using the highest frequencies possible while maintaining pH and $Paco_2$ within an acceptable range, the roundtable discussion provided 2 approaches to the management of mean P_{aw} and oxygenation. One approach used up to 2 recruitment maneuvers at HFOV initiation followed by adjustments up and down a mean P_{aw}:F_{IO_2} table. The alternate approach advocated a more aggressive recruitment strategy at initiation—maintenance of relatively high airway pressures until F_{IO_2} could be titrated down to 0.40, after which airway pressure would be decreased.

Recently, 2 large multicenter trials of HFOV versus conventional lung protective ventilation were conducted. These were the "Oscillation for ARDS Treated Early Trial" (OSCILLATE) and the "High Frequency OSCillation in ARDS trial" (OSCAR).[46,47] In OSCILLATE, the patient with early ARDS (P/F ratio ≤ 200 on $F_{IO_2} \geq 0.6$ and PEEP of 10 cm H_2O for <72 hours) were randomly assigned to conventional lung protective ventilation versus HFOV using an oscillator with well-understood performance characteristics (Sensormedics 3100B, Loma Linda, CA).[46] Mean airway pressure and F_{IO_2} pairings were guided by a table reflective of the PEEP:F_{IO_2} table used by the ARDS Network.[9,46] Recruitment maneuvers were required at HFOV initiation and with escalations in mean P_{aw}. Frequency was increased provided pH remained between 7.25 and 7.35. Of a planned 1200 patients, only 548 were randomly assigned because of an interim analysis that found higher mortality in the HFOV group (47% vs 35%; $P = .005$). Patients randomly assigned to HFOV were also noted to have received more sedation, fluids, vasopressors, and neuromuscular blockers.

In the OSCAR study, patients on PEEP ≥ 5 cm H_2O with a P/F ratio less than 200 were randomly assigned to a conventional lung protective strategy or HFOV using the Novalung Vision-α (Hechingen, Germany), a ventilator with less well-understood performance characteristics.[47] Mean airway pressure was increased as needed until Fio_2 could be decreased to 0.60, after which Fio_2 was decease until it reached 0.40. Thereafter, mean P_{aw} was decreased. Recruitment maneuvers were allowed, but not required. Ventilator frequency was adjusted to maintain pH between 7.25 and 7.40. Seven hundred and ninety-five patients were randomly assigned without a significant difference in outcomes.

Both studies had limitations. The OSCILLATE study used a high airway pressure strategy with frequent recruitment maneuvers that may have been injurious to patients whose lungs were not recruitable,[19,20,34,46] and could have contributed to hemodynamic compromise via right heart failure.[48] The increased use of sedation and neuromuscular blockers in the HFOV group may not have been necessary and may have increased the need for hemodynamic support in the form of vasopressors. Further, oscillator frequency on days 1 and 3 were only 5.5 Hz and 6.8 Hz, respectively. Many patients tolerate much higher frequencies.[44] For these reasons, the use of the protocol and the clinical management of the patients in this study could have been better. In the OSCAR study, average tidal volume in the control arm was high at 8.3 mL/kg ideal body weight (IBW), enrolling centers had limited experience using HFOV before the study, and the ventilator used for oscillation has not been well characterized.[47] Higher frequencies were used during HFOV (mean 7.8 Hz ± 1.8 on day 1) than in the OSCILLATE study, but with the Novalung Vision-α, this corresponded to an estimated Vt of 3.4 mL/kg IBW. A similar tidal volume is delivered at 3 Hz by the 3100B.[45] For these reasons, the OSCAR study seems to be a comparison of 2 suboptimal ventilator strategies.

Until better HFOV protocols are found to improve patient outcomes, HFOV should be limited to patients that have not responded to other rescue interventions, such as neuromuscular blockade and prone positioning. To facilitate HFOV protocols, the technology could be improved. The machine currently available in North America, the Sensormedics 3100B, was developed in the 1980s with little modification. Although small inspiratory efforts associated with small changes in circuit pressure are usually tolerated, more vigorous efforts disrupt circuit pressure, trigger alarms, interrupt oscillations, and can lead to dumping of the circuit pressure with associated alveolar derecruitment and hypoxia. In the laboratory setting, demand flow systems have been developed to respond to spontaneous respiratory efforts during ventilation with the 3100B.[49] These systems can restore mean P_{aw} to prescribed levels within 115 milliseconds of a simulated inspiration. In the clinical setting, this modification would likely lead to significant reductions in sedation, paralytics, and potentially vasopressors and fluids for patients during HFOV. Whether ventilator manufacturers will pursue modifications like this, that would improve HFOV technology and potentially patient outcomes, remains to be seen.

Airway Pressure Release Ventilation

During airway pressure release ventilation (APRV), a relatively high airway pressure is maintained (P-high: 20–30 cm H_2O) for most of the ventilator cycle.[50] Patients may breathe spontaneously at this pressure, but ventilation requires supplementation via brief (0.4–0.8 seconds) pressure releases (P-low: 0–10 cm H_2O). The number of releases per minute is equal to the ventilator rate. A sensitive demand flow and valve system maintains airway pressure at prescribed levels (P-high or P-low), irrespective of patient inspiratory or expiratory efforts.[51,52] Patient-ventilator dyssynchrony, breath stacking, and associated agitation are said to be minimal, sedation requirements low, and paralysis unnecessary. Advocates of APRV also suggest that it is lung protective because (1) adequate oxygenation and ventilation can be achieved with lower peak airway pressures, reducing the likelihood of barotrauma and overdistention injury; (2) extended exposure to P-high (long T-high) recruits atelectatic lung tissue, improving oxygenation; and (3) very brief exposure to P-low (short T-low) will prevent injury from cyclic derecruitment.[50] Further, the preservation of spontaneous breathing during APRV is thought to (1) enhance hemodynamic performance by increasing venous return, (2) improve ventilation perfusion matching through recruitment of posterior and inferior regions of the lung by the contracting diaphragm, and (3) limit the potential for ventilator-induced diaphragm dysfunction when compared with conventional modes.[53,54]

Although these reported aspects of APRV are attractive, few have been rigorously studied. The available literature is complicated by inconsistencies in nomenclature, making comparison of different studies difficult. Importantly, APRV has not been shown to improve outcomes among patients with ARDS when compared with the current standard of care. Which patients may benefit from

APRV and how best to optimize APRV settings are also not clear. Despite these issues, APRV is widely available and is even used exclusively in some centers. Based on the limited literature and lack of comparison to the current conventional standard of care, APRV, like HFOV, would be better used when other rescue measures (paralytics and prone positioning) have failed.

NONVENTILATOR THERAPIES OF BENEFIT

Irrespective of mechanical ventilation mode or approach to tidal volume and PEEP, additional interventions have been used with varying success in the management of ARDS.

Paralytics

Neuromuscular blockers (NMB) have been used in up to 55% of patients enrolled in randomized studies of ARDS patients in recent years.[55] NMBs are more commonly used in patients treated with nonconventional approaches such as HFOV or prone positioning.[56] NMBs improve patient–ventilator synchrony and frequently oxygenation.[57,58] Two putative mechanisms are thought to improved oxygenation. First, atelectasis that occurs because of dyssynchrony is avoided, and, as a result, there is less shunt-related hypoxemia. Second, NMBs allow the use of lung protective ventilatory strategies in patients who exhibit high respiratory rates and airway pressures despite adequate sedation leading to less inflammation. This latter hypothesis was suggested by the observation of improved oxygenation and decreased inflammatory mediators found in the bronchoalveolar lavage (BAL) fluid of ARDS patients that were paralyzed for 48 hours compared with those that were not paralyzed.[59] Two small studies (n = 56 and n = 36) and one large randomized, controlled trial of 340 patients showed improvements in P/F ratio at 48 hours among patients treated with NMBs during that time versus placebo.[58–60] Of note, the larger study also found a significant reduction in mortality at 28 days. At 90 days, the hazard ratio for death was 0.68 (95% CI, 0.48–0.98) after adjusting for baseline P/F ratio, P_{plat}, and SAPS II score.[60] There were no differences in ICU-acquired weakness, one of the main objections to the use of NMBs.

Not all NMBs are the same. Benzylisoquolinium compounds (eg, cisatracurium), as used in the studies referenced above, are eliminated by Hofmann degradation with an average recovery time of 70 minutes.[61] By contrast, aminosteroids (eg, pancuronium, vecuronium, rocuronium) are eliminated by the liver and kidney. Average

recovery time is longer (ie, vecuronium ∼400 minutes).[61] It has been suggested that the aminosteroids may increase the risk of ICU-acquired weakness compared with the benzylisoquoliniums.[57,62] Currently, it is not the standard of care to paralyze patients with ARDS. However, given the results above, it is a very reasonable approach in patient with refractory hypoxemia.

Prone Positioning

In the prone position, P_{pl} is more evenly distributed than in the supine position,[63] resulting in more homogeneous ventilation,[64] and improved ventilation–perfusion matching. Further, end-expiratory lung volume may be increased because of recruitment of otherwise atelectatic basilar lung regions. The result is improved oxygenation when compared with in the supine position. In animal models, prone positioning also reduces ventilator-induced injury.[65] These observations have led many to use prone positioning as a rescue measure for patients with refractory hypoxemia. However, some randomized, controlled trials of prone versus supine positioning in patients with ARDS show trends toward improved outcomes in post hoc analyses,[66,67] and suggest that this intervention may be beneficial as a standard measure. One such analysis suggests a benefit to prone positioning in the more severely ill,[66] whereas another suggests benefit in the less severely ill.[67]

In a recent study, patients with severe ARDS, defined by a P/F ratio ≤150 on standardized ventilator settings for 12 hours with F_{IO_2} of ≥0.60 and a PEEP of ≥5 cm H_2O, were randomly assigned to prone positioning for ≥16 consecutive hours daily versus continued supine positioning.[68] All patients were treated with a standard lung protective ventilator strategy. Mortality at day 28 was 16% and 32% in the prone and supine patients, respectively. After adjusting for severity of illness, the hazard of death for patients treated with prone positioning was 0.42 (95% CI, 0.26–0.66). More recently, a systematic review and meta-analysis limited to studies using lung protective ventilatory strategies with tidal volume reduction showed a mortality risk ratio of 0.74 (95% CI, 0.59–0.95) for patients treated in the prone position provided they were prone for ≥16 hours per day, received a lung protective ventilator strategy, and had severe ARDS. Of note, pressure ulcers, facial edema, endotracheal tube obstruction, and inadvertent dislodgement of chest tubes were more common events among prone patients. These events speak to the need for well-developed local pronation protocols and training programs in centers that plan to use prone positioning. Like NMBs, prone positioning has not yet become a standard. However, these data support that it is a safe and reasonable approach in a patient with refractory hypoxemia.

Fluid Balance

In the setting of nonhydrostatic pulmonary edema, as is the case with ARDS, animal studies suggest that furosemide infusions decrease shunt fraction, although not solely owing to mobilization of fluid from the lungs.[69–71] There is also a direct vasoactive effect that directs blood away from edematous regions, decreasing microvascular hydrostatic pressures. Early observational studies correlated positive fluid balance in ARDS with increased mortality,[72,73] whereas others have suggested improved outcomes when fluid balance is negative or even.[74,75] More recently, a randomized, controlled trial of 37 patients with ARDS and hypoproteinemia found that albumin replacement paired with a furosemide infusion resulted in significant weight loss over 5 days ($P = .04$) and a significant increase in P/F ratio compared with placebo.[76]

A larger study by the ARDS Network randomly assigned patients to a fluid conservative or fluid liberal strategy. At 7 days the fluid conservative group had a mean ($\pm$SE) fluid balance of -136 (±491) mL compared with 6992 (±502) mL in the fluid liberal group. Although there was no difference in mortality, ventilator-free days at day 28 after randomization were greater in the fluid conservative group (14.6 $\pm$ 0.5 days vs 12.1 $\pm$ 0.5 days, $P<.001$) and patients spent more days outside the ICU (13.4 $\pm$ 0.4 days vs 11.2 $\pm$ 0.4, $P<.001$). Of note, there was a trend toward an increased need for dialysis among survivors in the fluid liberal group. These findings strongly support the use of a fluid-conservative strategy in ARDS. A significant limitation of the fluid conservative strategy is the complexity of the protocol executed in the study. Fortunately, a simplified protocol used in subsequent ARDS Network studies was compared retrospectively with the original fluid-conservative protocol.[77] Although patients treated with the simplified protocol had greater fluid accumulation at 28 days (1918 $\pm$ 323 mL), ventilator-free days were similar to those on the more complex protocol, and there was no difference in mortality. The authors conclude that the simplified protocol is a reasonable alternative. A second limitation of the fluid-conservative approach that warrants mention is the post hoc observation that patients in the fluid-conservative arm were at greater risk for long-term neurocognitive impairment.[78] This finding will require further consideration and study.

NONVENTILATOR THERAPIES OF UNCERTAIN BENEFIT
Steroids

The use of corticosteroids in the management of ARDS remains of uncertain value, although the rationale seems sound. ARDS is a highly inflammatory state, and measured inflammatory cytokines in bronchoalveolar lavage fluid, many of which are dependent on NF-$\kappa\beta$, correlate with ARDS outcome.[79,80] Corticosteroids, when bound to glucocorticoid receptors, suppress transcription of many such cytokines by direct inhibition of transcription machinery in the nucleus.[81] Further, corticosteroids inhibit collagen deposition in the healing lung by disrupting fibroblast proliferation.[82] However, early studies of corticosteroids in patients at risk for ARDS,[83–86] and in those with early ARDS,[87] did not favor their use. A potential significant limitation of these studies was the short duration of therapy used (≤48 hours of corticosteroids). More recently, it was observed that patients that received longer courses of steroids may have improved outcomes.[88,89] In a study of patients with septic shock randomly assigned to 7 days of hydrocortisone therapy versus placebo, patients with adrenal insufficiency and ARDS were less likely to die (hazard ratio, 0.57; 95% CI, 0.36–0.89; $P = .013$) and had more ventilator-free days (5.7 vs 2.6, $P = .006$).[89]

The use of corticosteroids has also been studied for late-phase ARDS, which has been defined as lack of improvement 7 days after meeting criteria for the syndrome.[90,91] In the smaller of 2 studies, 28 patients were randomly assigned 2:1 to methylprednisolone 2 mg/kg/d for 14 days followed by a slow taper ending at 32 days of treatment versus placebo. Patients not improving at 10 days were crossed over to the alternate therapy. Patients in the treatment arm had significant improvements in P/F ratio, were more quickly extubated, and had better survival. Of note, 4 patients in the placebo arm were crossed over to receive methylprednisolone at day 10. All 4 died, raising concern for the very late use of corticosteroids in ARDS. The ARDS Network conducted a similar study for late-phase ARDS.[91] They randomly assigned 180 patients with persistent ARDS with a P/F ratio ≤200 between days 7 and 28 to methylprednisolone versus placebo. Methylprednisolone at 2 mg/kg/d was administered for 14 days, then 1 mg/kg for 7 days followed by a taper. If a patient was extubated before completing this regimen, and remained extubated for 48 hours, steroids were tapered over a 2-day period. Although there were no differences in the primary outcome of mortality at 60 days, patients that received corticosteroids had more ventilator-free days (11.2 vs 6.8; $P<.001$) and ICU-free days (8.9 vs 6.2; $P<.02$). However, among those extubated, reintubation was more common, as were complications related to myopathy or neuropathy (9 vs 0, $P = .008$). Lastly, in a post hoc analysis, it was observed that mortality was significantly higher in patients that were randomly assigned to the treatment arm more than 14 days after onset of ARDS (44% vs 12%; $P = .01$). Based on these mixed results, it is reasonable to consider use of corticosteroids between days 7 and 14 for patients with refractory ARDS. It would also seem reasonable to use a longer course of steroids with a slow taper. Additional study is warranted.

Inhaled Nitric Oxide

Inhaled nitric oxide (iNO) has been studied extensively in the setting or ARDS. However, randomized, controlled trials have not been able to find a mortality benefit.[92-97] Although iNO does seem to improve oxygenation during the first 48 to 72 hours, it has not been found to improve survival. More recently, a systematic review with meta-analysis that included 14 trials confirmed prior observations of improved oxygenation in the iNO groups and no mortality benefit. However, a greater risk of renal insufficiency among patients receiving iNO was observed with a relative risk of 1.59 (95% CI, 1.17–2.16). Despite these data, it is likely the iNO will get continued use in difficult-to-oxygenate patients with the hope that it will buy time for other therapies, such as antibiotics, to work. One important limitation of iNO is the high cost. As a result, other inhaled agents have been considered, such as inhaled prostaglandins. In a study that randomly assigned 105 patients with ARDS to iNO or inhaled epoprostenol (iEPO), P/F ratios increased in both groups, but there was no difference in the magnitude of the change or differences in adverse events.[98] However, iNO was estimated to be 4.5 to 17 times as costly as iEPO. As a result, many institutions are developing protocols for the use of iEPO in patient with refractory hypoxemia.

Statins

Two large randomized, controlled trials considered the use of statins in the setting of ARDS based on preliminary animal and human data that showed decreased lung inflammation after administration.[99-102] Neither study showed differences in the outcomes of mortality, ventilator-free days, or ICU-free days. However, the larger of the 2, which enrolled only sepsis-related ARDS, suggested an association between the use of statins and renal and hepatic injury. Based on the results of both studies, it is unlikely there will be further consideration of statins in this setting.

Extracorporeal Life Support

The early experience with ECLS in patients with ARDS was disappointing. In an early study; 90 patients with severe ARDS were randomly assigned to venoarterial ECLS or conventional mechanical ventilation (no specific ventilator protocol).[103] Survival was poor in each group (9.5% vs 8.3%; P value not significant). A subsequent observational study in which extracorporeal CO_2 removal ($ECCO_2$-R) was paired with low-frequency positive-pressure ventilation suggested improved outcomes with a survival rate of almost 50%.[104] However, in the mid-1990s, when $ECCO_2$-R was compared with conventional mechanical ventilation, mortality was higher in patients randomly assigned to $ECCO_2$-R.[105] Since then, it is thought by many that ECLS technology has improved significantly; better pumps, oxygenators, biocompatible circuits, and single site dual lumen catheters that are placed in the internal jugular vein have been developed.[106] The most recent study of ECLS randomly assigned patients with ARDS to treatment at a center in which ECLS was available and use of a lung protective ventilator protocol was standard or to usual care without transfer.[107] Although this study suggested improved outcomes in the group that was considered for ECLS with a relative risk for death at 6 months of 0.69 (95% CI, 0.05–0.97; $P = .03$), only 75% of the study group actually got ECLS, and lung protective ventilation was achieved in only 70% of the control group. It is, therefore, difficult to determine whether it was the use of ECLS or transfer to a specialty center capable of ECLS that improved outcomes.[106] Currently, the Extracorporeal Membrane Oxygenation for Severe Acute Respiratory Distress Syndrome (EOLIA) trial is underway (ClinicalTrials.gov NCT01470703).[108] In this phase 3, multicenter international study, the early use of venovenous ECLS is being compared with the current standard of care for severe ARDS. It is anticipated that enrollment of a planned 331 patients and the associated data collection for this study will be complete in October of 2015. The outcomes will likely determine the future use of this technology in the setting of severe ARDS.

FUTURE DIRECTIONS

Three general topics for future consideration are prevention, early identification, and novel therapies. Although a discussion of novel therapies is beyond the scope of this article, there is evidence that preventative strategies can significantly reduce the incidence of ARDS. Likewise, approaches to early identification have been developed and are likely to be further refined and integrated into electronic health records.

Prevention

The ability to reduce incident cases of ARDS has been shown with the use of simple best practice approaches. In one study, large baseline tidal volume was found to be an independent risk factor for subsequent ARDS.[109] In a study of esophagectomy, patients randomly assigned to single lung ventilation with 9 mL/kg IBW versus 5 mL/kg IBW with PEEP of 5 cm H_2O, inflammatory mediators in BAL and plasma were higher in patients ventilated with the larger tidal volume and no PEEP.[110] More recently, in patients presenting without lung injury randomly assigned to 10 mL/kg versus 6 mL/kg PBW, BAL inflammatory mediators were higher in those receiving the large tidal volume, as were rates of new acute lung injury (13.5% vs 2.6%, $P = .001$).[111] Lastly, in a meta-analysis of 20 studies that included data from 2822 patients comparing higher versus lower tidal volumes in patients without ARDS, the risk of ARDS and risk of death were higher in patients that were treated with higher tidal volumes.[112]

Prophylactic tidal volume reduction is not the only form of prevention. It has also been shown that blood products, including red cells, plasma, and platelets, especially from female donors, can all trigger ARDS.[113,114] A common event leading to ARDS is aspiration, and precautions against this have also reduced incident cases of ARDS.[6] These and other best practices, such as fluid management and early antibiotics in the setting of sepsis can be bundled into a Checklist for Lung Injury Prevention.[6,115]

Early Identification

As previously described, much of the reduction in incident cases of ARDS over time has been caused by reductions of nosocomial ARDS.[6] However, approaches that identify patients with or those who are likely to develop ARDS early could provide new opportunities not only for prevention but also to limit syndrome severity when it does occur. Two such systems have been developed.[116,117] The first is calculated from 22 variables, including predisposing conditions, physiologic data, and other risk modifiers.[117] This scoring system distinguished patients in whom ARDS developed from those in whom it did not with an area under the receiver operating

characteristic of 0.8 (95% CI, 0.78–0.82). Although the score performs reasonably well, it is labor intensive, and unless automated in an electronic health record, it will be challenging to use clinically. By contrast, the Early Acute Lung Injury Score exhibits comparable performance and may have greater clinical usefulness.[116] The calculation is only dependent on oxygen requirement, respiratory rate, and baseline immune suppression but requires screening for patients with new bilateral infiltrates on chest radiography. It has an area under the receiver operating characteristic of 0.85 (95% CI, 0.80–0.91). Regardless of which score is used, earlier identification will trigger care providers to consider changes to treatment plans as appropriate with the hope of mitigating the severity of impending ARDS.

SUMMARY

ARDS is a prevalent syndrome with many causes and high morbidity and mortality. Management of patients with this syndrome has changed dramatically over the last 20 years because of a systematic study of its causes and management options. Key advances are the use of low tidal volumes and a conservative fluid strategy. How best to prescribe PEEP remains to be determined. The recent evidence supporting an approach that minimized driving pressure is promising but will require further study. Whereas 10 years ago many clinicians would use HFOV as a first-line rescue mode for refractory hypoxemia, recent data strongly suggest that NMBs and prone positioning are better choices. Initiating corticosteroids for refractory ARDS between days 7 and 14 seems reasonable, but this should be done with careful consideration and acknowledgment of possible infectious and neuromuscular complications. Data determining the relative value of ECLS in severe ARDS should be available in the coming year. Lastly, as electronic health records become more sophisticated, care bundles that reduce risk factors for ARDS should be incorporated into ordersets, and tools predicting progression to ARDS should be built into clinical workflows. It is likely these interventions will further reduce the incidence, morbidity, and mortality of this syndrome.

REFERENCES

1. Ashbaugh DG, Bigelow DB, Petty TL, et al. Acute respiratory distress in adults. Lancet 1967; 2(7511):319–23.
2. Bernard GR, Artigas A, Brigham KL, et al. The American-European Consensus Conference on

ARDS. Definitions, mechanisms, relevant out-comes, and clinical trial coordination. Am J Respir Crit Care Med 1994;149(3 Pt 1):818–24.

3. Ferguson ND, Kacmarek RM, Chiche JD, et al. Screening of ARDS patients using standardized ventilator settings: influence on enrollment in a clinical trial. Intensive Care Med 2004;30(6):1111–6.

4. Force ADT, Ranieri VM, Rubenfeld GD, et al. Acute respiratory distress syndrome: the Berlin definition. JAMA 2012;307(23):2526–33.

5. Rubenfeld GD, Caldwell E, Peabody E, et al. Incidence and outcomes of acute lung injury. N Engl J Med 2005;353(16):1685–93.

6. Li G, Malinchoc M, Cartin-Ceba R, et al. Eight-year trend of acute respiratory distress syndrome: a population-based study in Olmsted County, Minnesota. Am J Respir Crit Care Med 2011;183(1):59–66.

7. Hernu R, Wallet F, Thiolliere F, et al. An attempt to validate the modification of the American-European consensus definition of acute lung injury/acute respiratory distress syndrome by the Berlin definition in a university hospital. Intensive Care Med 2013;39(12):2161–70.

8. Caser EB, Zandonade E, Pereira E, et al. Impact of distinct definitions of acute lung injury on its incidence and outcomes in Brazilian ICUs: prospective evaluation of 7,133 patients*. Crit Care Med 2014;42(3):574–82.

9. Ventilation with lower tidal volumes as compared with traditional tidal volumes for acute lung injury and the acute respiratory distress syndrome. The Acute Respiratory Distress Syndrome Network. N Engl J Med 2000;342(18):1301–8.

10. Hager DN, Krishnan JA, Hayden DL, et al. Tidal volume reduction in patients with acute lung injury when plateau pressures are not high. Am J Respir Crit Care Med 2005;172(10):1241–5.

11. Fan E, Needham DM, Stewart TE. Ventilatory management of acute lung injury and acute respiratory distress syndrome. JAMA 2005;294(22):2889–96.

12. Putensen C, Theuerkauf N, Zinserling J, et al. Meta-analysis: ventilation strategies and outcomes of the acute respiratory distress syndrome and acute lung injury. Ann Intern Med 2009;151(8):566–76.

13. Petrucci N, Iacovelli W. Lung protective ventilation strategy for the acute respiratory distress syndrome. Cochrane Database Syst Rev 2007;(3):CD003844.

14. Petrucci N, De Feo C. Lung protective ventilation strategy for the acute respiratory distress syndrome. Cochrane Database Syst Rev 2013;(2):CD003844.

15. Brower RG, Lanken PN, MacIntyre N, et al. Higher versus lower positive end-expiratory pressures in patients with the acute respiratory distress syndrome. N Engl J Med 2004;351(4):327–36.

16. Meade MO, Cook DJ, Guyatt GH, et al. Ventilation strategy using low tidal volumes, recruitment maneuvers, and high positive end-expiratory pressure for acute lung injury and acute respiratory distress syndrome: a randomized controlled trial. JAMA 2008;299(6):637–45.

17. Mercat A, Richard JC, Vielle B, et al. Positive end-expiratory pressure setting in adults with acute lung injury and acute respiratory distress syndrome: a randomized controlled trial. JAMA 2008; 299(6):646–55.

18. Briel M, Meade M, Mercat A, et al. Higher vs lower positive end-expiratory pressure in patients with acute lung injury and acute respiratory distress syndrome: systematic review and meta-analysis. JAMA 2010;303(9):865–73.

19. Grasso S, Stripoli T, De MM, et al. ARDSnet ventilatory protocol and alveolar hyperinflation: role of positive end-expiratory pressure. Am J Respir Crit Care Med 2007;176(8):761–7.

20. Grasso S, Fanelli V, Cafarelli A, et al. Effects of high versus low positive end-expiratory pressures in acute respiratory distress syndrome. Am J Respir Crit Care Med 2005;171(9):1002–8.

21. Gattinoni L, Caironi P, Cressoni M, et al. Lung recruitment in patients with the acute respiratory distress syndrome. N Engl J Med 2006;354(17): 1775–86.

22. Nieszkowska A, Lu Q, Vieira S, et al. Incidence and regional distribution of lung overinflation during mechanical ventilation with positive end-expiratory pressure. Crit Care Med 2004;32(7): 1496–503.

23. Amato MB, Barbas CS, Medeiros DM, et al. Beneficial effects of the "open lung approach" with low distending pressures in acute respiratory distress syndrome. A prospective randomized study on mechanical ventilation. Am J Respir Crit Care Med 1995;152(6 Pt 1):1835–46.

24. Harris RS, Hess DR, Venegas JG. An objective analysis of the pressure-volume curve in the acute respiratory distress syndrome. Am J Respir Crit Care Med 2000;161(2 Pt 1):432–9.

25. Amato MB, Barbas CS, Medeiros DM, et al. Effect of a protective-ventilation strategy on mortality in the acute respiratory distress syndrome. N Engl J Med 1998;338(6):347–54.

26. Grasso S, Terragni P, Mascia L, et al. Airway pressure-time curve profile (stress index) detects tidal recruitment/hyperinflation in experimental acute lung injury. Crit Care Med 2004;32(4): 1018–27.

27. Ranieri VM, Giuliani R, Fiore T, et al. Volume-pressure curve of the respiratory system predicts effects of PEEP in ARDS: "occlusion" versus "constant flow" technique. Am J Respir Crit Care Med 1994;149(1):19–27.

28. Ranieri VM, Zhang H, Mascia L, et al. Pressure-time curve predicts minimally injurious ventilatory

strategy in an isolated rat lung model. Anesthesiology 2000;93(5):1320–8.

29. Milic-Emili J, Mead J, Turner JM, et al. Improved technique for estimating pleural pressure from esophageal balloons. J Appl Physiol 1964;19: 207–11.

30. Hager DN, Brower RG. Customizing lung-protective mechanical ventilation strategies. Crit Care Med 2006;34(5):1554–5.

31. Talmor DS, Fessler HE. Are esophageal pressure measurements important in clinical decision-making in mechanically ventilated patients? Respir Care 2010;55(2):162–72 [discussion: 172–4].

32. Talmor D, Sarge T, Malhotra A, et al. Mechanical ventilation guided by esophageal pressure in acute lung injury. N Engl J Med 2008;359(20):2095–104.

33. Fish E, Novack V, Banner-Goodspeed VM, et al. The Esophageal Pressure-Guided Ventilation 2 (EPVent2) trial protocol: a multicentre, randomised clinical trial of mechanical ventilation guided by transpulmonary pressure. BMJ Open 2014;4(9): e006356.

34. Amato MB, Meade MO, Slutsky AS, et al. Driving pressure and survival in the acute respiratory distress syndrome. N Engl J Med 2015;372(8): 747–55.

35. Slutsky AS. Mechanical ventilation. American College of Chest Physicians' Consensus Conference. Chest 1993;104(6):1833–59.

36. Krishnan JA, Brower RG. High-frequency ventilation for acute lung injury and ARDS. Chest 2000; 118(3):795–807.

37. Fort P, Farmer C, Westerman J, et al. High-frequency oscillatory ventilation for adult respiratory distress syndrome–a pilot study. Crit Care Med 1997;25(6):937–47.

38. Mehta S, Lapinsky SE, Hallett DC, et al. Prospective trial of high-frequency oscillation in adults with acute respiratory distress syndrome. Crit Care Med 2001;29(7):1360–9.

39. Chiche JD, Boukef R, Laurent I, et al. High frequcency oscillatory ventilation (HFOV) improves oxygenation in patients with severe ARDS. Am J Respir Crit Care Med 2000;161:48.

40. David M, Weiler N, Heinrichs W, et al. High-frequency oscillatory ventilation in adult acute respiratory distress syndrome. Intensive Care Med 2003; 29(10):1656–65.

41. Derdak S, Mehta S, Stewart TE, et al. High-frequency oscillatory ventilation for acute respiratory distress syndrome in adults: a randomized, controlled trial. Am J Respir Crit Care Med 2002; 166(6):801–8.

42. Fessler HE, Derdak S, Ferguson ND, et al. A protocol for high-frequency oscillatory ventilation in adults: results from a roundtable discussion. Crit Care Med 2007;35(7):1649–54.

43. Froese AB. The incremental application of lung-protective high-frequency oscillatory ventilation. Am J Respir Crit Care Med 2002;166(6):786–7.

44. Fessler HE, Hager DN, Brower RG. Feasibility of very high-frequency ventilation in adults with acute respiratory distress syndrome. Crit Care Med 2008; 36(4):1043–8.

45. Hager DN, Fessler HE, Kaczka DW, et al. Tidal volume delivery during high-frequency oscillatory ventilation in adults with acute respiratory distress syndrome. Crit Care Med 2007;35(6):1522–9.

46. Ferguson ND, Cook DJ, Guyatt GH, et al. High-frequency oscillation in early acute respiratory distress syndrome. N Engl J Med 2013;368(9): 795–805.

47. Young D, Lamb SE, Shah S, et al. High-frequency oscillation for acute respiratory distress syndrome. N Engl J Med 2013;368(9):806–13.

48. Guervilly C, Forel JM, Hraiech S, et al. Right ventricular function during high-frequency oscillatory ventilation in adults with acute respiratory distress syndrome. Crit Care Med 2012;40(5):1539–45.

49. Roubik K, Rafl J, van Heerde M, et al. Design and control of a demand flow system assuring spontaneous breathing of a patient connected to an HFO ventilator. IEEE Trans Biomed Eng 2011; 58(11):3225–33.

50. Frawley PM, Habashi NM. Airway pressure release ventilation: theory and practice. AACN Clin Issues 2001;12(2):234–46.

51. Downs JB, Stock MC. Airway pressure release ventilation: a new concept in ventilatory support. Crit Care Med 1987;15(5):459–61.

52. Rasanen J, Downs JB, Stock MC. Cardiovascular effects of conventional positive pressure ventilation and airway pressure release ventilation. Chest 1988;93(5):911–5.

53. Wrigge H, Zinserling J, Neumann P, et al. Spontaneous breathing with airway pressure release ventilation favors ventilation in dependent lung regions and counters cyclic alveolar collapse in oleic-acid-induced lung injury: a randomized controlled computed tomography trial. Crit Care 2005;9(6): R780–9.

54. Putensen C, Zech S, Wrigge H, et al. Long-term effects of spontaneous breathing during ventilatory support in patients with acute lung injury. Am J Respir Crit Care Med 2001;164(1):43–9.

55. Raoof S, Goulet K, Esan A, et al. Severe hypoxemic respiratory failure: part 2–nonventilatory strategies. Chest 2010;137(6):1437–48.

56. Sessler CN. Sedation, analgesia, and neuromuscular blockade for high-frequency oscillatory ventilation. Crit Care Med 2005;33(3 Suppl): S209–16.

57. Sessler CN. Train-of-four to monitor neuromuscular blockade? Chest 2004;126(4):1018–22.

58. Gainnier M, Roch A, Forel JM, et al. Effect of neuromuscular blocking agents on gas exchange in patients presenting with acute respiratory distress syndrome. Crit Care Med 2004;32(1):113–9.

59. Forel JM, Roch A, Marin V, et al. Neuromuscular blocking agents decrease inflammatory response in patients presenting with acute respiratory distress syndrome. Crit Care Med 2006;34(11):2749–57.

60. Papazian L, Forel JM, Gacouin A, et al. Neuromuscular blockers in early acute respiratory distress syndrome. N Engl J Med 2010;363(12):1107–16.

61. Prielipp RC, Coursin DB, Scuderi PE, et al. Comparison of the infusion requirements and recovery profiles of vecuronium and cisatracurium 51W89 in intensive care unit patients. Anesth Analg 1995;81(1):3–12.

62. Hansen-Flaschen J, Cowen J, Raps EC. Neuromuscular blockade in the intensive care unit. More than we bargained for. Am Rev Respir Dis 1993;147(1):234–6.

63. Mutoh T, Guest RJ, Lamm WJ, et al. Prone position alters the effect of volume overload on regional pleural pressures and improves hypoxemia in pigs in vivo. Am Rev Respir Dis 1992;146(2):300–6.

64. Lamm WJ, Graham MM, Albert RK. Mechanism by which the prone position improves oxygenation in acute lung injury. Am J Respir Crit Care Med 1994;150(1):184–93.

65. Broccard A, Shapiro RS, Schmitz LL, et al. Prone positioning attenuates and redistributes ventilator-induced lung injury in dogs. Crit Care Med 2000;28(2):295–303.

66. Gattinoni L, Tognoni G, Pesenti A, et al. Effect of prone positioning on the survival of patients with acute respiratory failure. N Engl J Med 2001;345(8):568–73.

67. Mancebo J, Fernandez R, Blanch L, et al. A multicenter trial of prolonged prone ventilation in severe acute respiratory distress syndrome. Am J Respir Crit Care Med 2006;173(11):1233–9.

68. Guerin C, Reignier J, Richard JC, et al. Prone positioning in severe acute respiratory distress syndrome. N Engl J Med 2013;368(23):2159–68.

69. Geer RT, Soma LR, Barnes C, et al. Effects of albumin and/or furosemide therapy on pulmonary edema induced by hydrochloric acid aspiration in rabbits. J Trauma 1976;16(10):788–91.

70. Ali J, Chernicki W, Wood LD. Effect of furosemide in canine low-pressure pulmonary edema. J Clin Invest 1979;64(5):1494–504.

71. Reising CA, Chendrasekhar A, Wall PL, et al. Continuous dose furosemide as a therapeutic approach to acute respiratory distress syndrome (ARDS). J Surg Res 1999;82(1):56–60.

72. Simmons RS, Berdine GG, Seidenfeld JJ, et al. Fluid balance and the adult respiratory distress syndrome. Am Rev Respir Dis 1987;135(4):924–9.

73. Schuster DP. The case for and against fluid restriction and occlusion pressure reduction in adult respiratory distress syndrome. New Horiz 1993;1(4):478–88.

74. Humphrey H, Hall J, Sznajder I, et al. Improved survival in ARDS patients associated with a reduction in pulmonary capillary wedge pressure. Chest 1990;97(5):1176–80.

75. Mitchell JP, Schuller D, Calandrino FS, et al. Improved outcome based on fluid management in critically ill patients requiring pulmonary artery catheterization. Am Rev Respir Dis 1992;145(5):990–8.

76. Martin GS, Mangialardi RJ, Wheeler AP, et al. Albumin and furosemide therapy in hypoproteinemic patients with acute lung injury. Crit Care Med 2002;30(10):2175–82.

77. Grissom CK, Hirshberg EL, Dickerson JB, et al. Fluid management with a simplified conservative protocol for the acute respiratory distress syndrome*. Crit Care Med 2015;43(2):288–95.

78. Mikkelsen ME, Christie JD, Lanken PN, et al. The adult respiratory distress syndrome cognitive outcomes study: long-term neuropsychological function in survivors of acute lung injury. Am J Respir Crit Care Med 2012;185(12):1307–15.

79. Barnett N, Ware LB. Biomarkers in acute lung injury–marking forward progress. Crit Care Clin 2011;27(3):661–83.

80. Ware LB, Koyama T, Billheimer DD, et al. Prognostic and pathogenetic value of combining clinical and biochemical indices in patients with acute lung injury. Chest 2010;137(2):288–96.

81. Thompson BT. Corticosteroids for ARDS. Minerva Anestesiol 2010;76(6):441–7.

82. Thompson BT. Glucocorticoids and acute lung injury. Crit Care Med 2003;31(4 Suppl):S253–7.

83. Weigelt JA, Norcross JF, Borman KR, et al. Early steroid therapy for respiratory failure. Arch Surg 1985;120(5):536–40.

84. Schein RM, Bergman R, Marcial EH, et al. Complement activation and corticosteroid therapy in the development of the adult respiratory distress syndrome. Chest 1987;91(6):850–4.

85. Luce JM, Montgomery AB, Marks JD, et al. Ineffectiveness of high-dose methylprednisolone in preventing parenchymal lung injury and improving mortality in patients with septic shock. Am Rev Respir Dis 1988;138(1):62–8.

86. Bone RC, Fisher CJ Jr, Clemmer TP, et al. A controlled clinical trial of high-dose methylprednisolone in the treatment of severe sepsis and septic shock. N Engl J Med 1987;317(11):653–8.

87. Bernard GR, Luce JM, Sprung CL, et al. High-dose corticosteroids in patients with the adult respiratory

distress syndrome. N Engl J Med 1987;317(25): 1565–70.

88. Confalonieri M, Urbino R, Potena A, et al. Hydrocortisone infusion for severe community-acquired pneumonia - a preliminary randomized study. Am J Respir Crit Care Med 2005;171(3):242–8.

89. Annane D, Sebille V, Bellissant E. Ger-Inf-05 Study G: effect of low doses of corticosteroids in septic shock patients with or without early acute respiratory distress syndrome. Crit Care Med 2006; 34(1):22–30.

90. Meduri GU, Headley AS, Golden E, et al. Effect of prolonged methylprednisolone therapy in unresolving acute respiratory distress syndrome: a randomized controlled trial. JAMA 1998;280(2): 159–65.

91. Steinberg KP, Hudson LD, Goodman RB, et al. Efficacy and safety of corticosteroids for persistent acute respiratory distress syndrome. N Engl J Med 2006;354(16):1671–84.

92. Taylor RW, Zimmerman JL, Dellinger RP, et al. Inhaled nitric oxide in ASG: low-dose inhaled nitric oxide in patients with acute lung injury: a randomized controlled trial. JAMA 2004;291(13):1603–9.

93. Dellinger RP, Zimmerman JL, Taylor RW, et al. Effects of inhaled nitric oxide in patients with acute respiratory distress syndrome: results of a randomized phase II trial. Inhaled Nitric Oxide in ARDS Study Group. Crit Care Med 1998;26(1): 15–23.

94. Rossaint R, Falke KJ, Lopez F, et al. Inhaled nitric oxide for the adult respiratory distress syndrome. N Engl J Med 1993;328(6):399–405.

95. Michael JR, Barton RG, Saffle JR, et al. Inhaled nitric oxide versus conventional therapy: effect on oxygenation in ARDS. Am J Respir Crit Care Med 1998;157(5 Pt 1):1372–80.

96. Troncy E, Collet JP, Shapiro S, et al. Inhaled nitric oxide in acute respiratory distress syndrome: a pilot randomized controlled study. Am J Respir Crit Care Med 1998;157(5 Pt 1):1483–8.

97. Lundin S, Mang H, Smithies M, et al. Inhalation of nitric oxide in acute lung injury: results of a European multicentre study. The European Study Group of Inhaled Nitric Oxide. Intensive Care Med 1999; 25(9):911–9.

98. Torbic H, Szumita PM, Anger KE, et al. Inhaled epoprostenol vs inhaled nitric oxide for refractory hypoxemia in critically ill patients. J Crit Care 2013;28(5):844–8.

99. McAuley DF, Laffey JG, O'Kane CM, et al. Simvastatin in the acute respiratory distress syndrome. N Engl J Med 2014;371(18):1695–703.

100. National Heart L, Blood Institute ACTN, Truwit JD, et al. Rosuvastatin for sepsis-associated acute respiratory distress syndrome. N Engl J Med 2014; 370(23):2191–200.

101. Jacobson JR, Barnard JW, Grigoryev DN, et al. Simvastatin attenuates vascular leak and inflammation in murine inflammatory lung injury. Am J Physiol Lung Cell Mol Physiol 2005;288(6): L1026–32.

102. Shyamsundar M, McKeown ST, O'Kane CM, et al. Simvastatin decreases lipopolysaccharide-induced pulmonary inflammation in healthy volunteers. Am J Respir Crit Care Med 2009; 179(12):1107–14.

103. Zapol WM, Snider MT, Hill JD, et al. Extracorporeal membrane oxygenation in severe acute respiratory failure. A randomized prospective study. JAMA 1979;242(20):2193–6.

104. Gattinoni L, Pesenti A, Mascheroni D, et al. Low-frequency positive-pressure ventilation with extracorporeal CO_2 removal in severe acute respiratory failure. JAMA 1986;256(7):881–6.

105. Morris AH, Wallace CJ, Menlove RL, et al. Randomized clinical trial of pressure-controlled inverse ratio ventilation and extracorporeal CO_2 removal for adult respiratory distress syndrome. Am J Respir Crit Care Med 1994;149(2 Pt 1):295–305.

106. Brodie D, Bacchetta M. Extracorporeal membrane oxygenation for ARDS in adults. N Engl J Med 2011;365(20):1905–14.

107. Peek GJ, Mugford M, Tiruvoipati R, et al. Efficacy and economic assessment of conventional ventilatory support versus extracorporeal membrane oxygenation for severe adult respiratory failure (CESAR): a multicentre randomised controlled trial. Lancet 2009;374(9698):1351–63.

108. Combes A. Extracorporeal Membrane Oxygenation for Severe Acute Respiratory Distress Syndrome (EOLIA). Available at: https://clinicaltrials.gov/ct2/show/NCT01470703. Accessed April 05, 2015.

109. Gajic O, Frutos-Vivar F, Esteban A, et al. Ventilator settings as a risk factor for acute respiratory distress syndrome in mechanically ventilated patients. Intensive Care Med 2005;31(7):922–6.

110. Michelet P, D'Journo XB, Roch A, et al. Protective ventilation influences systemic inflammation after esophagectomy: a randomized controlled study. Anesthesiology 2006;105(5):911–9.

111. Determann RM, Royakkers A, Wolthuis EK, et al. Ventilation with lower tidal volumes as compared with conventional tidal volumes for patients without acute lung injury: a preventive randomized controlled trial. Crit Care 2010;14(1):R1.

112. Serpa Neto A, Cardoso SO, Manetta JA, et al. Association between use of lung-protective ventilation with lower tidal volumes and clinical outcomes among patients without acute respiratory distress syndrome: a meta-analysis. JAMA 2012;308(16): 1651–9.

113. Gajic O, Rana R, Winters JL, et al. Transfusion-related acute lung injury in the critically ill:

prospective nested case-control study. Am J Respir Crit Care Med 2007;176(9):886–91.

114. Gajic O, Yilmaz M, Iscimen R, et al. Transfusion from male-only versus female donors in critically ill recipients of high plasma volume components. Crit Care Med 2007;35(7):1645–8.

115. Kor DJ, Talmor DS, Banner-Goodspeed VM, et al, US Critical Illness and Injury Trials Group, Lung Injury Prevention with Aspirin Study Group (USCIIT-G:LIPS-A). Lung Injury Prevention with Aspirin (LIPS-A): a protocol for a multicentre randomised clinical trial in medical patients at high risk of acute lung injury. BMJ Open 2012;2(5) [pii:e001606].

116. Levitt JE, Calfee CS, Goldstein BA, et al. Early acute lung injury: criteria for identifying lung injury prior to the need for positive pressure ventilation*. Crit Care Med 2013;41(8):1929–37.

117. Gajic O, Dabbagh O, Park PK, et al. Early identification of patients at risk of acute lung injury: evaluation of lung injury prediction score in a multicenter cohort study. Am J Respir Crit Care Med 2011; 183(4):462–70.

Critically Ill Patients with Interstitial Lung Disease

Ryan Hadley, MD*, Robert Hyzy, MD

KEYWORDS

- Intensive care unit • Interstitial lung disease • Idiopathic pulmonary fibrosis

KEY POINTS

- Clinically significant interstitial lung disease (ILD) impairs pulmonary mechanics and gas exchange, which affects mechanical ventilatory strategies.
- Low tidal volume ventilation, to minimize volutrauma, in patients with ILD who require mechanical ventilation is recommended, although this has been extrapolated from data in acute respiratory distress syndrome (ARDS).
- Exacerbations of idiopathic pulmonary fibrosis (IPF), which lead to respiratory failure, are devastating with poor prognosis and can be incited by pulmonary surgery. Short-term survival may provide a window for lung transplantation.
- For patients with suspected, undiagnosed ILD in the intensive care unit, evaluation by an experienced pulmonologist, review of previous imaging, detailed medication and occupational history, and consideration of surgical lung biopsy are recommended.

INTRODUCTION

Interstitial lung disease (ILD) is a clinical syndrome of various etiologies and histopathologic categorization that when clinically significant, impair respiratory function. Progressive inflammation and scarring of the pulmonary parenchyma generate degradation of pulmonary mechanics and/or gas exchange. Eventual respiratory failure is the driving factor in mortality in some forms of ILD.[1] Often patients with ILD require intensive care for respiratory failure, surgical or medical procedures, or nonrespiratory organ failure. Underling impairment in pulmonary function necessitates alteration of ventilatory strategies. Knowledge of ILD comorbidities and exacerbation syndromes is requisite for the intensivist to provide accurate prognosis and potentially limit futile care.

EPIDEMIOLOGY

Variability in exposure to risk factors for ILD (smoking, occupation, and age) leads to regional variability in phenotypes and incidence of ILD.[2] Accurate identification and reporting bias significantly limit precise estimates of incidence and prevalence.[2] Compared with chronic obstructive lung disease ILD is uncommon, which can lead to lack of familiarity in centers not experienced with the care and diagnosis of ILD. In the United States the estimated prevalence of ILD is 81 and 67 per 100,000 in males and females, respectively, which is derived from a population-based study from New Mexico.[3] This is in stark contrast to the prevalence of chronic obstructive lung disease at 6700 per 100,000 (6.7%).[3,4] Autopsy reports from the same study indicate preclinical or

Division of Pulmonary & Critical Care Medicine, University of Michigan Health System, 1500 East Medical Center Drive, 3916 Taubman Center, SPC 5360, Ann Arbor, MI 48109, USA
* Corresponding author.
E-mail address: hadleyr@med.umich.edu

Clin Chest Med 36 (2015) 497–510
http://dx.doi.org/10.1016/j.ccm.2015.05.012
0272-5231/15/$ – see front matter Published by Elsevier Inc.

undiagnosed ILD in 1.8% of patients.[3] Seven percent of patients in the Framingham Heart Study were found to have interstitial abnormalities on chest computed tomography (CT), suggesting a large spectrum of undiagnosed subclinical ILD.[5]

In total there are more than 200 types of ILD.[2] ILD is separated into lung diseases of known causes, such as from occupation (pneumoconiosis), drug exposure, and other systemic disease[3] (rheumatologic syndromes), versus those that are idiopathic interstitial pneumonias. A full description of all of the types of ILD is outside the scope of this article, although some key clinical findings can be found in **Table 1**.

UNDERLYING PHYSIOLOGY

Pulmonary function tests (PFTs) and oxygen requirement measurements performed before intensive care unit (ICU) admission, should they be available, are invaluable. Generally, patients with ILD have restrictive physiology, which is typified by decreased forced vital capacity, total lung capacity, and increased ratio of forced expiratory volume in 1 second to forced vital capacity.[6] These changes on PFTs correlate with poor pulmonary compliance during mechanical ventilation, which impacts mechanical ventilatory strategy by elevating airway pressures needed to provide adequate tidal volumes (TVs). The PFTs may be pseudonormalized if concomitant emphysema coexists.[6]

Gas exchange is impaired almost universally in patients with clinically significant ILD,[6] often requiring ambulatory supplemental oxygen. In the ambulatory setting, gas exchange is measured by the lung's ability to take up carbon monoxide relative to the underlying hemoglobin content (diffusion capacity of lung for carbon monoxide [D_{LCO}]). D_{LCO} may be decreased out of proportion to the pulmonary mechanics if comorbid conditions of continued tobacco abuse, emphysema, or pulmonary hypertension are present. Ambulatory measurements of arterial blood gases are useful to determine baseline level of hypoxemia and acid-base status.

RESPIRATORY FAILURE

Acute or acute on chronic respiratory failure is a common presentation of patients with ILD to the ICU. Usually, this is caused by hypoxemic respiratory failure. General strategies for the treatment of this include exclusion of potentially reversible causes, such as pneumothorax, infection, pulmonary embolus, and left or right heart failure.

Outcomes

Most outcome data reported are from patients with idiopathic pulmonary fibrosis (IPF), the most common and most deadly ILD. The prognosis for patients with IPF who require mechanical ventilation for nonoperative respiratory failure is extremely poor, although mortality is not absolute.[7–11] Mallick[12] recently reviewed all reported available data of patients with IPF who were mechanically ventilated and found a hospital mortality of 87% and a 3-month mortality of 94%. This has led some to consider mechanical ventilation in patients with IPF with nonoperative respiratory failure futile,[8,11,12] although any survival window may potentially allow for lung transplantation.[9] A specific syndrome causing respiratory failure in IPF, acute exacerbation, is discussed later in this article.

Data from the poor outcomes associated with patients with IPF who require mechanical ventilation are often incorrectly assigned to all patients with ILD.[13] However, regardless of the cause of the ILD, a patient with severely degraded pulmonary compliance and/or gas exchange at baseline who is admitted with respiratory failure is likely to do poorly unless the cause of the respiratory failure is easily and quickly reversible. Respiratory failure caused by progressive worsening of ILD despite appropriate treatment is, in most cases, futile unless pulmonary transplantation is possible. Mechanical ventilatory and other organ support may be needed to allow for the appropriate diagnostic evaluation to ensure no reversible causes of deterioration are found. Critical care support for patients with respiratory failure from end-stage fibrosis that is not treatable pharmacologically or surgically should not be continued.

VENTILATORY STRATEGIES
Noninvasive Ventilation

Given reduced baseline pulmonary function and potentially disastrous outcome from endotracheal intubation, avoidance of intubation to prevent complications, such as ventilator-associated pneumonia, intensive care myopathy or neuropathy, and catheter-associated infections, is desirable whenever possible. Small, retrospective studies have reported some success with noninvasive positive pressure ventilation (NIV) with improved mortality compared with invasive mechanical ventilation (IMV) with survival in responders to NIV of around 40%.[14–17] As with most data in ILD, these studies are predominantly done with patients with IPF, because it is the most common ILD. Additionally, a selection bias for less

Table 1
Clinical pearls for ILD in the intensive care unit

Disease	Key Points for the Intensivist
Idiopathic pulmonary fibrosis (idiopathic usual interstitial pneumonia)	• Restrictive physiology • Honeycombing, reticular abnormalities, and minimal ground glass is classic, but not universal • New ground glass is acute exacerbation, infection, or left heart failure • Prognosis after acute exacerbation is dismal • Overall poor prognosis
Nonspecific interstitial pneumonia	• Restrictive physiology • Frequently associated with rheumatologic disease • CT can be diffuse ground glass or similar to IPF without honeycombing • More likely to respond to treatment than IPF • Better prognosis than IPF
Sarcoid	• Restrictive, obstructive, or combined physiology • Usually peribronchovascular nodules and/or thoracic lymphadenopathy on CT • May respond to treatment (steroids) • Myriad of extrapulmonary manifestations exist • Usually good prognosis

Connective tissue disease–associated ILD	• Restrictive physiology, except for obliterative bronchiolitis, which is obstructive
	• Common diseases
	  ○ Rheumatoid arthritis
	  ○ Systemic sclerosis
	  ○ Sjögren syndrome
	  ○ Dermatomyositis/polymyositis
	  ○ Mixed connective tissue disease
	• Varied histopathology patterns
	  ○ UIP
	  ○ Nonspecific interstitial pneumonia
	  ○ Organizing pneumonia
	  ○ Lymphocytic interstitial pneumonia
	  ○ Obliterative bronchiolitis
	• If on immunosuppression, consider opportunistic infection as a cause of decline
	• Pulmonary hypertension can complicate
	• Prognosis variable

Acute interstitial pneumonia	• Restrictive physiology
	• Essentially, idiopathic ARDS
	• Requires exclusion of
	  ○ Infection
	  ○ Inhalational exposure
	  ○ Medication
	  ○ Aspiration
	  ○ Acute eosinophilic pneumonia
	  ○ Diffuse alveolar hemorrhage
	  ○ Other causes of ARDS

Pneumoconiosis (occupational lung disease)	• Restrictive physiology
	• Occupational history is key
	• Most common are
	  ○ Asbestos
	    ■ CT may appear similar to IPF/UIP
	  ○ Silica and coal
	    ■ Progressive massive fibrosis (upper lobe coalescing masses)
	    ■ Increases risk for tuberculosis

(continued on next page)

Table 1 (continued)	
Disease	**Key Points for the Intensivist**

Hypersensitivity pneumonitis	• Restrictive, obstructive, or combined physiology
	• Antigen not always apparent
	• Include
	  ○ Farmer's lung
	  ○ Hot tub lung
	  ○ Bird fancier's lung
	• Typically treatment responsive (steroids)
	  ○ Withdrawal of offending agent essential
	• IgG to suspected antigen supports diagnosis
	• Acute form treated with high-dose steroids

Drug related	• Common culprits
	  ○ Various chemotherapeutics
	  ○ Amioderone
	  ○ Nitrofurantoin
	  ○ Methotrexate
	• Myriad of histopathologic patterns reported
	• Withdrawal of offending agent essential
	• www.pneumotox.com is an excellent resource for reported pulmonary toxicities
	• We recommend higher doses of steroid than that of AE-IPF

Smoking-related ILD	• Restrictive physiology, usually, but may coexist with chronic obstructive pulmonary disease
	• Respiratory bronchiolitis–ILD
	  ○ Ground glass and centrilobulare nodules in a smoker
	  ○ Smokers' macrophages on biopsy or bronchoalveolar lavage
	• Desquamative interstitial pneumonitis
	  ○ Ground glass in a smoker
	• Langerhan histiocytosis
	  ○ Oddly shaped cysts and nodules

Lymphangioleiomyomatosis	• Often obstructive physiology
	• Unexplained cysts of various sizes
	• Nodules and ground glass conspicuously absent
	• Spontaneous form only seen in women
	• Can be complicated by
	  ○ Pneumothorax
	  ○ Chylothorax
	  ○ Renal angiomyolipoma
	  ○ Tuberous sclerosis

Cryptogenic organizing pneumonia	• Usually restrictive physiology • Migratory infiltrates • Symptoms may mimic lower respiratory infection • Exclusion of infection, medication reaction is needed • Can be associated with rheumatologic conditions • Responds well to steroids

Abbreviations: ARDS, acute respiratory distress syndrome; IPF, idiopathic pulmonary fibrosis; UIP, usual interstitial pneumonia.

severely afflicted patients may be present in those who are able to be supported by NIV as compared with those who ultimately require IMV. Indeed, in two studies all patients who failed NIV died[14,15] and another reported a mortality rate of 85% in NIV failure.[17]

High-Flow Nasal Cannula

High-flow nasal cannula is a relatively new technology that has been used in patients without ILD admitted with hypoxemic respiratory failure, including those with acute respiratory distress syndrome (ARDS).[18–21] In contrast to traditional oxygen delivery devices that limit flow to less than 15 L/min, high-flow nasal cannula can provide up to 60 L/min oxygen flow, which provides better matching of flow requirement for patients with increased inspiratory flow demands from high minute ventilation.[22] When applied to ambulatory patients with IPF not in acute respiratory failure, a decrease in minute ventilation, breathing rate, capillary partial pressure of carbon dioxide, and small increases in airway pressure has been observed.[23] A single case report of successful use on high-flow nasal cannula in amiodarone-induced pulmonary fibrosis has been described, but further reported evidence specifically with patients with ILD with hypoxemic respiratory failure is lacking.[24]

Despite the lack of present published evidence, we have found high-flow nasal cannula use offers a potentially useful modality for treating patients with ILD with hypoxemia in the ICU who do not require immediate intubation. Although large prospective interventional studies are lacking, if no contraindications exist, NIV or high-flow nasal cannula are viable initial ventilatory support strategies for patients with ILD who present with respiratory failure. Additionally, stabilization of respiratory status without the need for sedation may allow for discussion of goals of care if prognosis is poor or provide time for other diagnostic or therapeutic interventions to determine prognosis.

Invasive Mechanical Ventilation

Appropriate, evidence-based strategies for IMV in patients with ILD have not been established. Lung protective ventilation (LPV) using a low TV is assumed to be beneficial to prevent volutrauma, although this has not been evaluated specifically in patients with ILD. Most of the initial studies that show a poor prognosis of patients with IPF receiving IMV were done in an era before routine use of LPV. Gaudry and colleagues[9] evaluated the prognosis of patients with fibrosing interstitial pneumonia (either IPF or fibrosing nonspecific interstitial pneumonia) presenting with respiratory failure in the LPV era. Unfortunately, despite an LPV strategy, with an average of 6 mL per kilogram ideal body weight, patients with fibrosing interstitial pneumonias admitted with respiratory failure continued to have a poor prognosis with only 22% surviving to ICU discharge.[9]

Because of underlying poor baseline lung compliance and possible additional pulmonary insults leading to respiratory failure, elevated plateau pressures are often tolerated to adequately ventilate patients with ILD who require IMV. Furthermore, the desired TV may be reached

very early in respiratory cycle. Additionally, increased recoil leads to a rapid exhalation phase. From this, higher respiratory rates can be used to maintain minute ventilation because of the underlying pathophysiology.

Permissive hypercapnia can be used until reversal of the acute process is sustained; however, the intensivist should recognize the potential difficulty of successfully managing acid-base status in a patient with baseline impaired respiratory status and possibly limits in dead space and V/Q matching once permissive hypercapnia ensues.

Little data exist regarding optimal ventilator settings. A single, retrospective study found an association with elevated positive end-expiratory pressures and worse outcomes.[7] This may simply be a marker of worse respiratory failure and hypoxemia requiring elevated mean airway pressures, although multiple markers of disease severity were controlled for in the multivariate analysis.[7] As proposed by the authors, the physiology of ILD may not improve with the addition of positive end-expiratory pressures because of the fibrotic nature of this condition, which has relatively little recruitable lung when compared with ARDS. Here, positive end-expiratory pressures may lead to worsened hemodynamics, V/Q matching, and ventilator-induced lung injury specifically in patients with ILD.[7] Data are not currently to the level to dictate treatment, and prospective studies are needed.

Extubation parameters for patients with ILD do not exist. Values used for patients in respiratory failure without ILD, such as rapid shallow breathing index,[25] may not be appropriate for patients with ILD given the physiologic need for tachypnea. Additionally, alterations in V/Q mismatch and gas exchange may lead to higher minute ventilation and fraction of inspired oxygen at the time of extubation. Thus, if a patient seems comfortable, is not hypercapnic, and level of inspired fraction of inspired oxygen can be supplied noninvasively (such as with high-flow nasal cannula) a trial of liberation from mechanical ventilation is likely warranted following a spontaneous breathing trial, even though the patient may be tachypneic to an extent (ie, >30 breaths per minute) not normally associated with a planned extubation.

Although data specifically for patients with ILD do not exist, LPV with TVs of 4 to 6 mL/kg ideal body weight, a plateau pressure less than 30 cm H_2O, minimization of inhaled oxygen content, and restrictive fluid balance similar to treatment of ARDS are advised.[26,27] Unfortunately, because of poor lung compliance, these settings are not always compatible with the patient's physiologic need for ventilation and toleration of higher respiratory rates and/or plateau pressures may be needed.[9]

WORSENING OF ESTABLISHED DIAGNOSIS

Underlying histopathology of the patient's ILD may or may not be known at the time of admission to the ICU. Exacerbation syndromes unique to specific interstitial lung diagnoses have been described.[28–31] It is important for the intensivist to identify the syndromes for prognosis and appropriate treatment, and to counsel patients and family about limiting futile interventions.

Acute Exacerbation of Idiopathic Pulmonary Fibrosis

IPF, the most common and deadly idiopathic interstitial pneumonia, often results in a measured and continued progression to respiratory failure and death (**Fig. 1**).[32] In the past two decades, acute, idiopathic worsening of respiratory function in patients with IPF, termed acute exacerbation of IPF (AE-IPF), has been identified as a particularly morbid event[33] causing abrupt and irreversible clinical worsening and placing the patient on a new trajectory (see **Fig. 1**).[32] Symptoms mimic viral

lower respiratory tract infection with cough, fever, leukocytosis, flulike symptoms, and worsening gas exchange, although not all of these need be present for diagnosis (**Box 1**).[28,29] Based on prospective clinical trials the annual incidence of acute exacerbations in patients with known IPF is 2% to 14%.[34–36] Exclusion of treatable causes of worsening is of utmost importance and is requisite for a diagnosis of AE-IPF (see **Box 1**).[28,29] Accurate diagnosis of AE-IPF is needed because it is often a terminal event with 78% to 86% mortality if mechanical ventilation is required.[9,37]

Patients with IPF who present with acute worsening of respiratory symptoms require cross-sectional imaging to evaluate for causes of respiratory embarrassment if not diagnosed by a chest radiograph. Pulmonary embolism should be evaluated because patients with pulmonary fibrosis are at elevated risk of venous thromboembolic disease.[38] A CT scan with pulmonary angiogram has the advantage of identifying in situ pulmonary embolus in patients without deep venous thrombosis and evaluation of the lung parenchyma for consolidation, although subtle ground glass may not be identifiable because of lack of breath-holding technique and

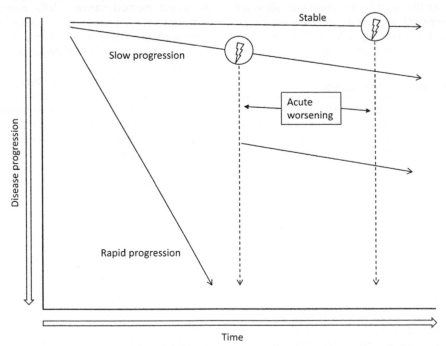

Fig. 1. Clinical course of idiopathic pulmonary fibrosis. Some patients develop slow decline in lung function, whereas others rapidly decline. Acute worsening, usually an exacerbation, causes rapid decline and places a patient on a new trajectory, if they survive. (*Reprinted with permission of* the American Thoracic Society. Copyright © 2015 American Thoracic Society. *From* Raghu G, Collard HR, Egan JJ, et al. An official ATS/ERS/JRS/ALAT statement: idiopathic pulmonary fibrosis: evidence-based guidelines for diagnosis and management. Am J Respir Crit Care Med 2011;183(6):798. Official journal of the American Thoracic Society. This document was published in 2011. Certain aspects of this document may be out of date and caution should be used when applying the information in clinical practice and other usages.)

administration of intravenous radiopaque contrast and thus an additional high-resolution CT scan may be required. Representative images of a high-resolution CT from a patient with IPF with acute exacerbation are seen in **Fig. 2**.

Given the significant overlap between symptoms of AE-IPF and infection, differentiation between these two entities is difficult. Consolidation on CT scan may be from acute exacerbation, but if it is focal and unilateral, pneumonia should be considered. Sampling with bronchoalveolar lavage is helpful in differentiation, but severe hypoxemia may preclude performing bronchoscopy. Ground

glass opacities may likewise be from infection, cardiogenic pulmonary edema, or ARDS from a known pulmonary or extrapulmonary cause and need to be excluded.[29] Additionally, comparison with prior cross-sectional imaging is needed to ensure the ground glass opacities are, in fact, new.

When histologic examination of pulmonary tissue is performed in patients with AE-IPF, often at autopsy, diffuse alveolar damage (DAD) is the most commonly described abnormality.[29] DAD is also the classic finding described in ARDS.

Considerable physiologic and histologic overlap exists between ARDS and AE-IPF. Namely, underlying pathologic injury of DAD, poor lung compliance, and severe hypoxemia are shared leading to similar behavior when receiving IMV. Avoidance of hyperoxia, barotrauma, and volutrauma is recommended with goals of arterial hemoglobin saturation of 88% or greater, plateau pressure less than 30, and TV of 6 mL/kg predicted body weight similar to ARDS,[26,28] although this is not evidence based.

No treatment has been proved to be effective for AE-IPF. Presumptive treatment with antibacterial antibiotics, anticoagulation, and diuretics is often attempted to correct potentially reversible causes of deterioration. Evaluation for infection with bronchoalveolar lavage is indicated if the patient can withstand bronchoalveolar lavage without life-threatening hypoxemia. Exclusion of elevated left heart filling pressures or heart failure, such as with an echocardiogram, BNP (brain natriuretic peptide), and clinical examination, is also requisite in patients with presumed AE-IPF. Use of diuretics may be attempted in patients admitted with AE-IPF with normal blood pressure and normal renal function. Benefit of minimizing positive fluid balance can be extrapolated from the data in ARDS, but data specifically in patients with AE-IPF are absent.[27]

If pulmonary embolism cannot be excluded because of inability to perform CT pulmonary

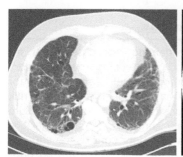 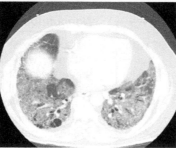

Fig. 2. Imaging from acute exacerbation of IPF. A 63-year-old man with biopsy-proved usual interstitial pneumonia and diagnosis of IPF transferred to our institution with acute (<2 week) worsening of chronic dyspnea and hypoxia without evidence of infection or heart failure. Representative images show new, diffuse, bilateral ground glass infiltrates with a background of known interstitial thickening and honeycombing (*right*) when compared with prior imaging from 1 year ago (*left*). The radiologic findings are consistent with acute exacerbation of IPF.

angiogram from clinical instability or renal failure, we suggest presumptive anticoagulation until embolism is excluded. Ventilation/perfusion scan is likely not useful because of underlying anatomic parenchymal destruction. Lower extremity Doppler is inadequate to completely exclude a pulmonary embolism, although if positive can be helpful because it would be an indication for anticoagulation.

Pharmacologic therapies directed toward the pathologic insult of AE-IPF have not been studied in randomized trials. Despite the lack of evidence, corticosteroids are typically used[9,28] with dosages of methylprednisolone ranging from 2 mg/kg/day to "pulse" methylprednisolone of 500 to 1000 mg per day. Administration of systemic corticosteroids is recommended by a consensus of experts, although dosage recommendations were not made.[32] To the extent that the histopathology of AE-IPF is DAD superimposed on usual interstitial pneumonia (UIP) and not capillaritis, we prefer a dose of 2 mg/kg/day of methylprednisolone in divided doses. Retrospective and anecdotal reports of treatment with cyclophosphamide[39–43] and cyclosporine A[44–46] are in the published literature, but are not at substantial size to make recommendation on their routine use. Use of anticoagulation in patients with AE-IPF without documented venous thromboembolism have some supportive data, but is not recommended at this time.[47]

In sum, for AE-IPF, we recommend exclusion and/or presumptive treatment of volume overload, bacterial pneumonia, including pseudomonas coverage and atypical coverage, with administration of ARDS doses of a total of 2 mg/kg per day methylprednisolone (**Box 2**). Cyclophosphamide, 2 mg/kg intravenously daily, can be considered on a case-by-case basis. Accurate diagnosis is of utmost importance given the poor prognosis of AE-IPF and the relatively good prognosis of reversible causes of respiratory failure, such as lower respiratory tract infection or pulmonary edema.

Acute Exacerbation of Non–Idiopathic Pulmonary Fibrosis Interstitial Lung Disease

Exacerbations of patients with ILD other than IPF have been reported.[30,31,48,49] Accurate prognostication cannot be made for non-IPF acute exacerbations because of the dearth of reported cases, although the largest series indicates an improved prognosis of non-IPF exacerbations as compared with IPF exacerbations with mortalities of 33% and 69% ($P = .04$), respectively.[49]

In contrast to IPF, ambulatory immunosuppressive medications may be indicated for patients with non-IPF ILD. Because of this a whole host of opportunistic infections or medication reactions need to be considered in an acute exacerbation of patients on immunosuppression. Bronchoscopy for exclusion of typical and atypical infections is recommended. Other pulmonary processes associated with the underlying systemic disease (eg, diffuse alveolar hemorrhage with lupus) may need to be considered.

Similar to AE-IPF, if other concomitant factors of respiratory demise have been excluded, increased immunosuppression with systemic corticosteroids or other agents is often used.[30,31,49] We recommend higher dosages of corticosteroids (methylprednisolone, 1 g per day for at least 3 days) for patients with rheumatologic disease as compared with IPF because of the possibility of capillaritis.

PERIOPERATIVE

ILD is associated with advanced age and significant comorbidities can exist. Many of these conditions may require operative management. Additionally, biopsy of lung tissue may be needed to determine the underlying ILD. Careful attention to patients with ILD during pulmonary and nonpulmonary surgical procedures is vital for the intensivist.

Nonpulmonary Procedures

No data exist regarding risk assessment for patients with ILD undergoing nonpulmonary surgery. Use of preoperative PFTs specifically for patients with ILD has not been studied for risk stratification for postoperative respiratory failure after nonpulmonary surgeries,[50,51] although it is assumed patients with poor compliance and gas exchange are at higher risk. There are no published guidelines for PFT values for which nonpulmonary surgery is contraindicated in patients with ILD. A risk-benefit analysis of the advantages of

---

Box 2
Suggested treatment of patients with IPF with acute respiratory failure

Antibacterials to include atypical (eg, mycoplasma, chlamydia) and pseudomonas

Diuretics

Presumptive anticoagulation or exclusion of pulmonary embolus

Corticosteroids (methylprednisolone, 2 mg/kg in divided doses twice a day)

operative management versus the risk of postoperative respiratory complications is required for any patient with ILD for whom surgery is recommended, such that elective and cosmetic procedures may be postponed or not performed and emergent procedures for life-threatening complications should proceed if no medical treatment options exist. AE-IPF has only been reported once in nonpulmonary surgery, and was recently reviewed.[52] Low TVs (LPV) is advised during surgery for minimization of lung injury, such as has been seen in recent data of patients without ILD undergoing high-risk surgery.[53]

Often, patients with ILD require diagnostic or therapeutic procedures with moderate sedation (eg, age-determined colonoscopy for cancer screening). Many patients who are nonhypercapnic can tolerate these procedures if adequate supplemental oxygen is supplied; however, a low threshold for consideration of support by an anesthesiologist is warranted.

Pulmonary Surgery

Lung cancer

Non–small cell lung cancer occurs in patients with ILD and at an increased rate.[54,55] Many patients with ILD cannot undergo operative therapy secondary to poor respiratory function.[56] No specific guidelines exist for surgical resection of non–small cell lung cancer in patients with ILD, although postoperative forced expiratory volume in 1 second and D_{LCO} should be calculated similar to other patients undergoing pulmonary resection.[57] Worse outcomes for patients with ILD have been described for those with worse preoperative dyspnea, a $Paco_2/Pao_2$ ratio of greater than 0.72, and other preoperative medical comorbidities.[58] Patients with IPF have higher perioperative complications and mortality when operated on with non–small cell lung cancer when their vital capacity is low.[59–62]

Patients with underlying IPF are at risk of developing an acute exacerbation after operation for lung cancer with rates varying from 7% to 27%[59,61,63,64] and mortality of 80% to 100% if an exacerbation occurs.[59,63,64] It is unclear what causes postoperative acute exacerbations, although trauma caused by mechanical ventilation has been suggested by evidence that the nonoperative lung shows more radiographic evidence of injury, likely from overdistention during single lung ventilation.[65] Patients with a composite physiologic index score of greater than 40 (see calculation in **Box 3**) have a 50% chance of developing ARDS/acute lung injury, which in current literature is best classified as AE-IPF.[64]

Box 3
Composite physiologic index

$$91 - (0.65 \times \%\ predicted\ D_{LCO}) - (0.53 \times \%\ predicted\ FVC) + (0.34 \times \%\ predicted\ FEV_1)$$

Abbreviations: DLCO, diffusion capacity of lung for carbon monoxide; FEV_1, forced expiratory volume in 1 second; FVC, forced vital capacity.
Data from Wells AU, Desai SR, Rubens MB, et al. Idiopathic pulmonary fibrosis: a composite physiologic index derived from disease extent observed by computed tomography. Am J Respir Crit Care Med 2003;167(7):962–9.

Similar to ARDS[27] a restrictive fluid strategy has been associated with decreased risk of perioperative lung injury in patients with IPF undergoing resection for lung cancer, and minimization of perioperative fluid administration is advised.[63]

Open lung biopsy for diagnosis of interstitial lung disease

Biopsy to determine underlying histopathology is, at times, needed to establish underlying histopathology in the undifferentiated ILD.[66] It is not known what threshold of impairment in PFTs should prohibit diagnostic open lung biopsy, and evaluation should be made on a case-to-case basis.[32]

Similar to pulmonary operations for lung cancer, AE-IPF has been reported.[65,67] Lung biopsy for patients with undifferentiated ILD has low mortality at 5% or less.[67–70] Park and colleagues[67] demonstrated performing biopsies in the midst of an AE-IPF had a particularly poor outcome with mortality of 28% compared with those with stable IPF, which had a mortality of 3%. Others have reported high rates of mortality when UIP is found, although the indication for many biopsies in this particular study was acute worsening of symptoms and therefore possibly in the midst of an acute exacerbation.[71] In one series, all patients who expired after surgery had DAD superimposed on UIP on autopsy, which is the pathologic finding of AE-IPF, suggesting that these patients has sustained an AE-IPF before surgery.[70] In sum, surgical lung biopsy in patients with stable respiratory function has low mortality, although those in AE-IPF or with worsening physiology likely have a much higher operative mortality.

NEW DIAGNOSIS OF INTERSTITIAL LUNG DISEASE IN THE INTENSIVE CARE UNIT

Often, ILD is known at the time of admission to the ICU. However, if the patient does not receive regular medical care, ILD may not be known at the time of admission. Alternatively, patients may present with acute exacerbation of underlying subclinical disease.[72] Additionally, acute reactions to medications or inhaled substances can induce ILD.

ILD is difficult to accurately diagnose, even for physicians trained in pulmonary medicine in a non-emergent context.[73] Added difficulty is encountered in determining a new diagnosis of ILD in patients admitted to the ICU, because many of the radiologic findings (ground glass opacities), physical examination findings (rales), and clinical syndromes (respiratory failure) overlap with other more common scenarios, such as lower respiratory tract infection or congestive heart failure. Findings used to differentiate underlying ILD from an acute syndrome are listed in **Box 4**. Attention to clinical scenarios that may predispose a patient to ILD are listed in **Box 5**.

In patients in whom ILD is suspected, consultation with a pulmonologist familiar with ILD is recommended. Diagnostic accuracy improves if the patient is evaluated by radiology, pathology, and pulmonary clinicians familiar with ILD.[73] If high-resolution CT imaging is classic for UIP, the underlying histopathology of IPF, lung biopsy is not required.[32] A surgical lung biopsy may be needed to determine the underlying pathology if a diagnosis cannot be reached clinically.[66]

It is particularly critical to identify and exclude certain diagnoses in the differential of undiagnosed ILD. Acute hypersensitivity pneumonitis and drug reactions, and ILD "mimics" acute eosinophilic pneumonia and diffuse alveolar hemorrhage, are important to identify because of their sensitivity to steroids, and possibly need for higher (500–1000 mg/day methylprednisolone) steroid dosages. Classically, hypersensitivity pneumonitis

---

Box 5
Predisposition to ILD

- Rheumatologic diagnosis
  - Scleroderma
  - Rheumatoid arthritis
  - Polymyositis/dermatomyositis
  - Sjögren syndrome
- Exposure to
  - Chemotherapy
  - Amioderone
  - Chronic nitrofurantoin
  - Sulfasalazine
  - Bird antigens (hypersensitivity pneumonitis)
  - Molds or hay (hypersensitivity pneumonitis)
  - Prior occupational exposure (eg, asbestos)
  - Other suspicious medications (a list can be found at www.pneumotox.com)

---

is thought of as an exuberant immune reaction to an inhaled protein (eg, bird antigens, mold, baker's yeast), often occupationally. A full discussion of hypersensitivity pneumonitis is outside the scope of this article, but was recently reviewed.[74]

PULMONARY HYPERTENSION

Because of parenchymal destruction, hypoxia, and shared molecular pathogenic mechanisms, pulmonary arterial hypertension can complicate ILD.[75,76] The degree to which pulmonary arterial hypertension impacts patients with ILD admitted to the ICU is unclear. Patients with signs of right ventricular heart failure should obviously be evaluated for pulmonary arterial hypertension. Transthoracic echocardiogram is the preferred first test, and can show signs of right ventricular overload, although it may not be completely sensitive or specific for pulmonary arterial hypertension,[75,76] especially if poor acoustic windows are encountered, such as with patients on IMV.

Pulmonary hypertension in patients with ILD admitted to the ICU, as diagnosed by echocardiogram, has been shown to be a poor prognostic indicator.[77] That being said, none of the patients in this study required treatment with vasoactive agents directed toward the pulmonary vasculature.[77] New-onset right ventricular embarrassment should prompt evaluation of left ventricular systolic or diastolic dysfunction or pulmonary embolus. Should the patient have signs of right

---

Box 4
Clues toward ILD

- Structural destruction of underlying pulmonary anatomy on CT scan (honeycombing, traction bronchiectasis, upper to middle lobe band scarring of stage 4 pulmonary sarcoid)
- Persistence and progression of imaging abnormality, if previous images are available
- Velcro rales persistent for several months or rales without clinical heart failure or infection
- Subacute to chronic worsening of exertional capacity

ventricular failure not caused by left ventricular dysfunction, pharmacologic agents directed toward the pulmonary vasculature can be considered if refractory to volume management and oxygen supplementation, although this is not evidence-based[75] and is not reported in the literature.

EXTRACORPOREAL LIFE SUPPORT

Extracorporeal life support (ECLS) has been used with success in patients with reversible pulmonary or cardiopulmonary failure, such as ARDS.[78] Use of ECLS as a bridge to recovery for patients with acute exacerbation of ILD, to our knowledge, has not been reported.

Venovenous ECLS support in patients with isolated respiratory failure allows for minimization or elimination of sedation, ability to exercise and therefore maintain musculoskeletal fitness, and concomitant support of severe hypoxemic or hypercarbic pulmonary failure.[79,80] Venoarterial ECLS can be used in patients with both cardiac and pulmonary failure, as opposed to isolated pulmonary failure. Both venovenous and venoarterial ECLS have been used as a support for ILD as a bridge to lung transplant.[79–84]

In our opinion, ECLS for patients with ILD should only be used if respiratory failure is believed to be reversible or if the patient is being evaluated for pulmonary transplant. Use of ECLS for a patient not previously evaluated for pulmonary transplant may be difficult because of the logistics of diagnostics needed before transplant listing and the questionable ability to obtain prior true informed consent to this life-altering therapy, although this has been reported with successful outcomes.[83] ECLS should not be used for AE-IPF if the patient is not a candidate for lung transplant because of the high morbidity and lack of effective therapeutic options.

LUNG TRANSPLANT

Pulmonary transplantation is a viable treatment of patients with ILD and irreversible respiratory failure without other significant nonpulmonary organ failure, chronic untreatable infectious disease, advanced age, and who are neither underweight nor overweight.[85] Mechanical ventilation and ECLS are no longer considered absolute contraindications to pulmonary transplantation. If no contraindications exist, consideration of transfer to a transplant center for evaluation is advised.

SUMMARY

ILD is a challenging entity when encountered in the ICU. Often alteration of ventilatory strategies is needed to combat poor compliance and gas exchange. Exclusion of reversible causes of respiratory failure while administering supportive care are the bedrocks of treating patients with ILD admitted with respiratory failure.

For patients with suspected undiagnosed ILD, evaluation by an experienced pulmonologist, review of previous imaging, detailed medication and occupational history, and consideration of surgical lung biopsy is recommended.

If an exacerbation syndrome is identified, corticosteroids are advised. AE-IPF has abysmal outcomes and the utility of supporting these patients in the ICU has been debated. Exacerbations can be provoked by diagnostic or therapeutic surgical procedures.

Despite these challenges, mortality for patients with ILD admitted to the ICU is not absolute. Additionally, even short-term recovery can provide a window for a life-saving transplantation in appropriate patients with ILD.[9]

REFERENCES

1. Olson AL, Swigris JJ, Lezotte DC, et al. Mortality from pulmonary fibrosis increased in the United States from 1992 to 2003. Am J Respir Crit Care Med 2007;176(3):277–84.
2. Demedts M, Wells AU, Antó JM, et al. Interstitial lung diseases: an epidemiological overview. Eur Respir J Suppl 2001;32:2s–16s.
3. Coultas DB, Zumwalt RE, Black WC, et al. The epidemiology of interstitial lung diseases. Am J Respir Crit Care Med 1994;150(4):967–72.
4. Centers for Disease Control and Prevention (CDC). Chronic obstructive pulmonary disease among adults—United States, 2011. MMWR Morb Mortal Wkly Rep 2012;61(46):938–43.
5. Hunninghake GM, Hatabu H, Okajima Y, et al. MUC5B promoter polymorphism and interstitial lung abnormalities. N Engl J Med 2013;368(23):2192–200.
6. Martinez FJ, Flaherty K. Pulmonary function testing in idiopathic interstitial pneumonias. Proc Am Thorac Soc 2006;3(4):315–21.
7. Fernandez-Perez ER, Yilmaz M, Jenad H, et al. Ventilator settings and outcome of respiratory failure in chronic interstitial lung disease. Chest 2008;133(5):1113–9.
8. Blivet S, Philit F, Sab JM, et al. Outcome of patients with idiopathic pulmonary fibrosis admitted to the ICU for respiratory failure. Chest 2001;120(1):209–12.
9. Gaudry S, Vincent F, Rabbat A, et al. Invasive mechanical ventilation in patients with fibrosing interstitial pneumonia. J Thorac Cardiovasc Surg 2014;147(1):47–53.

10. Saydain G, Islam A, Afessa B, et al. Outcome of patients with idiopathic pulmonary fibrosis admitted to the intensive care unit. Am J Respir Crit Care Med 2002;166(6):839–42.

11. Stern JB, Mal H, Groussard O, et al. Prognosis of patients with advanced idiopathic pulmonary fibrosis requiring mechanical ventilation for acute respiratory failure. Chest 2001;120(1):213–9.

12. Mallick S. Outcome of patients with idiopathic pulmonary fibrosis (IPF) ventilated in intensive care unit. Respir Med 2008;102(10):1355–9.

13. Vial-Dupuy A, Sanchez O, Douvry Et Al B, et al. Outcome of patients with interstitial lung disease admitted to the intensive care unit. Sarcoidosis Vasc Diffuse Lung Dis 2013;30(2):134–42.

14. Vianello A, Arcaro G, Battistella L, et al. Noninvasive ventilation in the event of acute respiratory failure in patients with idiopathic pulmonary fibrosis. J Crit Care 2014;29(4):562–7.

15. Yokoyama T, Kondoh Y, Taniguchi H, et al. Noninvasive ventilation in acute exacerbation of idiopathic pulmonary fibrosis. Intern Med 2010; 49(15):1509–14.

16. Tomii K, Tachikawa R, Chin K, et al. Role of non-invasive ventilation in managing life-threatening acute exacerbation of interstitial pneumonia. Intern Med 2010;49(14):1341–7.

17. Gungor G, Tatar D, Saltürk C, et al. Why do patients with interstitial lung diseases fail in the ICU? a 2-center cohort study. Respir Care 2013;58(3):525–31.

18. Sztrymf B, Messika J, Mayot T, et al. Impact of high-flow nasal cannula oxygen therapy on intensive care unit patients with acute respiratory failure: a prospective observational study. J Crit Care 2012; 27(3):324.e9–13.

19. Roca O, de Acilu MG, Caralt B, et al. Humidified high flow nasal cannula supportive therapy improves outcomes in lung transplant recipients readmitted to the intensive care unit because of acute respiratory failure. Transplantation 2015;99(5): 1092–8.

20. Messika J, Ben Ahmed K, Gaudry S, et al. Use of high-flow nasal cannula oxygen therapy in subjects with ARDS: a 1-year observational study. Respir Care 2015;60(2):162–9.

21. Roca O, Riera J, Torres F, et al. High-flow oxygen therapy in acute respiratory failure. Respir Care 2010;55(4):408–13.

22. El-Khatib MF. High-flow nasal cannula oxygen therapy during hypoxemic respiratory failure. Respir Care 2012;57(10):1696–8.

23. Braunlich J, Beyer D, Mai D, et al. Effects of nasal high flow on ventilation in volunteers, COPD and idiopathic pulmonary fibrosis patients. Respiration 2013;85(4):319–25.

24. Boyer A, Vargas F, Delacre M, et al. Prognostic impact of high-flow nasal cannula oxygen supply in an ICU patient with pulmonary fibrosis complicated by acute respiratory failure. Intensive Care Med 2011;37(3):558–9.

25. Yang KL, Tobin MJ. A prospective study of indexes predicting the outcome of trials of weaning from mechanical ventilation. N Engl J Med 1991;324(21): 1445–50.

26. The acute respiratory distress syndrome Network. Ventilation with lower tidal volumes as compared with traditional tidal volumes for acute lung injury and the acute respiratory distress syndrome. N Engl J Med 2000;342(18):1301–8.

27. National Heart, Lung, and Blood Institute Acute Respiratory Distress Syndrome (ARDS) Clinical Trials Network, Wiedemann HP, Wheeler AP, et al. Comparison of two fluid-management strategies in acute lung injury. N Engl J Med 2006;354(24):2564–75.

28. Hyzy R, Huang S, Myers J, et al. Acute exacerbation of idiopathic pulmonary fibrosis. Chest 2007;132(5): 1652–8.

29. Collard HR, Moore BB, Flaherty KR, et al. Acute exacerbations of idiopathic pulmonary fibrosis. Am J Respir Crit Care Med 2007;176(7):636–43.

30. Park IN, Kim DS, Shim TS, et al. Acute exacerbation of interstitial pneumonia other than idiopathic pulmonary fibrosis. Chest 2007;132(1):214–20.

31. Suda T, Kaida Y, Nakamura Y, et al. Acute exacerbation of interstitial pneumonia associated with collagen vascular diseases. Respir Med 2009; 103(6):846–53.

32. Raghu G, Collard HR, Egan JJ, et al. An official ATS/ ERS/JRS/ALAT statement: idiopathic pulmonary fibrosis: evidence-based guidelines for diagnosis and management. Am J Respir Crit Care Med 2011;183(6):788–824.

33. Kondoh Y, Taniguchi H, Kawabata Y, et al. Acute exacerbation in idiopathic pulmonary fibrosis. Analysis of clinical and pathologic findings in three cases. Chest 1993;103(6):1808–12.

34. Azuma A, Nukiwa T, Tsuboi E, et al. Double-blind, placebo-controlled trial of pirfenidone in patients with idiopathic pulmonary fibrosis. Am J Respir Crit Care Med 2005;171(9):1040–7.

35. Idiopathic Pulmonary Fibrosis Clinical Research Network, Martinez FJ, de Andrade JA, et al. Randomized trial of acetylcysteine in idiopathic pulmonary fibrosis. N Engl J Med 2014;370(22):2093–101.

36. Richeldi L, du Bois RM, Raghu G, et al. Efficacy and safety of nintedanib in idiopathic pulmonary fibrosis. N Engl J Med 2014;370(22):2071–82.

37. Kim DS, Park JH, Park BK, et al. Acute exacerbation of idiopathic pulmonary fibrosis: frequency and clinical features. Eur Respir J 2006;27(1):143–50.

38. Sprunger DB, Olson AL, Huie TJ, et al. Pulmonary fibrosis is associated with an elevated risk of thromboembolic disease. Eur Respir J 2012;39(1): 125–32.

39. Song JW, Hong SB, Lim CM, et al. Acute exacerbation of idiopathic pulmonary fibrosis: incidence, risk factors and outcome. Eur Respir J 2011; 37(2):356–63.

40. Simon-Blancal V, Freynet O, Nunes H, et al. Acute exacerbation of idiopathic pulmonary fibrosis: outcome and prognostic factors. Respiration 2012; 83(1):28–35.

41. Okamoto T, Ichiyasu H, Ichikado K, et al. Clinical analysis of the acute exacerbation in patients with idiopathic pulmonary fibrosis. Nihon Kokyuki Gakkai Zasshi 2006;44(5):359–67 [in Japanese].

42. Ambrosini V, Cancellieri A, Chilosi M, et al. Acute exacerbation of idiopathic pulmonary fibrosis: report of a series. Eur Respir J 2003;22(5):821–6.

43. Parambil JG, Myers JL, Ryu JH. Histopathologic features and outcome of patients with acute exacerbation of idiopathic pulmonary fibrosis undergoing surgical lung biopsy. Chest 2005;128(5): 3310–5.

44. Inase N, Sawada M, Ohtani Y, et al. Cyclosporin A followed by the treatment of acute exacerbation of idiopathic pulmonary fibrosis with corticosteroid. Intern Med 2003;42(7):565–70.

45. Sakamoto S, Homma S, Miyamoto A, et al. Cyclosporin A in the treatment of acute exacerbation of idiopathic pulmonary fibrosis. Intern Med 2010; 49(2):109–15.

46. Homma S, Sakamoto S, Kawabata M, et al. Cyclosporin treatment in steroid-resistant and acutely exacerbated interstitial pneumonia. Intern Med 2005;44(11):1144–50.

47. Kubo H, Nakayama K, Yanai M, et al. Anticoagulant therapy for idiopathic pulmonary fibrosis. Chest 2005;128(3):1475–82.

48. Churg A, Müller NL, Silva CI, et al. Acute exacerbation (acute lung injury of unknown cause) in UIP and other forms of fibrotic interstitial pneumonias. Am J Surg Pathol 2007;31(2):277–84.

49. Tachikawa R, Tomii K, Ueda H, et al. Clinical features and outcome of acute exacerbation of interstitial pneumonia: collagen vascular diseases-related versus idiopathic. Respiration 2012;83(1):20–7.

50. Qaseem A, Snow V, Fitterman N, et al. Risk assessment for and strategies to reduce perioperative pulmonary complications for patients undergoing noncardiothoracic surgery: a guideline from the American College of Physicians. Ann Intern Med 2006;144(8):575–80.

51. Bapoje SR, Whitaker JF, Schulz T, et al. Preoperative evaluation of the patient with pulmonary disease. Chest 2007;132(5):1637–45.

52. Ghatol A, Ruhl AP, Danoff SK. Exacerbations in idiopathic pulmonary fibrosis triggered by pulmonary and nonpulmonary surgery: a case series and comprehensive review of the literature. Lung 2012; 190(4):373–80.

53. Futier E, Constantin JM, Paugam-Burtz C, et al. A trial of intraoperative low-tidal-volume ventilation in abdominal surgery. N Engl J Med 2013;369(5): 428–37.

54. Le Jeune I, Gribbin J, West J, et al. The incidence of cancer in patients with idiopathic pulmonary fibrosis and sarcoidosis in the UK. Respir Med 2007; 101(12):2534–40.

55. Park J, Kim DS, Shim TS, et al. Lung cancer in patients with idiopathic pulmonary fibrosis. Eur Respir J 2001;17(6):1216–9.

56. Martinod E, Azorin JF, Sadoun D, et al. Surgical resection of lung cancer in patients with underlying interstitial lung disease. Ann Thorac Surg 2002; 74(4):1004–7.

57. Brunelli A, Kim AW, Berger KI, et al. Physiologic evaluation of the patient with lung cancer being considered for resectional surgery: diagnosis and management of lung cancer, 3rd ed: American College of Chest Physicians evidence-based clinical practice guidelines. Chest 2013;143(5 Suppl): e166S–90S.

58. Carrillo G, Estrada A, Pedroza J, et al. Preoperative risk factors associated with mortality in lung biopsy patients with interstitial lung disease. J Invest Surg 2005;18(1):39–45.

59. Shintani Y, Ohta M, Iwasaki T, et al. Predictive factors for postoperative acute exacerbation of interstitial pneumonia combined with lung cancer. Gen Thorac Cardiovasc Surg 2010;58(4):182–5.

60. Kawasaki H, Nagai K, Yoshida J, et al. Postoperative morbidity, mortality, and survival in lung cancer associated with idiopathic pulmonary fibrosis. J Surg Oncol 2002;81(1):33–7.

61. Kushibe K, Kawaguchi T, Takahama M, et al. Operative indications for lung cancer with idiopathic pulmonary fibrosis. Thorac Cardiovasc Surg 2007; 55(8):505–8.

62. Watanabe A, Higami T, Ohori S, et al. Is lung cancer resection indicated in patients with idiopathic pulmonary fibrosis? J Thorac Cardiovasc Surg 2008; 136(5):1357–63, 1363.e1–2.

63. Mizuno Y, Iwata H, Shirahashi K, et al. The importance of intraoperative fluid balance for the prevention of postoperative acute exacerbation of idiopathic pulmonary fibrosis after pulmonary resection for primary lung cancer. Eur J Cardiothorac Surg 2012;41(6):e161–5.

64. Kumar P, Goldstraw P, Yamada K, et al. Pulmonary fibrosis and lung cancer: risk and benefit analysis of pulmonary resection. J Thorac Cardiovasc Surg 2003;125(6):1321–7.

65. Kondoh Y, Taniguchi H, Kitaichi M, et al. Acute exacerbation of interstitial pneumonia following surgical lung biopsy. Respir Med 2006;100(10):1753–9.

66. American Thoracic Society, European Respiratory Society. American Thoracic Society/European

Respiratory Society International Multidisciplinary Consensus Classification of the Idiopathic Interstitial Pneumonias. This joint statement of the American Thoracic Society (ATS), and the European Respiratory Society (ERS) was adopted by the ATS board of directors, June 2001 and by the ERS Executive Committee, June 2001. Am J Respir Crit Care Med 2002;165(2):277–304.

67. Park JH, Kim DK, Kim DS, et al. Mortality and risk factors for surgical lung biopsy in patients with idiopathic interstitial pneumonia. Eur J Cardiothorac Surg 2007;31(6):1115–9.

68. Ayed AK, Raghunathan R. Thoracoscopy versus open lung biopsy in the diagnosis of interstitial lung disease: a randomised controlled trial. J R Coll Surg Edinb 2000;45(3):159–63.

69. Gaensler EA, Carrington CB. Open biopsy for chronic diffuse infiltrative lung disease: clinical, roentgenographic, and physiological correlations in 502 patients. Ann Thorac Surg 1980;30(5):411–26.

70. Tiitto L, Heiskanen U, Bloigu R, et al. Thoracoscopic lung biopsy is a safe procedure in diagnosing usual interstitial pneumonia. Chest 2005;128(4):2375–80.

71. Utz JP, Ryu JH, Douglas WW, et al. High short-term mortality following lung biopsy for usual interstitial pneumonia. Eur Respir J 2001;17(2):175–9.

72. Sakamoto K, Taniguchi H, Kondoh Y, et al. Acute exacerbation of idiopathic pulmonary fibrosis as the initial presentation of the disease. Eur Respir Rev 2009;18(112):129–32.

73. Flaherty KR, Andrei AC, King TE Jr, et al. Idiopathic interstitial pneumonia: do community and academic physicians agree on diagnosis? Am J Respir Crit Care Med 2007;175(10):1054–60.

74. Selman M, Pardo A, King TE Jr. Hypersensitivity pneumonitis: insights in diagnosis and pathobiology. Am J Respir Crit Care Med 2012;186(4):314–24.

75. Behr J, Ryu JH. Pulmonary hypertension in interstitial lung disease. Eur Respir J 2008;31(6):1357–67.

76. Caminati A, Cassandro R, Harari S. Pulmonary hypertension in chronic interstitial lung diseases. Eur Respir Rev 2013;22(129):292–301.

77. Zafrani L, Lemiale V, Lapidus N, et al. Acute respiratory failure in critically ill patients with interstitial lung disease. PLoS One 2014;9(8): e104897.

78. Peek GJ, Mugford M, Tiruvoipati R, et al. Efficacy and economic assessment of conventional ventilatory support versus extracorporeal membrane oxygenation for severe adult respiratory failure (CESAR): a multicentre randomised controlled trial. Lancet 2009;374(9698):1351–63.

79. Javidfar J, Brodie D, Iribarne A, et al. Extracorporeal membrane oxygenation as a bridge to lung transplantation and recovery. J Thorac Cardiovasc Surg 2012;144(3):716–21.

80. Nosotti M, Rosso L, Tosi D, et al. Extracorporeal membrane oxygenation with spontaneous breathing as a bridge to lung transplantation. Interact Cardiovasc Thorac Surg 2013;16(1):55–9.

81. Bermudez CA, Rocha RV, Zaldonis D, et al. Extracorporeal membrane oxygenation as a bridge to lung transplant: midterm outcomes. Ann Thorac Surg 2011;92(4):1226–31 [discussion: 1231–2].

82. Toyoda Y, Bhama JK, Shigemura N, et al. Efficacy of extracorporeal membrane oxygenation as a bridge to lung transplantation. J Thorac Cardiovasc Surg 2013;145(4):1065–70 [discussion: 1070–1].

83. Hoopes CW, Kukreja J, Golden J, et al. Extracorporeal membrane oxygenation as a bridge to pulmonary transplantation. J Thorac Cardiovasc Surg 2013;145(3):862–7 [discussion: 867–8].

84. Lang G, Taghavi S, Aigner C, et al. Primary lung transplantation after bridge with extracorporeal membrane oxygenation: a plea for a shift in our paradigms for indications. Transplantation 2012;93(7): 729–36.

85. Orens JB, Estenne M, Arcasoy S, et al. International guidelines for the selection of lung transplant candidates: 2006 update–a consensus report from the Pulmonary Scientific Council of the International Society for Heart and Lung Transplantation. J Heart Lung Transplant 2006;25(7): 745–55.

Management of Right Heart Failure in the Intensive Care Unit

Cyrus A. Kholdani, MD, Wassim H. Fares, MD, MSc*

KEYWORDS

- Right heart failure (RHF) • Right ventricular failure (RVF) • Pulmonary arterial hypertension (PAH)
- Pulmonary hypertension (PH) • Pulmonary vasodilators • Atrial septostomy • Potts shunt

KEY POINTS

- Right heart failure is a syndrome of multiple possible causes that can eventually result in circulatory failure and death.
- Hemodynamic support of a failing right ventricle must address its preload, contractile, and afterload states.
- Additional adjunctive support measures to optimize electromechanical coupling and ventilator support remain important interventions.
- Rescue interventions to offload a failing right ventricle continue to have a role in the management of this highly morbid syndrome.

INTRODUCTION

Right heart failure (RHF) is a clinical syndrome that arises from a disturbance of the right-sided circulatory system and results in elevated venous pressure and/or aberrant delivery of blood to the pulmonary circulation. It represents a pathologic disturbance of any component of the right heart circulatory system, which consists of the venous system up to the level of the pulmonary capillaries and, therefore, has both systemic (the systemic veins up to the level of the pulmonic valve) and pulmonary components (the precapillary pulmonary circulation).[1] Within this framework lies the more specific concept of right ventricular failure (RVF), which is often a major component of RHF. Conceptualized hemodynamically, RVF occurs at the point at which cardiac output (CO) and blood pressure drop despite an increased RV end-diastolic pressure (RVEDP).[2] It can be suspected when the right atrial pressure (RAP) to pulmonary artery occlusion pressure ratio is less than or equal

to 0.8 to 1, usually with a low cardiac index (CI).[3] Exacerbating this presentation is the negative impact of a failing, distended right ventricle (RV) on left ventricle (LV) function with further reduction of CO.[4] The RV may fail when subjected to pressure or volume overload, ischemia, intrinsic myocardial disease, or from pericardial limitation.[5]

DIAGNOSTIC CLUES

The classic physical examination findings in a patient in RVF include an elevated jugular venous pressure with a prominent v wave. On auscultation, one may note a prominent pulmonic component of the second heart sound and the holosystolic murmur of tricuspid regurgitation (TR). On palpation, one may note a right ventricular heave, hepatomegaly, ascites, and/or lower extremity edema. Although the pulmonary examination may point to underlying lung disease, the suggestion of pulmonary edema is not consistent with isolated RVF and suggests possibilities such

Pulmonary Vascular Disease Program, Pulmonary, Critical Care, & Sleep Medicine, Department of Internal Medicine, Yale School of Medicine, 15 York Street, LCI 105, New Haven, CT 06510, USA
* Corresponding author.
E-mail address: Wassim.Fares@yale.edu

Clin Chest Med 36 (2015) 511–520
http://dx.doi.org/10.1016/j.ccm.2015.05.015
0272-5231/15/$ – see front matter © 2015 Elsevier Inc. All rights reserved.

as left-sided heart disease or noncardiogenic causes.

Laboratory studies can help determine the underlying cause of RVF if it is indeed secondary to pulmonary arterial hypertension (PAH) with serologic markers of connective tissue disease, human immunodeficiency virus infection, and the viral hepatitides with concurrent assessment of liver function. Polycythemia, suggestive of chronic hypoxemia, can be associated with the World Health Organization Group 3 causes of pulmonary hypertension (PH), which can ultimately result in cor pulmonale. Both overdistension and ischemia of the RV predispose to elevations of cardiac enzymes and B-type or pro-B-type natriuretic peptide. Positive biomarkers are well-described in pulmonary embolism and confer greater mortality risk.[6,7]

Electrocardiography remains frequently used in the initial assessment of acute heart failure but is an insensitive test of PH, pulmonary embolism, or RVF. Nonetheless, one may see evidence of right axis deviation, an R:S wave of greater than 1 in V_1, an R wave greater than 0.5 mV in V_1 and electrocardiographic signs of right atrial enlargement (p pulmonale) with P wave amplitude greater than 2.5 mm in leads II, III, and aVF; or greater than 1.5 mm in V_1.[8] The qR pattern in lead V_1, in which one sees the negative deflection of a q wave immediately followed by an upward R wave, has also been associated with RV strain and adverse outcomes in patients presenting with acute pulmonary embolism.[9]

ASSESSMENT OF RIGHT HEART FAILURE

The management of RVF should be predicated on an assessment of the preload, the RV contractility, and the afterload. The preload stress of RV is intimately tied with the volume status of the patient (see later discussion) (**Fig. 1**).

When suspecting the clinical syndrome of RVF, an assessment of the contractile state is essential. The right ventricular ejection fraction (RVEF) is a commonly used index for this. Nonetheless, its value depends highly on the loading conditions of the RV and may not provide an accurate reflection of contractility.[10] The RV chamber size is larger than the LV's, rendering the RVEF less than its counterpart and ranges from 40% to 76% depending on the method of its analysis, with MRI and radionuclide angiography being the most accurate. Unfortunately, neither modality is practical for assessing a critically ill patient.

Although different than contractility, CO is a relevant clinical parameter and can be obtained with placement of a pulmonary artery catheter (PAC). Given the absence of improved outcomes data in favor of empiric placement of PACs in the critically ill, its use must be considered in the context of the information it provides and how that might alter management.[11] Furthermore, different techniques used to measure CO are not necessarily equivalent; there can be significant discrepancy between sequentially obtained Fick and thermodilution measurements of CO.[12] Echocardiography, conversely, is a noninvasive test

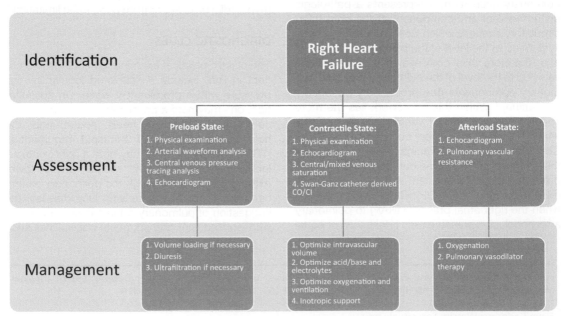

Fig. 1. Summarized assessment and management of the preload, contractile, and afterload states in the setting of right heart failure.

that can be performed at the bedside and provide crucial clinical and prognostic data in addition to its ability to demonstrate effects of therapeutic maneuvers. Tricuspid annular plane systolic excursion is an echocardiographic-derived variable that can serve as a quantitative crude measure of RV systolic performance.[13] Other echocardiographic findings that can help guide therapy include distortion of the short-axis view of the LV with either flattening or even reversal of the interventricular septum curvature during systole or diastole that may signify pressure or volume overload respectively.[14]

Assessing RV afterload is complicated by the challenges of determining the pulmonary input impedance.[15] Simplified, this parameter is composed of the pulmonary arterial compliance, inductance, and pulmonary vascular resistance (PVR). The pulmonary artery compliance is based on the elastic properties of the pulmonary circulation and is defined as the change in volume for a given change in pressure. The compliance of the pulmonary vasculature determines how the ejected load of the RV is buffered and can be approximated as the ratio of the stroke volume to the pulse pressure.[16] The inductance, a dynamic property, is the response of the vasculature to changes in blood flow. The PVR is defined as the mean reduction in pressure between the main pulmonary artery and the left atrium divided by the CO. Clinically, it is the most straightforward of the aforementioned parameters to measure and generally depends on the resistance conferred by small vessels.

In addition to tachycardia, the initial response of the RV to an acute increase in afterload stress will be rapid augmentation of its contractile state to improve stroke volume, also known as homeometric autoregulation or the Anrep effect.[17] Although initially accomplished through altered cellular calcium dynamics, it is perpetuated by neurohormonal activation.[18] The initial increase in PA pressures is well-tolerated in a normal ventricle. Further rise of the PVR results in heterometric autoregulation with RV dilatation. It is beyond this point when continued elevation of the PVR can result in hemodynamic collapse and cardiac arrest.[19] Consequently, promptly assessing afterload stress is vital to the management of RVF because decompensation can occur precipitously.

MANAGEMENT
Intravascular Volume Management

Assessing the preload state of the RV is intimately tied with intravascular volume management. Traditionally, the management of hypotension was volume expansion. Human studies using fluid challenges demonstrate that the normal RV output depends on preload.[20] With excessive volume loading, however, myocardial distension will result in increased wall tension and, in keeping with the Frank-Starling mechanism, leads to disadvantageous stretching of muscle fibers that culminates in ventricular function failure. This scenario is of particular importance in the setting of PH when there may already be a basal component of RVF. Patients with PH who have an elevated plasma volume, who also have higher RAPs, have worse outcomes.[21] Prompt identification of RV volume overload is crucial in the management of RVF.

Although there is no definitive single test to prove volume overload, there are several findings that are suggestive. The analogous findings of a rising V-wave on a central venous pressure (CVP) tracing or worsening TR on echocardiography may herald worsening volume overload.[22] Echocardiographic evidence of an increased right ventricular dimension index and paradoxic septal motion during diastole are classic, albeit nonspecific, findings consistent with volume overload.[23] With progressive RV dilatation there will be progressive shifting of the interventricular septum and worsening TR that will reduce LV preload and thus CO.

Vasoactive Support

When using vasoactive agents in the management of RVF there are several key principles that inform their use (**Box 1**). The primary goal of vasoactive support in the management of RVF is the maintenance of adequate perfusion, including RV perfusion. The driving pressure for coronary perfusion is the difference between the aortic root pressure and the intraventricular pressure of the ventricle. For the LV, the aortic root pressure will not exceed the intraventricular pressure in early systole and, consequently, the chamber receives its coronary flow primarily during diastole. In contrast, the normal RV has intraventricular pressures consistently below that of the aortic root and thus is perfused throughout the cardiac cycle. This pressure gradient will decrease as pulmonary artery pressure (PAP) and thus PVR rise.[24] In acute PH, the increased RVEDP can ultimately result in right coronary blood flow occurring solely during systole due to the altered pressure gradient between the aorta and RV.[2] This switch heralds the onset of RV ischemia, which portends imminent hemodynamic collapse.[2,25] Therefore, vasoactive agents that maintain an adequate aortic root pressure help maximize RV function through maintenance of its normal pattern of perfusion.

Box 1
Vasoactive agents in right heart failure

Vasopressors:

Norepinephrine[a]

Vasopressin

Phenylephrine

Epinephrine[a]

Dopamine[a]

Inotropes:

Dobutamine

Milrinone

Pulmonary vasodilators:

Inhaled nitric oxide

Epoprostenol

Treprostinil

Sildenafil

[a] Additional inotropic properties.

Vasoactive agents that lower the ratio of the PVR to the systemic vascular resistance (SVR) favor adequate perfusion without excessively adding to the burden of RV afterload.

The sympathomimetic vasopressors

The sympathomimetic vasopressors, norepinephrine (NE) and phenylephrine, have variable effects on both the pulmonary and systemic circulations. These 2 agents have varied dose-related effects on both α- and β-adrenergic receptors in chronic PH.[26] NE stimulates both the $\alpha1$ and $\beta1$ receptors and, through them, exerts its systemic vasopressor and inotropic or chronotropic effects, respectively. Although stimulation of the $\alpha1$ receptor can lead to pulmonary vascular vasoconstriction, an actual increase in the PVR is only likely to occur at higher doses with data from animal studies only demonstrating this phenomenon at doses above 0.5 μg/kg/min.[27] In chronic PH, NE decreases the PVR/SVR ratio.[26] Importantly, through its inotropic actions, NE can result in improved RV performance and the improved CO may be present without any concurrent increase in PVR.[28]

Phenylephrine acts solely through direct stimulation of the α-receptor. When used in RVF, phenylephrine has been shown to improve RV myocardial perfusion.[2] However, this effect is at the expense of increased PAP and thus PVR with decreased RV performance.[26,29] In patients with clinically significant PH, the use of phenylephrine should generally be avoided.

Vasopressin

Vasopressin, a nonsympathomimetic vasoconstrictor, functions through stimulation of V1 receptor. Through a nitric oxide–dependent mechanism, vasopressin's stimulation of the V1 receptor can also result in a PVR reduction.[30,31] In the process, vasopressin can help reduce the PVR/SVR ratio.[32] When inodilator therapy results in systemic hypotension, vasopressin can be used as an adjunctive therapy to raise SVR without having an effect on the CO.[33] Whereas doses in animal models in significant excess of what is prescribed clinically can result in an increase in PVR, decreased RV performance, and possibly bradycardia, vasopressin maintains a favorable hemodynamic profile in RVF.[34,35] Doses in excess of 0.08 U/min can potentially have a detrimental effect on the CO.[36]

Dopamine

Dopamine, a sympathomimetic inotrope and catecholamine, can act through stimulation of the D1, $\alpha1$- and $\beta1$-receptors with variable regional and systemic hemodynamic effects. In patients with PH, dopamine will increase the CO but with tachycardia as a frequent side effect.[37] In animal models, when administered at doses less than or equal to 10 μg/kg/min, dopamine does not increase the PVR.[38] Compared with NE in the treatment of shock, however, it was associated with more adverse events, particularly tachyarrhythmia, and an increased frequency of death among the subset with cardiogenic shock in a large multicenter, randomized trial.[39]

Epinephrine

Epinephrine, a potent $\beta1$-agonist that also stimulates the $\beta2$- and $\alpha1$-receptors, is poorly studied in the setting of PH. Epinephrine has a positive effect on RV output at the expense of an increased mean PAP (mPAP) and, in animal studies, a more favorable effect on the PVR/SVR relationship than dopamine has been noted.[40,41]

Inotropic therapy

The sympathomimetic inotrope dobutamine and the inodilator milrinone are both used in the treatment of congestive heart failure (CHF). Dobutamine stimulates the $\beta1$-adrenergic receptor and improves myocardial contractility.[42] Compared with dopamine, it is less likely to cause tachyarrhythmia and, when administered at doses less than or equal to 5 ug/kg/min, can decrease the PVR.[27] Based on animal models of PH, however, doses exceeding 10 μg/kg/min predispose to tachyarrhythmia, systemic hypotension, and worsening PVR.[43] When used in combination with inhaled nitric oxide, dobutamine infusion at a rate of 10 μg/kg/min resulted in an increased

CI, decreased PVR, and an improvement in gas transfer parameters.[44] Nonetheless, doses in excess of 5 to 7.5 µg/kg/min may necessitate concurrent use of a systemic vasoconstrictor to combat any reductions in SVR.

Milrinone, a bipyridine phosphodiesterase (PDE)-3 inhibitor, inhibits the degradation of cyclic adenosine monophosphate with an eventual increase in intracellular calcium influx to improve myocyte contractility while serving as a vasodilator.[45] In animal models of chronic PH, milrinone improves RV function and reduces PVR.[46] RVF is a relatively common complication of end-stage CHF and can be present in 20% to 40% of patients undergoing left ventricular assist device (LVAD) placement, with milrinone having beneficial effects on RV function, pulmonary hemodynamics, and LVAD flow.[47] Given its vasodilator properties, milrinone often needs to be paired with a vasopressor, with vasopressin having a more favorable effect on the PVR/SVR than NE.[48] Nebulized milrinone, which is not approved by the Food and Drug Administration (FDA), also has a potential role in the treatment of RVF.[49]

Levosimendan functions through the inhibition of PDE3 and sensitization of troponin-C to calcium. It has demonstrated an ability to reduce the PVR while increasing RV efficiency.[50,51] Because it does not have FDA approval in the United States, its use is limited.

Pulmonary Vasodilators

When increases in PVR ultimately result in CO impairment, it is crucial to use pulmonary vasodilator therapy to interrupt a vicious cycle. The decreased CO and systemic hypotension beget not only acidosis and desaturation of mixed venous blood but also reduced RV perfusion and progressive reduction in CO. Pulmonary vasodilators reduce RV afterload and increase RV stroke volume while minimizing the deleterious effects of systemic hypotension and hypoxemia. These agents include prostanoids, endothelin receptor antagonists, or mediators of cyclic guanosine monophosphate (including PDE5 inhibitors or guanylate cyclase stimulators). Although all of these classes have developed well-described roles in the management of chronic PAH, their use in the management of acute RVF is more limited in both scope and available data.

Inhaled nitric oxide

Inhaled nitric oxide (iNO) is a potent vasodilator with a short half-life secondary to its prompt inactivation by hemoglobin that, consequently, minimizes any effects beyond the pulmonary vasculature and mandates its continuous administration.[52] In patients with PH and acute pulmonary embolism, iNO has been shown to rapidly reduce PVR, thereby improving the RVEF.[53,54] Furthermore, iNO has additive effects on pulmonary hemodynamics when combined with epoprostenol.[55] Prolonged use of iNO is associated with a dose-dependent development of methemoglobinemia.[56] Withdrawal ought to be done carefully given the risk of rebound RV dysfunction, an effect that can be potentially assuaged with use of PDE5 inhibitors.[57]

Prostanoid analogue therapy

Prostanoid analogues include prostacyclin (epoprostenol), its related analogue (iloprost), treprostinil, and prostaglandin-E_1. In chronic PAH, intravenous epoprostenol, compared with conventional therapy, reduces mortality while improving CO and pulmonary hemodynamics.[58] It is limited by its 3 to 6 minute half-life and dose-dependent side effects, which includes systemic hypotension. Use of intravenous epoprostenol in the acute setting has been described primarily in cardiac surgery patients. In such clinical circumstances, intravenous epoprostenol shows effective acute PVR reduction.[59] Among patients with acute respiratory distress syndrome (ARDS), inhaled epoprostenol has similar effects on hemodynamics and gas transfer as iNO.[60] Although not FDA-approved, inhaled epoprostenol use in RVF reduces mPAP without altering the systemic mean arterial pressure.[61] In patients undergoing heart or lung transplantation, inhaled epoprostenol demonstrated similar reductions in mPAP and CVP with comparable improvements in CI compared with iNO.[62] As is the case with iNO, abrupt discontinuation of any prostanoid analogue, including epoprostenol, carries the risk of rebound PH and RVF.

Phosphodiesterase-5 inhibitors

Sildenafil is an FDA-approved PDE5 inhibitor with a potential role in the management of RVF.[63] Its efficacy is in part related to the reduced levels of endothelial nitric oxide and increased PDE5 expression in patients with PAH.[64,65] Although it has the theoretic possibility of systemic hypotension, sildenafil acutely reduces PVR and further augments the ability of iNO to do so as well.[66] Use of sildenafil also is supported by some potential theoretic advantages. PDE5 inhibition may mechanically improve RV contractility and improve myocardial perfusion.[65,67,68] Being available in intravenous form also makes it a good option for therapy in these critically ill RVF patients who often times may not be able to take pills.

SUMMARY OF VASOACTIVE SUPPORT

Vasoactive support in RHF should first focus on ensuring adequate perfusion with vasopressor support with NE being favored given its additional inotropic properties. Then RV function should be supported through both a reduction in PVR with a pulmonary vasculature selective agent and additional inotropic support as necessary.

Adjunctive Support

Hypoxemia may lead to pulmonary vasoconstriction and, therefore, increase RV afterload. Oxygen therapy has demonstrably reduced PVR and improved CI in subjects with all varieties of PH.[69] Consequently, oxygen therapy is an important component to the management of RVF.

Digitalis has been used for centuries as a treatment of CHF.[70] In cor pulmonale, however, it is not a recommended intervention.[71] When acutely used in the setting of RV dysfunction in the setting of PAH, however, digitalis can result in an increased CO with an improved neurohormonal profile.[72]

Maintenance of Sinus Rhythm

Sinus rhythm is of particular importance in the setting of RV dysfunction with its absence increasing the likelihood of an adverse outcome in cases of chronic RVF.[73] Retrospective studies in subjects with PAH or inoperable chronic thromboembolic PH demonstrated a higher risk of clinical deterioration in subjects who had supraventricular tachycardias (SVTs).[74] Of the observed SVTs, atrial fibrillation and atrial flutter were equally present and both were 4 times more common than atrioventricular nodal reentrant tachycardia. Restoration of sinus rhythm invariably resulted in clinical improvement.

Dyssynchrony of the RV is a potential sign of more severe dysfunction.[75] Pressure-overloaded myocytes will have prolonged action potential and contraction time, which will ultimately predispose to dyssynchronous ventricles, a state that will increase the RV wall stress.[76]

Ventilator Strategies

Given the intimate relationship between intrathoracic pressure and hemodynamics, ventilator strategies must be tailored in RHF. The deleterious effects of cyclic tidal ventilation and positive end-expiratory pressure on ventricular function are well-established.[77] PVR is determined by the cumulative tone of the alveolar and extra-alveolar, or parenchymal, vasculature. Classic physiologic teaching suggested that as the lung reaches total lung capacity (TLC), alveolar vessels lengthen and narrow, whereas extra-alveolar vessels widen. Whereas the former results in an increased PVR, the latter results in its reduction such that the net result on PVR as the lung approaches TLC cannot necessarily be predicted based on the volume of blood in the pulmonary circuit. Because lung volume increasingly exceeds functional residual capacity, there is progressive alveolar distension with alveolar vessel compression, thereby increasing the PVR.

Prospective studies evaluating the consequences of mechanical ventilation on RV function generally involve patients with ARDS. Doppler echocardiographic assessment of RV output impedance demonstrates cyclic changes in the setting of mechanical ventilation.[78] In vivo studies using live dogs have demonstrated that PVR is at relative high values at both low-lung volumes and high-lung volumes, resulting in a U-shaped relationship between tidal volume and PVR.[79] Consequently, the appropriate ventilator settings for a patient in RVF mimic those that are used for ARDS with 2 notable exceptions: avoidance of permissive hypercapnia and higher oxygen saturation goals.

Doppler echocardiographic studies demonstrate prompt pulmonary circulatory responses manifested as increases in the maximum systolic tricuspid pressure gradient to both acute increases in the P_{CO_2} and decreases in P_{O_2}.[80] Canine studies have demonstrated that inadequate oxygen delivery can result in decreasing contractility, depressed CO, and consequent coronary hypoperfusion, which perpetuate a cycle that can ultimately lead to cardiac arrest.[81] Consequently, it is important to avoid myocardial acidosis and the subsequent impairment of the effect of intracellular calcium on myocardial contractile proteins, leading to contractile impairment.[82]

Rescue Interventions

Atrial septostomy
Atrial septostomy was first described in a 22-year-old patient with PAH given the data suggesting that patients with PAH and patent foramen ovales (PFO) had better functional status than those without the shunt.[83] The PFO provides an offloading mechanism for the failing RV and can be safely generated through percutaneous interventions in experienced hands when appropriate patients are selected.[84] Despite generation of a shunt, there may be improved systemic oxygen delivery with improved RV function and CO.[85] Contraindications to atrial septostomy include impending death in the context of RVF, mean RAP greater

than 20 mm Hg, PVR greater than 15 Wood units, or a blood oxygen saturation of less than 90% on room air at rest. Even when appropriate candidates are selected, the short-term mortality rates after atrial septostomy can range from 15% to 23% at 1 month.[84] Furthermore, spontaneous closure of the generated shunt is possible.[84]

Potts shunt

In cases of severe PH with RVF when a septostomy would be poorly tolerated owing to massive right-to-left shunt physiology, a Potts shunt can be considered. Like atrial septostomy, a Potts shunt generates features that are characteristic of Eisenmenger syndrome. In this procedure, an anastomosis is generated between the left pulmonary artery and the descending aorta. In contrast to atrial septostomy, a Potts shunt will avoid exposing the brain and myocardium to desaturated blood and the risk of paradoxic emboli are only prone to affect the lower body. Transcatheter generation of a Potts shunt also offers the possibility of generating a pressure-restrictive shunt, which could potentially be closed later.[86]

SUMMARY

Despite improvements in the care of patients with RHF over the last 20 years, there still remains a paucity of robust studies demonstrating clear roles and mortality benefits for any particular intervention. Available data drawn from smaller human studies emphasize the importance of addressing the intravascular volume status, supporting RV contractility, and reducing the afterload when indicated. Simultaneous supportive care to address conditions that commonly afflict critically ill patients remains vital to the management of RHF. Nonetheless, the persistently high mortality and morbidity rates of RHF underscore the need for strong prospective studies.

REFERENCES

1. Mehra MR, Park MH, Landzberg MJ, et al. Right heart failure: toward a common language. Pulm Circ 2013;3(4):963–7.
2. Vlahakes GJ, Turley K, Hoffman JI. The pathophysiology of failure in acute right ventricular hypertension: hemodynamic and biochemical correlations. Circulation 1981;63(1):87–95.
3. Zochios V, Jones N. Acute right heart syndrome in the critically ill patient. Heart Lung Vessel 2014; 6(3):157–70.
4. Bemis CE, Serur JR, Borkenhagen D, et al. Influence of right ventricular filling pressure on left ventricular pressure and dimension. Circ Res 1974; 34(4):498–504.
5. Haddad F, Doyle R, Murphy DJ, et al. Right ventricular function in cardiovascular disease, part II: pathophysiology, clinical importance, and management of right ventricular failure. Circulation 2008;117(13): 1717–31.
6. Mehta NJ, Jani K, Khan IA. Clinical usefulness and prognostic value of elevated cardiac troponin I levels in acute pulmonary embolism. Am Heart J 2003;145(5):821–5.
7. La Vecchia L, Ottani F, Favero L, et al. Increased cardiac troponin I on admission predicts in-hospital mortality in acute pulmonary embolism. Heart 2004;90(6):633–7.
8. Murphy ML, Thenabadu PN, de Soyza N, et al. Reevaluation of electrocardiographic criteria for left, right and combined cardiac ventricular hypertrophy. Am J Cardiol 1984;53(8):1140–7.
9. Kucher N, Walpoth N, Wustmann K, et al. QR in V1– an ECG sign associated with right ventricular strain and adverse clinical outcome in pulmonary embolism. Eur Heart J 2003;24(12):1113–9.
10. Haddad F, Hunt SA, Rosenthal DN, et al. Right ventricular function in cardiovascular disease, part I: anatomy, physiology, aging, and functional assessment of the right ventricle. Circulation 2008; 117(11):1436–48.
11. Hadian M, Pinsky MR. Evidence-based review of the use of the pulmonary artery catheter: impact data and complications. Crit Care 2006;10:S8.
12. Fares WH, Blanchard SK, Stouffer GA, et al. Thermodilution and Fick cardiac outputs differ: impact on pulmonary hypertension evaluation. Can Respir J 2012;19(4):261–6.
13. Ueti OM, Camargo EE, Ueti Ade A, et al. Assessment of right ventricular function with Doppler echocardiographic indices derived from tricuspid annular motion: comparison with radionuclide angiography. Heart 2002;88(3):244–8.
14. Louie EK, Rich S, Levitsky S, et al. Doppler echocardiographic demonstration of the differential effects of right ventricular pressure and volume overload on left ventricular geometry and filling. J Am Coll Cardiol 1992;19(1):84–90.
15. Brimioulle S, Maggiorini M, Stephanazzi J, et al. Effects of low flow on pulmonary vascular flow-pressure curves and pulmonary vascular impedance. Cardiovasc Res 1999;42(1):183–92.
16. Segers P, Brimioulle S, Stergiopulos N, et al. Pulmonary arterial compliance in dogs and pigs: the three-element windkessel model revisited. Am J Physiol 1999;277(2 Pt 2):H725–31.
17. Pawlush DG, Musch TI, Moore RL. Ca2+-dependent heterometric and homeometric autoregulation in hypertrophied rat heart. Am J Physiol 1989;256(4 Pt 2): H1139–47.
18. Nootens M, Kaufmann E, Rector T, et al. Neurohormonal activation in patients with right ventricular

failure from pulmonary hypertension: relation to hemodynamic variables and endothelin levels. J Am Coll Cardiol 1995;26(7):1581–5.

19. Guyton AC, Lindsey AW, Gilluly JJ. The limits of right ventricular compensation following acute increase in pulmonary circulatory resistance. Circ Res 1954; 2(4):326–32.

20. Reuse C, Vincent JL, Pinsky MR. Measurements of right ventricular volumes during fluid challenge. Chest 1990;98(6):1450–4.

21. James KB, Stelmach K, Armstrong R, et al. Plasma volume and outcome in pulmonary hypertension. Tex Heart Inst J 2003;30(4):305–7.

22. Price LC, Wort SJ, Finney SJ, et al. Pulmonary vascular and right ventricular dysfunction in adult critical care: current and emerging options for management: a systematic literature review. Crit Care 2010;14(5):R169.

23. Tajik AJ, Gau GT, Ritter DG, et al. Echocardiographic pattern of right ventricular diastolic volume overload in children. Circulation 1972;46(1):36–43.

24. Lowensohn HS, Khouri EM, Gregg DE, et al. Phasic right coronary artery blood flow in conscious dogs with normal and elevated right ventricular pressures. Circ Res 1976;39(6):760–6.

25. Gold FL, Bache RJ. Transmural right ventricular blood flow during acute pulmonary artery hypertension in the sedated dog. Evidence for subendocardial ischemia despite residual vasodilator reserve. Circ Res 1982;51(2):196–204.

26. Kwak YL, Lee CS, Park YH, et al. The effect of phenylephrine and norepinephrine in patients with chronic pulmonary hypertension*. Anaesthesia 2002;57(1):9–14.

27. Kerbaul F, Rondelet B, Motte S, et al. Effects of norepinephrine and dobutamine on pressure load-induced right ventricular failure. Crit Care Med 2004;32(4):1035–40.

28. Ducas J, Duval D, Dasilva H, et al. Treatment of canine pulmonary hypertension: effects of norepinephrine and isoproterenol on pulmonary vascular pressure-flow characteristics. Circulation 1987; 75(1):235–42.

29. Rich S, Gubin S, Hart K. The effects of phenylephrine on right ventricular performance in patients with pulmonary hypertension. Chest 1990;98(5): 1102–6.

30. Eichinger MR, Walker BR. Enhanced pulmonary arterial dilation to arginine vasopressin in chronically hypoxic rats. Am J Physiol 1994;267(6 Pt 2): H2413–9.

31. Evora PR, Pearson PJ, Schaff HV. Arginine vasopressin induces endothelium-dependent vasodilatation of the pulmonary artery. V1-receptor-mediated production of nitric oxide. Chest 1993;103(4):1241–5.

32. Tayama E, Ueda T, Shojima T, et al. Arginine vasopressin is an ideal drug after cardiac surgery for the management of low systemic vascular resistant hypotension concomitant with pulmonary hypertension. Interact Cardiovasc Thorac Surg 2007;6(6): 715–9.

33. Gold J, Cullinane S, Chen J, et al. Vasopressin in the treatment of milrinone-induced hypotension in severe heart failure. Am J Cardiol 2000;85(4):506–8. A11.

34. Leather HA, Segers P, Berends N, et al. Effects of vasopressin on right ventricular function in an experimental model of acute pulmonary hypertension. Crit Care Med 2002;30(11):2548–52.

35. Varma S, Jaju BP, Bhargava KP. Mechanism of vasopressin-induced bradycardia in dogs. Circ Res 1969;24(6):787–92.

36. Migotto WH, Simeone F, Dahi H. Effects of vasopressin on hemodynamics in cardiogenic shock. Chest 2005;128(4):168s.

37. Holloway EL, Polumbo RA, Harrison DC. Acute circulatory effects of dopamine in patients with pulmonary hypertension. Br Heart J 1975;37(5):482–5.

38. Lejeune P, Naeije R, Leeman M, et al. Effects of dopamine and dobutamine on hyperoxic and hypoxic pulmonary vascular tone in dogs. Am Rev Respir Dis 1987;136(1):29–35.

39. De Backer D, Biston P, Devriendt J, et al. Comparison of dopamine and norepinephrine in the treatment of shock. N Engl J Med 2010;362(9):779–89.

40. Le Tulzo Y, Seguin P, Gacouin A, et al. Effects of epinephrine on right ventricular function in patients with severe septic shock and right ventricular failure: a preliminary descriptive study. Intensive Care Med 1997;23(6):664–70.

41. Barrington KJ, Finer NN, Chan WK. A blind, randomized comparison of the circulatory effects of dopamine and epinephrine infusions in the newborn piglet during normoxia and hypoxia. Crit Care Med 1995;23(4):740–8.

42. Leier CV, Webel J, Bush CA. The cardiovascular effects of the continuous infusion of dobutamine in patients with severe cardiac failure. Circulation 1977; 56(3):468–72.

43. Bradford KK, Deb B, Pearl RG. Combination therapy with inhaled nitric oxide and intravenous dobutamine during pulmonary hypertension in the rabbit. J Cardiovasc Pharmacol 2000;36(2):146–51.

44. Vizza CD, Rocca GD, Roma AD, et al. Acute hemodynamic effects of inhaled nitric oxide, dobutamine and a combination of the two in patients with mild to moderate secondary pulmonary hypertension. Crit Care 2001;5(6):355–61.

45. Honerjager P. Pharmacology of bipyridine phosphodiesterase III inhibitors. Am Heart J 1991;121(6 Pt 2):1939–44.

46. Chen EP, Bittner HB, Davis RD Jr, et al. Milrinone improves pulmonary hemodynamics and right ventricular function in chronic pulmonary hypertension. Ann Thorac Surg 1997;63(3):814–21.

47. Kihara S, Kawai A, Fukuda T, et al. Effects of milrinone for right ventricular failure after left ventricular assist device implantation. Heart Vessels 2002; 16(2):69–71.

48. Jeon Y, Ryu JH, Lim YJ, et al. Comparative hemodynamic effects of vasopressin and norepinephrine after milrinone-induced hypotension in off-pump coronary artery bypass surgical patients. Eur J Cardiothorac Surg 2006;29(6):952–6.

49. Buckley MS, Feldman JP. Nebulized milrinone use in a pulmonary hypertensive crisis. Pharmacotherapy 2007;27(12):1763–6.

50. Ukkonen H, Saraste M, Akkila J, et al. Myocardial efficiency during levosimendan infusion in congestive heart failure. Clin Pharmacol Ther 2000;68(5): 522–31.

51. Slawsky MT, Colucci WS, Gottlieb SS, et al. Acute hemodynamic and clinical effects of levosimendan in patients with severe heart failure. Study Investigators. Circulation 2000;102(18):2222–7.

52. Griffiths MJ, Evans TW. Inhaled nitric oxide therapy in adults. N Engl J Med 2005;353(25):2683–95.

53. Pepkezaba J, Higenbottam TW, Dinhxuan AT, et al. Inhaled nitric-oxide as a cause of selective pulmonary vasodilatation in pulmonary-hypertension. Lancet 1991;338(8776):1173–4.

54. Capellier G, Jacques T, Balvay P, et al. Inhaled nitric oxide in patients with pulmonary embolism. Intensive Care Med 1997;23(10):1089–92.

55. Vater Y, Martay K, Dembo G, et al. Intraoperative epoprostenol and nitric oxide for severe pulmonary hypertension during orthotopic liver transplantation: a case report and review of the literature. Med Sci Monit 2006;12(12):CS115–8.

56. Weinberger B, Laskin DL, Heck DE, et al. The toxicology of inhaled nitric oxide. Toxicol Sci 2001; 59(1):5–16.

57. Atz AM, Wessel DL. Sildenafil ameliorates effects of inhaled nitric oxide withdrawal. Anesthesiology 1999;91(1):307–10.

58. Barst RJ, Rubin LJ, Long WA, et al. A comparison of continuous intravenous epoprostenol (prostacyclin) with conventional therapy for primary pulmonary hypertension. N Engl J Med 1996;334(5):296–301.

59. Kieler-Jensen N, Milocco I, Ricksten SE. Pulmonary vasodilation after heart transplantation. A comparison among prostacyclin, sodium nitroprusside, and nitroglycerin on right ventricular function and pulmonary selectivity. J Heart Lung Transplant 1993;12(2): 179–84.

60. Zwissler B, Kemming G, Habler O, et al. Inhaled prostacyclin (PGI2) versus inhaled nitric oxide in adult respiratory distress syndrome. Am J Respir Crit Care Med 1996;154(6 Pt 1):1671–7.

61. De Wet CJ, Affleck DG, Jacobsohn E, et al. Inhaled prostacyclin is safe, effective, and affordable in patients with pulmonary hypertension, right heart dysfunction, and refractory hypoxemia after cardiothoracic surgery. J Thorac Cardiovasc Surg 2004; 127(4):1058–67.

62. Khan TA, Schnickel G, Ross D, et al. A prospective, randomized, crossover pilot study of inhaled nitric oxide versus inhaled prostacyclin in heart transplant and lung transplant recipients. J Thorac Cardiovasc Surg 2009;138(6):1417–24.

63. Galie N, Ghofrani HA, Torbicki A, et al. Sildenafil citrate therapy for pulmonary arterial hypertension. N Engl J Med 2005;353(20):2148–57.

64. Giaid A, Saleh D. Reduced expression of endothelial nitric oxide synthase in the lungs of patients with pulmonary hypertension. N Engl J Med 1995;333(4):214–21.

65. Nagendran J, Archer SL, Soliman D, et al. Phosphodiesterase type 5 is highly expressed in the hypertrophied human right ventricle, and acute inhibition of phosphodiesterase type 5 improves contractility. Circulation 2007;116(3):238–48.

66. Preston IR, Klinger JR, Houtches J, et al. Acute and chronic effects of sildenafil in patients with pulmonary arterial hypertension. Respir Med 2005; 99(12):1501–10.

67. Halcox JP, Nour KR, Zalos G, et al. The effect of sildenafil on human vascular function, platelet activation, and myocardial ischemia. J Am Coll Cardiol 2002;40(7):1232–40.

68. Fung E, Fiscus RR, Yim AP, et al. The potential use of type-5 phosphodiesterase inhibitors in coronary artery bypass graft surgery. Chest 2005;128(4):3065–73.

69. Johnson MC, Kirkham FJ, Redline S, et al. Left ventricular hypertrophy and diastolic dysfunction in children with sickle cell disease are related to asleep and waking oxygen desaturation. Blood 2010; 116(1):16–21.

70. Withering W. An account of the foxglove. Printed by M. Swinney for GGJ. and J Robinson. London; Birmingham (United Kingdom): Classics of Medicine Library; 1979.

71. Green LH, Smith TW. The use of digitalis in patients with pulmonary disease. Ann Intern Med 1977;87(4): 459–65.

72. Rich S, Seidlitz M, Dodin E, et al. The short-term effects of digoxin in patients with right ventricular dysfunction from pulmonary hypertension. Chest 1998;114(3):787–92.

73. Goldstein JA, Harada A, Yagi Y, et al. Hemodynamic importance of systolic ventricular interaction, augmented right atrial contractility and atrioventricular synchrony in acute right ventricular dysfunction. J Am Coll Cardiol 1990;16(1):181–9.

74. Tongers J, Schwerdtfeger B, Klein G, et al. Incidence and clinical relevance of supraventricular tachyarrhythmias in pulmonary hypertension. Am Heart J 2007;153(1):127–32.

75. Marcus JT, Gan CT, Zwanenburg JJ, et al. Interventricular mechanical asynchrony in pulmonary

arterial hypertension: left-to-right delay in peak shortening is related to right ventricular overload and left ventricular underfilling. J Am Coll Cardiol 2008;51(7):750–7.

76. Vonk-Noordegraaf A, Haddad F, Chin KM, et al. Right heart adaptation to pulmonary arterial hypertension: physiology and pathobiology. J Am Coll Cardiol 2013;62(25 Suppl):D22–33.

77. Jardin F, Delorme G, Hardy A, et al. Reevaluation of hemodynamic consequences of positive pressure ventilation: emphasis on cyclic right ventricular afterloading by mechanical lung inflation. Anesthesiology 1990;72(6):966–70.

78. Vieillard-Baron A, Loubieres Y, Schmitt JM, et al. Cyclic changes in right ventricular output impedance during mechanical ventilation. J Appl Physiol (1985) 1999;87(5):1644–50.

79. Hakim TS, Michel RP, Chang HK. Effect of lung inflation on pulmonary vascular resistance by arterial and venous occlusion. J Appl Physiol Respir Environ Exerc Physiol 1982;53(5):1110–5.

80. Balanos GM, Talbot NP, Dorrington KL, et al. Human pulmonary vascular response to 4 h of hypercapnia and hypocapnia measured using Doppler echocardiography. J Appl Physiol (1985) 2003; 94(4):1543–51.

81. Walley KR, Becker CJ, Hogan RA, et al. Progressive hypoxemia limits left ventricular oxygen consumption and contractility. Circ Res 1988;63(5):849–59.

82. Endoh M. Acidic pH-induced contractile dysfunction via downstream mechanism: identification of pH-sensitive domain in troponin I. J Mol Cell Cardiol 2001;33(7):1297–300.

83. Rich S, Lam W. Atrial septostomy as palliative therapy for refractory primary pulmonary hypertension. Am J Cardiol 1983;51(9):1560–1.

84. Law MA, Grifka RG, Mullins CE, et al. Atrial septostomy improves survival in select patients with pulmonary hypertension. Am Heart J 2007;153(5):779–84.

85. Kerstein D, Levy PS, Hsu DT, et al. Blade balloon atrial septostomy in patients with severe primary pulmonary hypertension. Circulation 1995;91(7): 2028–35.

86. Esch JJ, Shah PB, Cockrill BA, et al. Transcatheter Potts shunt creation in patients with severe pulmonary arterial hypertension: initial clinical experience. J Heart Lung Transplant 2013;32(4):381–7.

Advances in Sepsis Research

Peter Bentzer, MD, PhD[a,b,c], James A. Russell, MD[a,b], Keith R. Walley, MD[a,b],*

KEYWORDS

- Sepsis • Innate immune receptors • Pathogen • Clearance • Edema • Vascular leak

KEY POINTS

- Treatment strategies targeting early pathophysiological alterations in sepsis improve outcomes.
- Pathogen toxins are triggers of inflammation in sepsis, and therapies aimed at enhancing toxin clearance represent potential complements to early antimicrobial therapy.
- The innate immune response is an early built-in host response to infecting pathogens. Treatments aimed at modifying this response have therapeutic potential.
- Vascular leak, secondary edema formation, and hypovolemia contribute to poor outcome in sepsis; several distinct pathophysiological mechanisms may be targeted to ameliorate this response.

INTRODUCTION

Of the World Health Organization top 10 causes of death, 4 fulfill the definition of sepsis (www.who.int). Sepsis occurs when infection results in systemic inflammation[1,2] and is termed severe sepsis when accompanied by new organ dysfunction. The 28-day mortality rate of severe sepsis is 15% to 30%,[3–6] which increases to 20% to 60% when complicated by arterial vasodilation and ventricular dysfunction, leading to septic shock.[7] The number of deaths due to severe sepsis and septic shock is greater than the number of deaths due to acute myocardial infarction, even in the Western world,[3] and continues to increase.[4] Effective treatment of severe sepsis can lead to complete resolution with no sequelae, whereas ineffective treatment is fatal or leads to long-term morbidities and increased long-term mortality rates; so timely effective therapy is crucial.[8]

Herein the authors consider aspects of the septic inflammatory response that provide novel targets for therapeutic intervention. Specifically, (1) clearance of inflammatory pathogen molecules from the circulation, (2) modulation of innate immune receptors and intracellular signaling, as well as (3) vascular leak are considered.

PATHOGENS AND PATHOGEN TOXINS

Targeting the host septic inflammatory response (eg, anti–tumor necrosis factor,[9] activated protein C [APC][5]) has not worked in more than 30 phase 3 randomized controlled trials (RCTs).[10–12] In contrast, simply targeting the pathogen by source control (draining the abscess, etc) and early broad-spectrum antibiotics is very effective. Kumar and colleagues[13] found that for every hour delay in antibiotic administration after onset of septic shock, mortality increased by 7%. Another

Disclosure statement: P. Bentzer has no competing interests to declare. K.R. Walley and J.A. Russell have founded Cyon Therapeutics, which has licensed intellectual property from the University of British Columbia related to PCSK9 in sepsis.
a Centre for Heart Lung Innovation, University of British Columbia, Vancouver, British Columbia, Canada; b Division of Critical Care Medicine, St. Paul's Hospital, University of British Columbia, 1081 Burrard Street, Vancouver, British Columbia V6Z 1Y6, Canada; c Department of Anesthesiology and Intensive Care, Lund University, Lund SE-221 85, Sweden
* Corresponding author. St. Paul's Hospital, University of British Columbia, 1081 Burrard Street, Vancouver, British Columbia V6Z 1Y6, Canada.
E-mail address: keith.walley@hli.ubc.ca

Clin Chest Med 36 (2015) 521–530
http://dx.doi.org/10.1016/j.ccm.2015.05.009

chestmed.theclinics.com

less-established approach targeting the pathogen is to enhance clearance of toxins. Whether alive or dead, pathogens elicit an inflammatory response by release of toxins such as lipopolysaccharide (LPS) from gram-negative bacteria; the structurally similar glycolipid, lipoteichoic acid (LTA) from gram-positive bacteria; and other glycolipids such as phospholipomannan (PLM) from fungal pathogens.[14] These toxins bind to innate immune receptors (see section on Innate Immune Signaling Induced by Pathogen Toxins) to trigger a septic inflammatory response. Accordingly, clearance of pathogen toxins is an important, underrecognized, and modifiable aspect of sepsis management that complements effective antimicrobial therapy.

Pathogen Toxins Induce an Inflammatory Response

Septic shock is primarily due to release of pathogen toxins.[8] The lipid A domain of LPS binds Toll-like receptor 4 (TLR4) expressed on many cell lines, thereby inducing nuclear factor (NF)-κB signaling and the subsequent proinflammatory and antiinflammatory cytokine response.[15] LTA of gram-positive bacterial cell membranes is composed of a polyglycerolphosphate chain connected by a glycolipid moiety[16] and binds TLR2 and TLR6 to induce NF-κB signaling.[17] Fungal PLM is composed primarily of C24 hydroxy fatty acids linked to phytoceramide and phytosphingosine, with a hydrophilic polysaccharide domain consisting of mannose residues.[18] PLM and related glycolipids are ligands for TLR2, TLR4, and TLR6.

Sequestration as the Initial Step in Limiting the Adverse Effects of Pathogen Toxins

Pathogen toxins in the aqueous phase are quickly bound by transfer proteins that bind lipid moieties.[19] When transfer protein availability is limited, LPS incorporation into lipoproteins is reduced and LPS toxicity is increased, thus transfer proteins are the first step in sequestering pathogen toxins. LPS binding protein (LBP) and bactericidal permeability-increasing protein are homologous to the endogenous lipid transfer protein phospholipid transfer protein (PLTP), and all bind pathogen toxins.[19] LBP and PLTP bind LPS and transfer it from micelles or from LPS aggregates in the aqueous phase to high-density lipoprotein (HDL)[20,21] and other lipoproteins.[22] While LBP can bind and additionally transfer LPS to CD14, a cofactor in subsequent signaling via TLR4, PLTP does not transfer LPS to CD14[20] and, thus, does not trigger downstream inflammatory

signaling. LBP more effectively transfers LPS from bacterial cell wall fragments to lipoproteins than PLTP.

Following binding by transfer proteins, LPS is transferred to and sequestered within HDL and, after LBP and PLTP-facilitated transfer, within low-density lipoprotein (LDL) and very-low-density lipoprotein (VLDL).[23] LPS, LTA, and even the LPS lipid A analog, eritoran,[24] are distributed primarily on HDL (~60%) with the remainder on LDL and VLDL particles. In sepsis, this distribution shifts from the predominant HDL carriage of LPS to increased LDL and VLDL carriage of LPS.

Subsequent Clearance of Pathogen Toxins from the Circulating Lipoprotein Compartment

Pathogen toxins are then cleared primarily by hepatic uptake and excretion in bile.[25] Characterization of the exact mechanisms of hepatic clearance of pathogen toxins is limited but likely involves the LDL receptor (LDLR). LDLR knockout mice have increased mortality after cecal ligation and puncture compared with mice with intact LDLR[26] suggesting a central LDLR role in pathogen toxin clearance.

Further support for the role of LDLR in pathogen toxin clearance is provided by recent observations that PCSK9 decreases LPS clearance and increases the innate immune response to pathogen toxins.[27] Circulating PCSK9, produced primarily by the liver, binds LDLR expressed on hepatocytes and, upon internalization of the LDLR complex, targets it for lysosomal degradation so that it is not recycled back to the hepatocyte cell surface (**Fig. 1**). Thus, increased PCSK9 activity decreases LDLR expression of hepatocytes, whereas reduced PCSK9 activity results in increased LDLR expression and increases pathogen toxin clearance, decreases cytokine inflammatory response, and improves survival from sepsis. This effect is lost in LDLR knockout in mice and by an LDLR genetic variant that interferes with binding of PCSK9 to the LDLR.[27] Taken together, these data support the hypothesis that pathogen toxin clearance depends substantially on PCSK9 and the LDLR.

How This Knowledge May Lead to Innovative Therapeutic Strategies

Mechanisms of pathogen toxin clearance may be novel targets for treatment. PCSK9 inhibition to increase pathogen toxin clearance conceivably could decrease the inflammatory response and improve survival in human sepsis. PCSK9 inhibition targets the pathogen and like antibiotics, may be particularly effective.

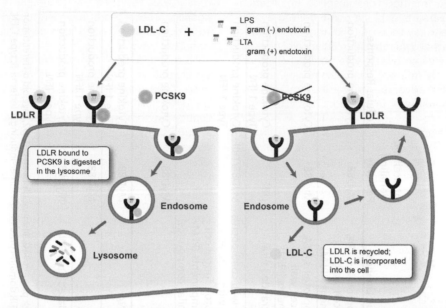

Fig. 1. Endocytosis of the LDLR/LDL cholesterol (LDL-C) complex in the presence and absence of PCSK9.

INNATE IMMUNE SIGNALING INDUCED BY PATHOGEN TOXINS
Innate Immune Receptors

Innate immune receptors, including TLRs, nucleotide-binding oligomerization domain (NOD)-like receptors (NLRs), and retinoic acid-inducible gene (RIG)-like receptors (RLRs), contribute to the myocardial, and other organ systems', response to danger signals. TLRs, NLRs, and RLRs are pattern recognition receptors that respond to exogenous ligands for pathogen-associated molecular patterns (PAMPs). Potentially more important, innate immune receptors also respond to endogenous ligands, damage-associated molecular patterns (DAMPs).

Toll-like receptors

TLRs are type I transmembrane receptors consisting of extracellular leucine-rich repeats linked to a cytoplasmic Toll/interleukin-1 receptor (TIR) homology domain.[28] Ten or more TLRs respond to endogenous and exogenous danger signals[28] (**Table 1**). TLRs 1, 2, 4, 5, and 6 are expressed on the cell surface. The response of TLR4 to gram-negative bacterial cell wall molecules such as LPS is best understood. TLR2 in concert with TLR1 or TLR6 recognizes bacterial cell wall components such as LTA, peptidoglycan, and yeast cell wall components.[28] TLR5 binds gram-negative bacterial flagellin. TLRs 3, 7, 8, and 9 are expressed mainly intracellularly; their predominantly nucleic acid ligands must be internalized into endosomes to initiate signaling.[28] TLR3 recognizes double-stranded (ds) viral RNA, TLR7

recognizes single-stranded viral RNA, and TLR9 recognizes unmethylated CpG bacterial DNA.[29] DAMPs have been identified for many TLRs including heat shock protein 60 (HSP60), HSP70, and Gp96. Endogenous ligands for TLR4 include fibrinogen[28] the fibronectin EDA (extra domain A) domain, and hyaluronan. Endogenous mRNA is a DAMP for TLR3.[30,31]

NOD-like receptors

NLRs can be grouped into 4 NOD receptors, which induce a proinflammatory response via NF-κB, and 14 NLR pyrin domain-containing receptors plus several NLR caspase recruitment domain-containing receptors,[32,33] which assemble the inflammasome. Inflammasomes involve multiple proteins, notably including caspases. The assembled inflammasome can then be activated by PAMPs and by endogenous activators (low intracellular K⁺ levels and reactive oxygen species). Subsequent inflammasome signaling involves caspase-mediated cleavage leading to processing and secretion of mature interleukin (IL)-1β and IL-18.[32] NLRs mediate tissue injury by their IL-1β and IL-18 signatures.[32] Compared with TLRs, much less is known about NLRs.

Retinoic acid-inducible gene-like receptors

RLRs are recently discovered cytosolic RNA helicases that act as innate immune receptors in sensing viral dsRNA by recognizing 5′-triphosphate ends, which characterize nonself RNA.[34] RLRs include RIG-1, melanoma differentiation-associated protein 5, and LGP2 (Laboratory of Genetics and Physiology). RIG-1 results in a type I

Table 1
Summary of endogenous and exogenous TLR receptor ligands described in humans

Receptor	Cell Types	Localization	Endogenous Ligands	Exogenous Ligands	Intracellular Signaling Pathway	Cellular Response
TLR1 + TLR2	B lymphocytes Dendritic cells, monocytes/ macrophages	Cell surface	β-Defensin, biglycan, HSP, HMGB1, hyaluronic acid	G (+) lipoproteins, LTA, fungal cell wall components (PLM)	MyD88	Cytokine production
TLR2 + TLR6	B lymphocytes Dendritic cells, monocytes/ macrophages	Cell surface	β-Defensin, biglycan, HSP, HMGB1, hyaluronic acid	G (+) lipoproteins, LTA, fungal cell wall components (PLM)	MyD88	Cytokine production
TLR3	B lymphocytes Dendritic cells	Endosomes/ lysosomes	mRNA	Double-stranded viral RNA	TRIF	Cytokine production Type 1 IFN
TLR4	B lymphocytes, dendritic cells, monocytes/macrophages Neutrophils, intestinal epithelium	Cell surface	β-Defensin, fibronectin, hyaluronic acid, heparan sulfate, fibrinogen, HMGB1, S100, oxidized LDL	G (−) cell wall components for LPS with MD2 as a coreceptor, fungal cell wall components (PLM and similar compounds)	MyD88/TRIF	Cytokine production Type 1 IFN
TLR5	Dendritic cells, monocytes/ macrophages, intestinal epithelium	Cell surface	—	Flagellin	MyD88	Cytokine production
TLR7	B lymphocytes, dendritic cells, monocytes/macrophages	Endosomes/ lysosomes	ssRNA	ss Viral RNA	MyD88	Cytokine production Type 1 IFN
TLR8	Dendritic cells, mast cells, monocytes/macrophages	Endosomes/ lysosomes	ssRNA	—	MyD88	Cytokine production Type 1 IFN
TLR9	B lymphocytes, dendritic cells, monocytes/macrophages	Endosomes/ lysosomes	IgG chromatin complex	Unmethylated CpG DNA	MyD88	Cytokine production Type 1 IFN

Abbreviations: G (−), gram negative; G (+), gram positive; HMGB1, high-mobility group box-1 protein; HSP, heat shock protein; IgG, immunoglobulin G; MD2, myeloid differentiation factor 2; mRNA, messenger RNA; MyD88, myeloid differentiation primary response gene 88; ss, single stranded; TRIF, TIR domain-containing adapter-inducing interferon-β; type 1 IFN, type 1 interferon.

interferon (IFN) response by signaling via interferon regulatory factor 3 (IRF3) and IRF7. IRF3 and IRF7 form homodimers and heterodimers, which form part of the transcription enhancer complex for IFN-β in the nucleus. RIG-1 also can signal via NF-κB.[35]

Nuclear factor-κB and alternative signaling pathways

Activation of most TLRs by ligand binding results in dimerization, a change in conformation, and recruitment of the adaptor protein myeloid differentiation primary response gene 88 (MyD88) to the cytoplasmic TIR domain.[36] MyD88 recruits IRAK4 (interleukin-1 receptor-associated kinase), which, with participation of TAK1 binding protein (TAB2) and TRAF6, leads to activation of TGF-Beta-Activated Kinase (TAK1). TAK1 activates IκB kinase (IKK) leading to liberation of NF-κB from its inhibitor, IκBα (nuclear factor of kappa light polypeptide gene enhancer in B-cells inhibitor, alpha), and subsequent translocation of NF-κB to the nucleus where it induces proinflammatory cytokine production. NF-κB is a critical mediator of several inflammatory pathways.

All TLRs except TLR3 signal via MyD88 to induce NF-κB activity. Increased NF-κB activity leads to different responses in different cell types, although all these responses are part of the complex inflammatory response that PAMPs initiate. Other TLR-initiated pathways have been identified. TIR domain-containing adapter-inducing interferon-β (TRIF), like MyD88, is an alternate adaptor protein that binds to the TIR domain of TLR3 and TLR4.[37] TRIF interacts with TRAF6, RIP1, and TAK1, leading to activation of NF-κB and IRF3. TAK1 can also activate mitogen-activated protein kinase kinase (MKK3/6) and MKK7, which signal via inflammatory gene transcription factors p38 and JNK (c-Jun N-terminal kinase).

NOD1 and NOD2 also signal via NF-κB independent of MyD88. Ligation of these NLRs results in activation of RIP2, which interacts with IKKγ to allow release of NF-κB and translocation into the nucleus.[32,33] RIP2 alternatively signals via TAK1, TAB1, and TAB2/3 to activate the p38 MAPK (mitogen-activated protein kinase) signaling pathway. NLR inflammasomes share caspase signaling pathways.[32]

An Example of Septic Organ Dysfunction: Proinflammatory and Antiinflammatory Responses in the Heart

Cardiomyocytes' primary function is contraction to provide the motive force that drives cardiac output and generates arterial pressure. Cardiomyocytes have key additional properties, analogous to innate immune antigen-presenting cells (eg, dendritic cells, tissue macrophages). Cardiomyocytes respond to PAMP-induced danger signals with complex inflammatory and functional responses.[38–51] In response to inflammatory stimuli, cardiomyocytes express proinflammatory and antiinflammatory cytokines (eg, IL-6, IL-10), which initiate a local inflammatory response, recruiting inflammatory cells necessary for repair, and increase expression of cell surface adhesion molecules (eg, intercellular adhesion molecule [ICAM-1]) allowing interaction and outside-in signaling from participating inflammatory cells and the extracellular matrix.[43,45,50–53] ICAM-1 expression and subsequent ligand binding decrease cardiomyocyte contractility by involving calcium channel-binding proteins S100A8/A9.[54] This complex response starts with binding of pathogen molecules to innate immune receptors.

How This Knowledge May Lead to Innovative Therapeutic Strategies

Sepsis therapies are most beneficial if initiated early, and the innate immune response (involves all tissues) is an early host response. Thus modifying the innate immune response could ameliorate multiple organ system dysfunction. Conceivably, early administration of therapies aimed at modulation of innate immunity may be beneficial. Thus innate immunity pathways are reasonable targets to consider as new therapeutic strategies for sepsis.

VASCULAR LEAK
Fluid Homeostasis in Sepsis

Hypovolemia secondary to vascular leakage is an important contributor to hemodynamic instability in sepsis and often leads to large-volume fluid resuscitation with ensuing edema formation and organ dysfunction. Observational studies show an association between fluid overload and outcome,[55] and RCTs suggest benefit from restrictive fluid administration.[56] Experimental studies showing that interventions specifically targeting vascular leakage increases survival without affecting markers of inflammatory response further support that vascular leakage is a determinant of outcome and not simply a marker of injury severity.[57]

Transvascular fluid transport depends on transcapillary hydrostatic and colloid osmotic pressures as well as permeability for fluid and macromolecules. Extravasation of macromolecules (eg, albumin) occurs by both diffusion and convection; thus, changes in both permeability and transcapillary hydrostatic pressure are of central importance for this process. In most organs, hydrostatic and osmotic pressures are unbalanced and net fluid filtration from circulation to tissue occurs. Normally, approximately 5% of the intravascular albumin leaves the circulation every hour and is returned to the circulation via the lymph. Inflammation-induced changes in the interstitial matrix and lymphatic function are potentially important contributors to hypovolemia in sepsis. However, most studies investigating disruptions in fluid homeostasis in sepsis have focused on pathways involved in increases in permeability such as the vascular endothelial growth factor as well as the angiopoietin and thrombin pathways.[58] In the following discussion, 2 other mechanisms and pathways, the sphingosine-1-phosphate (S1P) and vasopressin systems, are highlighted as potential therapeutic targets in sepsis. Both systems have been shown to influence plasma volume in whole animal models of sepsis, and drugs approved for human use are available.

Vascular Leak and the Vasopressin Axis in Sepsis

The initial phase of sepsis is characterized by vasodilatation secondary to increased production of vasodilatory substances (nitric oxide, prostacyclin), decreased production of vasoconstrictors (vasopressin), changed expression of vasoconstrictive receptors,[59] and disruption of myogenic control mechanisms responsible for autoregulation of capillary hydrostatic pressure[60] (**Fig. 2**). If

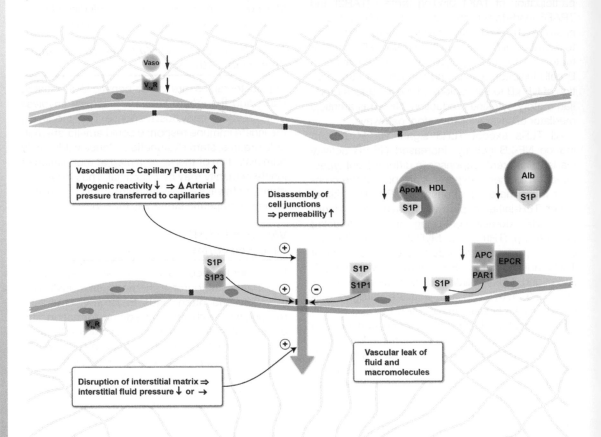

Fig. 2. Mechanisms involved in sepsis induced vascular leak. Vasodilation is partly due to changes in concentration of vasoconstricting agents such as vasopressin (Vaso) and decreased expression of vasopressin receptors ($V_{1a}R$) on smooth muscle cells as well as vasodilators such as nitric oxide. Precapillary arteriolar vasodilation increases capillary pressure. Decreased myogenic activity causes a change in arterial pressure that is transferred to the capillaries, the major site of vascular fluid exchange. Vascular endothelial permeability is increased through multiple mechanisms acting on intercellular junctions of endothelial cells. For example, decreased availability of spinogosine-1-phosphate (S1P) through decreased plasma levels of apolipoprotein M (ApoM) and albumin (Alb) will decrease permeability via decreased stimulation of S1P1 receptors (S1P1 in the figure). Decreased levels of activated protein C (APC) increase permeability through decreased endothelial synthesis of S1P because of decreased activation of the endothelial protein C receptor (EPCR)/protease-activated receptor (PAR)-1 receptor complex. S1P also increases permeability through activation of endothelial S1P3 receptors (S1P3 in the figure), but the importance of this pathway in sepsis is unclear. Sepsis-induced inflammation disrupts the interstitial matrix and transiently decreases interstitial pressure, which may contribute to early leak of fluid.

hypotension persists after fluid resuscitation, Surviving Sepsis guidelines[61] recommend norepinephrine to maintain mean arterial pressure above 65 mm Hg. However, norepinephrine may cause fluid filtration and decrease plasma volume in inflammatory conditions.[62,63] A tentative explanation of norepinephrine's effect is increased capillary pressure because of a change in the precapillary to postcapillary resistance ratio.[64] These observations raise the question whether other vasoconstrictors may have a more beneficial effect on fluid balance.

Vasopressin is recommended as a second-line treatment in septic shock. Vasopressin elicits vasoconstriction through the V_{1a} receptor on smooth muscle cells and has V_2-induced antidiuretic and procoagulant actions through stimulation of renal and endothelial V_2 receptors. Recently, animal studies have reported potentially important effects on vascular leakage of vasopressin derivatives highly selective for V_{1a} receptors (eg, selepressin). Selepressin reduced fluid requirements and protected against vascular leak when compared with noradrenalin or vasopressin.[65,66] A preliminary report from a phase 2 trial also suggested a dose-dependent limitation of positive fluid balance by selepressin compared with placebo in septic shock. The mechanisms of vascular leakage protection by V_{1a} agonism in sepsis is not known.

V_{1a} receptors are generally not expressed on endothelial cells; perhaps the beneficial effect of selective V_{1a} agonism on vascular leakage is mediated via a more favorable precapillary to postcapillary resistance ratio, decreased capillary hydrostatic pressure, and less vascular leakage compared with norepinephrine. Large RCTs are needed to determine whether selective V_{1a} receptor agonism improves outcomes of septic shock.

Sphingosine-1-Phosphate and Endothelial Permeability

S1P is a lipid with multiple functions including immune modulation and maintenance of endothelial barrier function. S1P binds to a series of G-protein-coupled receptors, S1P receptors 1–5; endothelial S1P receptor 1 (S1P1) decreases permeability primarily through AKT-1 and Rac-1 activation with the endothelial cytoskeleton and eNOS (endothelial nitric oxide synthase) as downstream targets. S1P2 and S1P3 increase permeability through RHO kinase activation. Erythrocytes are the major source of S1P in plasma, and most cell types have the ability to synthesize S1P. The concentration of S1P is higher in plasma than in lymph, which in turn is higher than in the interstitium, and maintenance of this S1P concentration gradient is important for maintenance of normal barrier function. In plasma, about 60% of S1P is bound to apolipoprotein M (ApoM) (in HDL particles) and about 35% is bound to albumin.

Maintenance of normal endothelial barrier function by S1P is mediated by S1P bound to both ApoM and albumin.[67,68] S1P synthesis and release from endothelial cells can be initiated through activation of protease-activated receptor-1 by a complex of APC bound to the endothelial protein C receptor.[69] The therapeutic potential of S1P/S1P1 is supported by studies showing that administration of S1P (or structurally similar drugs such as the precursor analog FTY 720) counteracts vascular leakage and hypovolemia in experimental sepsis.[70,71] Clinical application may be limited by a narrow therapeutic window above which increased vascular leakage through S1PR2 (S1P receptor) and S1PR3 stimulation may be seen. Furthermore, the immunomodulatory effects of nonselective S1PR agonist may limit efficacy and safety. Consequently, more specific S1PR1 receptor agonists or alternative approaches to increase S1PR signaling could be of interest. More specific agonists (FTY 720 (S)-phosphate, CYM 5452, SEW2871) show promising results in models of inflammation-induced lung and renal permeability.[72,73] Nonanticoagulant APC derivatives increase survival and decease vascular leakage in sepsis models and offer an alterative approach to decease vascular leakage through the S1PR1 pathway.[74] The observation that ApoM is the main carrier of S1P together with the observation that ApoM level is decreased in sepsis suggests that S1P's barrier protective effects may be enhanced by increasing plasma levels of ApoM in sepsis.[75]

How This Knowledge May Lead to Innovative Therapeutic Strategies

Disturbances in vascular leakage, fluid homeostasis with ensuing hypovolemia, and edema formation are important for outcome in sepsis. The vasopressin and S1P systems are promising targets to minimize vascular leakage; selective stimulation of $V1_a$ receptors and S1P1 receptors holds therapeutic promise. The importance of the interstitial matrix and the lymphatic system for hypovolemia and edema formation in sepsis represents a new frontier for sepsis research.

Why Have Most Sepsis Trials Failed?

Most pivotal phase 3 RCTs in sepsis have failed despite strong preclinical evidence and promising phase 2 RCTs. Why have so many RCTs missed the mark? There are several possible explanations. First, the drug targets are enmeshed in redundant pathways that respond to drug intervention to maintain the disorder of sepsis. Second, the preclinical models may not be appropriate in modeling human sepsis because most are simple, acute models in young animals without comorbidities, the opposite of many patients with sepsis. Third, the phase 2 RCTs are often small (n = 100–300), considerably smaller than phase 2 RCTs in other conditions such as heart disease. Fourth, sepsis is a heterogeneous condition that may be composed of responders and nonresponders according to genotype, gene expression, and clinical variables. Finally, the underlying mortality of sepsis has decreased to 20% to 30% because of earlier intervention with fluids, vasopressors, and antibiotics; thus, many RCTs are underpowered for these now lower mortality rates.

So the authors suggest that future programs should include more appropriate preclinical models, larger phase 2 RCTs, predictive biomarkers to test a more homogeneous patient sample, and composite outcome variables (eg, measures of organ dysfunction).

SUMMARY

Sepsis is a disease with a high short- and long-term mortality and morbidity. In this review, aspects of the septic inflammatory response that provide promising novel targets for therapeutic interventions are considered. Increased clearance of the bacterial toxin LPS by inhibition of PCSK9 suggests that clearance of pathogen toxins complements source control and early broad-spectrum antibiotics. The innate immune response is a key component in host defense, and signaling pathways (eg, TLRs) are potential therapeutic targets in sepsis. The observations that positive fluid balance is associated with poor outcome and that treatment strategies to limit fluid overload improve outcome suggest that disturbances in vascular leakage and fluid homeostasis are determinants of outcome in sepsis rather than simply markers of severity. The vasopressin and S1P pathways are promising targets to modulate vascular leakage.

REFERENCES

1. Bone RC. The sepsis syndrome. Definition and general approach to management. Clin Chest Med 1996;17:175–81.

2. Levy MM, Fink MP, Marshall JC, et al. 2001 SCCM/ESICM/ACCP/ATS/SIS international sepsis definitions conference. Crit Care Med 2003;31:1250–6.

3. Angus DC, Linde-Zwirble WT, Lidicker J, et al. Epidemiology of severe sepsis in the United States:

analysis of incidence, outcome, and associated costs of care. Crit Care Med 2001;29:1303–10.

4. Angus DC, Pereira CA, Silva E. Epidemiology of severe sepsis around the world. Endocr Metab Immune Disord Drug Targets 2006;6:207–12.

5. Bernard GR, Vincent JL, Laterre PF, et al. Efficacy and safety of recombinant human activated protein C for severe sepsis. N Engl J Med 2001;344:699–709.

6. Vincent JL, Sakr Y, Sprung CL, et al. Sepsis in European intensive care units: results of the SOAP study. Crit Care Med 2006;34:344–53.

7. Russell JA, Walley KR, Singer J, et al. Vasopressin versus norepinephrine infusion in patients with septic shock. N Engl J Med 2008;358:877–87.

8. Russell JA. Management of sepsis. N Engl J Med 2006;355:1699–713.

9. Morris PE, Zeno B, Bernard AC, et al. A placebo-controlled, double-blind, dose-escalation study to assess the safety, tolerability and pharmacokinetics/pharmacodynamics of single and multiple intravenous infusions of AZD9773 in patients with severe sepsis and septic shock. Crit Care 2012;16:R31.

10. Dubois MJ, Vincent JL. Clinically-oriented therapies in sepsis: a review. J Endotoxin Res 2000;6:463–9.

11. Eichacker PQ, Parent C, Kalil A, et al. Risk and the efficacy of antiinflammatory agents: retrospective and confirmatory studies of sepsis. Am J Respir Crit Care Med 2002;166:1197–205.

12. Vincent JL, Sun Q, Dubois MJ. Clinical trials of immunomodulatory therapies in severe sepsis and septic shock. Clin Infect Dis 2002;34:1084–93.

13. Kumar A, Roberts D, Wood KE, et al. Duration of hypotension before initiation of effective antimicrobial therapy is the critical determinant of survival in human septic shock. Crit Care Med 2006;34:1589–96.

14. Trinel PA, Plancke Y, Gerold P, et al. The Candida albicans phospholipomannan is a family of glycolipids presenting phosphoinositolmannosides with long linear chains of beta-1,2-linked mannose residues. J Biol Chem 1999;274:30520–6.

15. Gallay P, Heumann D, Le Roy D, et al. Mode of action of anti-lipopolysaccharide-binding protein antibodies for prevention of endotoxemic shock in mice. Proc Natl Acad Sci U S A 1994;91:7922–6.

16. Reichmann NT, Grundling A. Location, synthesis and function of glycolipids and polyglycerolphosphate lipoteichoic acid in gram-positive bacteria of the phylum Firmicutes. FEMS Microbiol Lett 2011; 319:97–105.

17. Kimbrell MR, Warshakoon H, Cromer JR, et al. Comparison of the immunostimulatory and proinflammatory activities of candidate gram-positive endotoxins, lipoteichoic acid, peptidoglycan, and lipopeptides, in murine and human cells. Immunol Lett 2008;118: 132–41.

18. Trinel PA, Maes E, Zanetta JP, et al. Candida albicans phospholipomannan, a new member of tho

fungal mannose inositol phosphoceramide family. J Biol Chem 2002;277:37260–71.

19. Azzam KM, Fessler MB. Crosstalk between reverse cholesterol transport and innate immunity. Trends Endocrinol Metab 2012;23:169–78.

20. Hailman E, Albers JJ, Wolfbauer G, et al. Neutralization and transfer of lipopolysaccharide by phospholipid transfer protein. J Biol Chem 1996;271:12172–8.

21. Gautier T, Klein A, Deckert V, et al. Effect of plasma phospholipid transfer protein deficiency on lethal endotoxemia in mice. J Biol Chem 2008;283:18702–10.

22. Vreugdenhil AC, Rousseau CH, Hartung T, et al. Lipopolysaccharide (LPS)-binding protein mediates LPS detoxification by chylomicrons. J Immunol 2003;170:1399–405.

23. Berbee JF, Havekes LM, Rensen PC. Apolipoproteins modulate the inflammatory response to lipopolysaccharide. J Endotoxin Res 2005;11:97–103.

24. Fleischer JG, Rossignol D, Francis GA, et al. Deactivation of the lipopolysaccharide antagonist eritoran (E5564) by high-density lipoprotein-associated apolipoproteins. Innate Immun 2012;18:171–8.

25. Harris HW, Grunfeld C, Feingold KR, et al. Chylomicrons alter the fate of endotoxin, decreasing tumor necrosis factor release and preventing death. J Clin Invest 1993;91:1028–34.

26. Lanza-Jacoby S, Miller S, Jacob S, et al. Hyperlipoproteinemic low-density lipoprotein receptor-deficient mice are more susceptible to sepsis than corresponding wild-type mice. J Endotoxin Res 2003;9:341–7.

27. Walley KR, Thain KR, Russell JA, et al. PCSK9 is a critical regulator of the innate immune response and septic shock outcome. Sci Transl Med 2014;6:258ra143.

28. Akira S, Uematsu S, Takeuchi O. Pathogen recognition and innate immunity. Cell 2006;124:783–801.

29. Akira S, Takeda K, Kaisho T. Toll-like receptors: critical proteins linking innate and acquired immunity. Nat Immunol 2001;2:675–80.

30. Nakada E, Nakada TA, Walley KR, et al. mRNA induces RANTES production in trophoblast cells via TLR3 only when delivered intracellularly using lipid membrane encapsulation. Placenta 2011;32:500–5.

31. Nakada E, Walley KR, Nakada T, et al. Toll-like receptor-3 stimulation upregulates sFLT-1 production by trophoblast cells. Placenta 2009;30:774–9.

32. Petrilli V, Dostert C, Muruve DA, et al. The inflammasome: a danger sensing complex triggering innate immunity. Curr Opin Immunol 2007;19:615–22.

33. Proell M, Riedl SJ, Fritz JH, et al. The nod-like receptor (NLR) family: a tale of similarities and differences. PLoS one 2008;3:e2119.

34. Hornung V, Ellegast J, Kim S, et al. 5'-Triphosphate RNA is the ligand for RIG-I. Science 2006;314:994–7.

35. Paz S, Sun Q, Nakhaei P, et al. Induction of IRF-3 and IRF-7 phosphorylation following activation of the RIG-I pathway. Cell Mol Biol 2006;52:17–28.

36. Slack JL, Schooley K, Bonnert TP, et al. Identification of two major sites in the type I interleukin-1 receptor cytoplasmic region responsible for coupling to proinflammatory signaling pathways. J Biol Chem 2000;275:4670–8.

37. Kumar H, Kawai T, Akira S. Pathogen recognition by the innate immune system. Int Rev Immunol 2011;30:16–34.

38. Goddard CM, Poon BY, Klut ME, et al. Leukocyte activation does not mediate myocardial leukocyte retention during endotoxemia in rabbits. Am J Physiol 1998;275:H1548–57.

39. Herbertson MJ, Werner HA, Goddard CM, et al. Anti-tumor necrosis factor-alpha prevents decreased ventricular contractility in endotoxemic pigs. Am J Respir Crit Care Med 1995;152:480–8.

40. Herbertson MJ, Werner HA, Studer W, et al. Decreased left ventricular contractility during porcine endotoxemia is not prevented by ibuprofen. Crit Care Med 1996;24:815–9.

41. Herbertson MJ, Werner HA, Walley KR. Nitric oxide synthase inhibition partially prevents decreased LV contractility during endotoxemia. Am J Physiol 1996;270:H1979–84.

42. McDonald TE, Grinman MN, Carthy CM, et al. Endotoxin infusion in rats induces apoptotic and survival pathways in hearts. Am J Physiol Heart Circ Physiol 2000;279:H2053–61.

43. Simms MG, Walley KR. Activated macrophages decrease rat cardiac myocyte contractility: importance of ICAM-1-dependent adhesion. Am J Physiol 1999;277:H253–60.

44. Walley KR, Hebert PC, Wakai Y, et al. Decrease in left ventricular contractility after tumor necrosis factor-alpha infusion in dogs. J Appl Physiol (1985) 1994;76:1060–7.

45. Davani EY, Dorscheid DR, Lee CH, et al. Novel regulatory mechanism of cardiomyocyte contractility involving ICAM-1 and the cytoskeleton. Am J Physiol Heart Circ Physiol 2004;287:H1013–22.

46. Boyd JH, Mathur S, Wang Y, et al. Toll-like receptor stimulation in cardiomyoctes decreases contractility and initiates an NF-kappaB dependent inflammatory response. Cardiovasc Res 2006;72:384–93.

47. Boyd JH, Chau EH, Tokunaga C, et al. Fibrinogen decreases cardiomyocyte contractility through an ICAM-1-dependent mechanism. Crit Care 2008;12:R2.

48. De Rossi M, Bernasconi P, Baggi F, et al. Cytokines and chemokines are both expressed by human myoblasts: possible relevance for the immune pathogenesis of muscle inflammation. Int Immunol 2000;12:1329–35.

49. Finkel MS, Oddis CV, Jacob TD, et al. Negative inotropic effects of cytokines on the heart mediated by nitric oxide. Science 1992;257:387–9.

50. Hattori Y, Kasai K. Induction of mRNAs for ICAM-1, VCAM-1, and ELAM-1 in cultured rat cardiac myocytes and myocardium in vivo. Biochem Mol Biol Int 1997;41:979–86.

51. Niessen HW, Krijnen PA, Visser CA, et al. Intercellular adhesion molecule-1 in the heart. Ann N Y Acad Sci 2002;973:573–85.

52. Raeburn CD, Dinarello CA, Zimmerman MA, et al. Neutralization of IL-18 attenuates lipopolysaccharide-induced myocardial dysfunction. Am J Physiol Heart Circ Physiol 2002;283:H650–7.

53. Raeburn CD, Calkins CM, Zimmerman MA, et al. ICAM-1 and VCAM-1 mediate endotoxemic myocardial dysfunction independent of neutrophil accumulation. Am J Physiol Regul Integr Comp Physiol 2002;283:R477–86.

54. Boyd JH, Kan B, Roberts H, et al. S100A8 and S100A9 mediate endotoxin-induced cardiomyocyte dysfunction via the receptor for advanced glycation end products. Circ Res 2008;102:1239–46.

55. Boyd JH, Forbes J, Nakada TA, et al. Fluid resuscitation in septic shock: a positive fluid balance and elevated central venous pressure are associated with increased mortality. Crit Care Med 2011;39:259–65.

56. National Heart, Lung, and Blood Institute Acute Respiratory Distress Syndrome (ARDS) Clinical Trials Network, Wiedemann HP, Wheeler AP, et al. Comparison of two fluid-management strategies in acute lung injury. N Engl J Med 2006;354:2564–75.

57. London NR, Zhu W, Bozza FA, et al. Targeting Robo4-dependent slit signaling to survive the cytokine storm in sepsis and influenza. Sci Transl Med 2010;2:23ra19.

58. Opal SM, van der Poll T. Endothelial barrier dysfunction in septic shock. J Intern Med 2015;277:277–93.

59. Schmidt C, Hocherl K, Kurt B, et al. Role of nuclear factor-kappaB-dependent induction of cytokines in the regulation of vasopressin V1A-receptors during cecal ligation and puncture-induced circulatory failure. Crit Care Med 2008;36:2363–72.

60. Favory R, Poissy J, Alves I, et al. Activated protein C improves macrovascular and microvascular reactivity in human severe sepsis and septic shock. Shock 2013;40:512–8.

61. Dellinger RP, Levy MM, Rhodes A, et al. Surviving sepsis campaign: international guidelines for management of severe sepsis and septic shock. Critical Care Medicine 2012;41(2):580–637.

62. Dubniks M, Persson J, Grande PO. Effect of blood pressure on plasma volume loss in the rat under increased permeability. Intensive Care Med 2007;33:2192–8.

63. Nygren A, Redfors B, Thoren A, et al. Norepinephrine causes a pressure-dependent plasma volume decrease in clinical vasodilatory shock. Acta anaesthesiologica Scand 2010;54:814–20.

64. Minnear FL, Barrie PS, Malik AB. Effects of epinephrine and norepinephrine infusion on lung fluid balance in sheep. J Appl Physiol Respir Environ Exerc Physiol 1981;50:1353–7.

65. Maybauer MO, Maybauer DM, Enkhbaatar P, et al. The selective vasopressin type 1a receptor agonist selepressin (FE 202158) blocks vascular leak in ovine severe sepsis*. Crit Care Med 2014;42:e525–33.

66. Rehberg S, Ertmer C, Vincent JL, et al. Role of selective V1a receptor agonism in ovine septic shock. Crit Care Med 2011;39:119–25.

67. Adamson RH, Clark JF, Radeva M, et al. Albumin modulates S1P delivery from red blood cells in perfused microvessels: mechanism of the protein effect. Am J Physiol Heart Circ Physiol 2014;306:H1011–7.

68. Christoffersen C, Obinata H, Kumaraswamy SB, et al. Endothelium-protective sphingosine-1-phosphate provided by HDL-associated apolipoprotein M. Proc Natl Acad Sci U S A 2011;108:9613–8.

69. Feistritzer C, Riewald M. Endothelial barrier protection by activated protein C through PAR1-dependent sphingosine 1-phosphate receptor-1 crossactivation. Blood 2005;105:3178–84.

70. Lundblad C, Axelberg H, Grande PO. Treatment with the sphingosine-1-phosphate analogue FTY 720 reduces loss of plasma volume during experimental sepsis in the rat. Acta anaesthesiologica Scand 2013;57:713–8.

71. Peng X, Hassoun PM, Sammani S, et al. Protective effects of sphingosine 1-phosphate in murine endotoxin-induced inflammatory lung injury. Am J Respir Crit Care Med 2004;169:1245–51.

72. Wang L, Sammani S, Moreno-Vinasco L, et al. FTY720 (s)-phosphonate preserves sphingosine 1-phosphate receptor 1 expression and exhibits superior barrier protection to FTY720 in acute lung injury. Crit Care Med 2014;42:e189–99.

73. Wang Z, Sims CR, Patil NK, et al. Pharmacologic targeting of sphingosine-1-phosphate receptor 1 improves the renal microcirculation during sepsis in the mouse. J Pharmacol Exp Ther 2015;352:61–6.

74. Kerschen EJ, Fernandez JA, Cooley BC, et al. Endotoxemia and sepsis mortality reduction by non-anticoagulant activated protein C. J Exp Med 2007;204:2439–48.

75. Kumaraswamy SB, Linder A, Akesson P, et al. Decreased plasma concentrations of apolipoprotein M in sepsis and systemic inflammatory response syndromes. Crit Care 2012;16:R60.

Management of Infections with Drug-Resistant Organisms in Critical Care: An Ongoing Battle

Sergio E. Trevino, MD, Marin H. Kollef, MD*

KEYWORDS

- Multidrug-resistant organisms • Carbapenem-resistant organisms
- Initial appropriate antimicrobial therapy • Adjunctive aerosolized antimicrobial therapy

KEY POINTS

- Infections with multidrug-resistant organisms (MDROs) are common in critically ill patients and are challenging to manage appropriately.
- Strategies that can be used in the treatment of MDRO infections in the intensive care unit (ICU) include combination therapy, adjunctive aerosolized therapy, and optimization of pharmacokinetics with higher doses or extended-infusion therapy as appropriate.
- Rapid diagnostic tests could assist in improving timely appropriate antimicrobial therapy for MDRO infections in the ICU.

INTRODUCTION

Patient care in intensive care units (ICUs) routinely includes diagnosing and managing infectious diseases. Infections can be either the immediate indication or the consequence of a patient requiring ICU care. ICUs are associated with a greatly increased risk of hospital-acquired infections. There is also an increased risk that the infection is caused by an organism that has acquired or developed resistance to most antibiotics; a multidrug-resistant organism (MDRO). Infections with MDROs are associated with increased morbidity and mortality. Among other factors, the delay in appropriate antibiotic therapy contributes significantly to the increased mortality of these infections. Prompt recognition and timely, appropriate treatment of infections caused by MDROs present a serious challenge to ICU providers. This article reviews recent literature on the management of difficult-to-treat organisms relevant to infections in the ICU.

TREATMENT

The decision to start antimicrobial therapy for a suspected infection in a critically ill patient is an important one. With the increasing prevalence of MDROs, providers are faced with the difficult situation of balancing the mortality benefit of early appropriate antibiotic therapy with the environmental damage (selection and development of such organisms) caused by unnecessary antimicrobial medications. In patients with septic shock, the delay of empiric antimicrobial therapy is associated with increased mortality.[1] The same applies to documented hospital-acquired infections, such as pneumonia or bloodstream infections, for which inappropriate or delayed empiric initial antibiotic therapy is associated with an increased risk of

Disclosures: None.
Pulmonary and Critical Care Division, Washington University School of Medicine, 660 South Euclid Avenue #8052, St Louis, MO 63110, USA
* Corresponding author.
E-mail address: mkollef@dom.wustl.edu

Clin Chest Med 36 (2015) 531–541
http://dx.doi.org/10.1016/j.ccm.2015.05.007
0272-5231/15/$ – see front matter © 2015 Elsevier Inc. All rights reserved.

death that is not attenuated by treatment escalation.[2,3] Thus, in the setting of documented infection or suspected infection with hemodynamic instability, appropriate empiric antimicrobials should be started promptly. In hemodynamically stable patients requiring critical care for noninfectious reasons with a suspicion of having acquired an infection that is not yet documented, the answer is not as clear. Hranjec and colleagues[4] suggest that, in this scenario, waiting for objective evidence of infection before starting empiric antimicrobials may not worsen outcomes. This possibility requires further research.

Antibiotic therapies in critically ill patients require specific considerations. They often have an altered volume of distribution of antibiotics, low plasma albumin concentrations that significantly affect pharmacokinetics, as well as altered renal excretion. It is widely known that patients in the ICU frequently develop acute kidney injury and require dose adjustment of antimicrobials; however, the opposite effect has been described as well. Patients in the ICU can develop a state of augmented renal clearance, with increased glomerular filtration, tubular secretion, and reabsorption.[5,6] The DALI (Defining Antibiotic Levels in Intensive Care Patients) study, a multinational pharmacokinetic analysis of β-lactam antibiotics, described how 20% of patients fail to achieve the minimum antibiotic concentration required for adequate treatment and up to 50% failed to meet the preferred level when standard recommended doses are used.[7] Insufficient antibiotic exposure leads to the development of antimicrobial resistance as well as worse clinical outcomes. The dosing of antibiotics in infected critically ill patients should be personalized to achieve optimal concentrations, and higher doses are often required.

The selection of an empiric antibiotic regimen that will reliably qualify as initially appropriate antibiotic therapy (IAAT) for patients with risk factors for MDROs is also challenging. It is widely recommended that the regimen include activity against both methicillin-resistant Staphylococcus aureus (MRSA) and resistant gram-negative organisms (eg, Pseudomonas aeruginosa). In the past, the use of an additional agent that covers gram-negative organisms (eg, an aminoglycoside, quinolone, or colistin) was recommended empirically in this specific population.[8] The current evidence, at least for ventilator-associated pneumonia (VAP), does not show any benefit and shows potential harm with this approach.[9,10] Despite this evidence, there might still be a role for this strategy in a specific population, such as patients with a history of carbapenem-resistant Enterobacteriaceae

(CRE), Pseudomonas spp, or Acinetobacter spp infections.

Gram-negative Infections

Infections caused by gram-negative MDROs are frequently seen in the ICU. The organisms encountered include Enterobacter spp (AmpC-type β-lactamase), extended-spectrum β-lactamase (ESBL)–producing Enterobacteriaceae, CRE, as well as Acinetobacter baumannii and P aeruginosa. These organisms can develop resistance to most commonly used antibiotics (so-called extensively drug-resistant [XDR] organisms) and occasionally become colistin-only susceptible (COS) or even pandrug resistant (PDR). There are limited therapeutic options for infections caused by gram-negative MDROs. A summary of therapeutic options is given in **Table 1**.

Enterobacter spp is commonly encountered in the ICU as the causal agent of nosocomial infections. Its treatment can be particularly challenging, because it is known to harbor AmpC-type β-lactamases and develop resistance during therapy with β-lactamase inhibitors. Historically, experts have recommended treatment with carbapenems, especially for bloodstream infections (BSIs). Cefepime is a poor inducer and more stable to AmpC-type β-lactamases, providing a therapeutic option that should be effective and also provide less environmental pressure for the development of carbapenem resistance. Siedner and colleagues[11] reported a retrospective analysis of 368 cases of Enterobacter spp bacteremia, in which cefepime was as effective as carbapenems for this particular infection. Cefepime can be used as a carbapenem-sparing agent for the treatment of Enterobacter spp bacteremia. This action is specific for this AmpC-type β-lactamase–producing organism and does not apply for ESBL-producing Enterobacteriaceae (Escherichia coli, Klebsiella spp, and so forth), in which cefepime is inferior to carbapenems.[12,13]

Once a rarity, infections with ESBL-producing Enterobacteriaceae have now become common in ICUs around the world. The mainstay of therapy for serious infections with ESBL-producing organisms is carbapenem monotherapy. An emerging challenge in the ICU setting is the treatment of infections with organisms that are now resistant to carbapenems (CRE, Pseudomonas spp, and Acinetobacter spp). Recently the US Centers for Disease Control and Prevention reported that the proportion of Enterobacteriaceae that were CRE increased from 1.2% in 2001 to 4.2% in 2011, with most of the increase observed in Klebsiella spp (from 1.6% to 10.4%).[14] Antibiotic treatment

Table 1
Antimicrobials frequently reported in the treatment of infections with MDRO

	Antibiotic	ICU/MDR Dose	Main Toxicities	Comments
Drug-resistant gram-negative organisms	Meropenem Imipenem Doripenem	1–2 g IV every 8 h 500–1000 mg every 6 h 500–1000 mg IV every 8 h	Seizures (imipenem>meropenem> doripenem), thrombocytopenia, drug fever	Consider carbapenems in combination therapy regimens for CRE infections. Consider extended infusion for MDROs
	Tigecycline	200 mg IV loading dose, followed by 100 mg IV every 12 h	Nausea, emesis	This dose is double the standard recommended dose (see text), exclusively for MDRO gram-negative infections
	Colistin IV	9 million units (720 mg) IV loading dose, followed by 9 million units IV/d divided in 2–3 doses	Reversible nephrotoxicity, neurotoxicity	This is a higher dose than indicated by the package insert to achieve appropriate plasma levels earlier
	Colistin inhaled	3 million units/d in divided doses	Airway irritation	No evidence of increased systemic toxicity
	Ampicillin/ sulbactam	9 g IV every 8 h	Rash, diarrhea, drug fever, leukopenia, thrombocytopenia, transaminitis, seizures	High dose for treatment of Acinetobacter spp
	Tobramycin inhaled Amikacin inhaled	300 mg every 12 h 300–400 mg every 12 h	Nephrotoxic, ototoxicity, and vestibular toxicity	Systemic absorption may occur and warrants close monitoring for toxicities
Gram-positive organisms	Vancomycin	15–20 mg/kg IV every 8–12 h	Nephrotoxicity, neutropenia, thrombocytopenia	Consider alternative therapy if MRSA MIC ≥2 mg/L
	Daptomycin	6–10 mg/kg or 750 mg IV every 24 h	Transaminitis, reversible CPK level increase, myopathy, falsely increased INR, eosinophilic pneumonia	Not appropriate for pneumonia. High doses may be required in critically ill patients (see text)
	Linezolid	600 mg IV or PO every 12 h	Reversible myelosuppression, serotonin syndrome, lactic acidosis, optic neuritis, peripheral neuropathy	Benefit in toxin-producing strains and MRSA pneumonia. Activity against VRE, VISA
	Ceftaroline	800 mg IV every 8 h	Interstitial nephritis, neutropenia, thrombocytopenia	Higher dose (every 8 vs 12 h) in critically ill patients may be required
	Telavancin	10 mg/kg IV every 24 h	Nephrotoxicity, taste disturbance, nausea, emesis	Avoid in patients with renal insufficiency if possible

The antibiotics (with dose and off-label use) represent the most commonly reported in the literature in the treatment of MDRO infections. This list is not meant to be comprehensive.
Abbreviations: CPK, creatine phosphokinase; INR, International Normalized Ratio; IV, intravenous; MDR, multidrug resistant; MIC, minimum inhibitory concentration; PO, per oral; VISA, vancomycin-intermediate S aureus; VRE, vancomycin-resistant Enterococcus.

options are limited and include tigecycline, fosfomycin, colistin, and aminoglycosides. At present there are many questions regarding the optimal therapeutic approach but no published randomized controlled trials to answer them. Falagas and colleagues[15,16] and Tzouvelekis and colleagues[17] recently published detailed analyses of the available literature on clinical experience treating CRE infections. It must be stressed that this is not equivalent to randomized controlled trials and has many limitations, but it is the best guidance that is available at this point to treat infections that have a reported mortality of around 40%. Tzouvelekis and colleagues[17] reported that monotherapy with an in vitro active agent resulted in high mortalities when using carbapenem (40.1%), tigecycline (41.1%), or colistin (42.8%). This finding was comparable with the mortality with therapy that did not include active agents (46.1%). The exact reason for monotherapy having such a high mortality in this population is unknown. It is likely multifactorial, including a combination of inappropriate dosing, the rapid induction of resistance, or the presence of unrecognized polymicrobial infections. Combination therapy showed a lower mortality than monotherapy, especially with carbapenem-containing regimens (18.8%) versus carbapenem-sparing regimens (30.7%). The survival benefit of carbapenem-containing combination regimens remained regardless of the infection site. When choosing a regimen, clinicians must keep in mind that the positive effect of carbapenems in a combination regimen is mostly seen against organisms with minimum inhibitory concentration (MIC) less than or equal to 8 mg/L, and possibly up to 16 mg/L if used in triple combination therapy.[18,19] There is not enough evidence to help determine whether there is differential efficacy between colistin, tigecycline, or aminoglycosides. Selection should be based on susceptibility patterns. When selecting colistin as therapy, a higher loading dose equivalent to 9 million IU should be considered to achieve steady state earlier and avoid plasma levels less than the MIC.[20] A similar dose increase should be recommended when using tigecycline. Current standard dosing recommendations are about half of the original planned dose because of perceived unacceptable nausea and emesis with higher doses. This recommendation resulted in serum concentrations that are lower than the MICs of most gram-negative pathogens. A loading dose of 200 mg followed by 100 mg every 12 hours should be considered in these patients, with close monitoring for toxicity.[21,22] Extensive clinical experience with aminoglycosides and the potential in vitro synergic effect with carbapenems make

them a reasonable choice when appropriate.[23] If triple therapy is desired or there is a need for concomitant administration of systemic colistin and aminoglycosides, close monitoring of renal function should occur for possible additive nephrotoxic effects.

Another strategy that should be considered is extended infusion of β-lactams for the treatment of MDROs. β-Lactams' ability to kill bacteria is related to the time bacteria are exposed to a concentration of the antibiotic that exceeds the MIC. Changing the method of infusion from intermittent to continuous intravenous (IV) infusion achieves higher plasma antibiotic concentration. Despite showing improved mortality in retrospective studies,[24,25] this did not translate into improved mortality when evaluated in severe sepsis in a multicenter, prospective, randomized, double-blind trial.[26] The study was underpowered to evaluate improved survival but did show higher clinical cure rates. Recently, an Australian multicenter randomized controlled trial was completed and again failed to show benefit in outcomes from prolonged infusion. The results will be published shortly (Jeffrey Lipman, personal communication, 2015). Despite the evidence, there may still be a role of extended-infusion β-lactams for certain MDROs or organisms with higher MICs when used in combination therapy.

Fosfomycin has been used for treatment of ESBL Enterobacteriaceae. Reported susceptibility of ESBL-producing E coli and Klebsiella pneumoniae to fosfomycin is 96.8% and 81.3%, respectively.[27] Fosfomycin has been used for a wide range of infections with success,[28] but most of the recent experience is with urinary tract infections. Although anecdotal and observational success has been reported, further research is required to evaluate fosfomycin as an alternative for systemic infections with MDROs (including Pseudomonas spp) not involving the urinary tract.

Colistin has reemerged as an alternative therapy and occasionally as a last resort for some infections. Studies evaluating the efficacy of IV colistin for COS gram-negative infections exist mostly as cohort studies. The predominant infection studied is VAP, the most common infectious complication of ICU care and frequently caused by gram-negative MDROs. Cohort studies support the finding that treating COS P aeruginosa and A baumannii with IV colistin is as effective as alternative therapy (ie, carbapenem) for a susceptible organism showing comparable mortality.[29–32] This is despite the fact that colistin was usually used as a last-resort option and the timing to appropriate antibiotic was longer with colistin than with the control group.[33]

Acinetobacter spp is a less frequently encountered organism with multiple treatment options that include sulbactam, antipseudomonal β-lactams, tetracycline, tigecycline, quinolones, aminoglycosides, and polymyxins. The problem with this organism is that it easily acquires resistance mechanisms, with a much higher likelihood of developing carbapenem resistance than *Pseudomonas* spp or Enterobacteriaceae. Because carbapenems are often last-resort empiric therapy, non-IAAT rates are very high with infections with this organism, directly contributing to increased mortality.[34] Although colistin resistance has been reported, it remains an infrequent occurrence.[35] The most commonly used therapies for multidrug-resistant or XDR *Acinetobacter* spp include high-dose ampicillin/sulbactam, tigecycline, and colistin. It is unclear whether there is a benefit from combination therapy compared with monotherapy, but carbapenems, aminoglycosides, and rifampicins have been used as adjunctive therapy.[36] Combination therapy may be favored because, in critically ill patients, *Acinetobacter* spp infections are commonly polymicrobial.

A strategy that clinicians often use is adjunctive aerosolized (AS) antibiotics for pneumonia with MDROs. Tumbarello and colleagues[37] reported a retrospective analysis of patients with VAP caused by COS gram-negative organisms (*P aeruginosa* and *Acinetobacter* spp), which suggested that AS colistin might be beneficial to IV colistin. The use of AS and IV colistin was associated with higher cure rates, organism eradication, and fewer days requiring mechanical ventilation than IV colistin alone, without any increase in systemic toxicity. There was no difference in mortality or ICU length of stay. Many recent observational and small randomized trials have shown encouraging results with less toxicity using adjunctive inhaled therapy (mostly with aminoglycosides or colistin) for the treatment of ventilated patients with pneumonia caused by gram-negative MDRO.[38] Combination inhaled therapy with amikacin and fosfomycin seems promising as adjunctive therapy in VAP because of an observed in vitro synergistic effect against gram-negative bacteria with documented resistance to aminoglycosides.[39,40] A randomized controlled trial designed to evaluate this strategy is currently underway. Adjunctive inhaled therapy should not be implemented routinely for VAP, but can be considered when resistant organisms are involved. Inhaled monotherapy (ie, inhaled colistin without concomitant IV antimicrobials) for MDRO respiratory tract infections, including ventilator-associated tracheobronchitis, has been reported in small observational studies and requires further investigation. At this time, it should be avoided because it carries the risk of treatment failure and the further development of resistance in organisms that already have limited therapeutic options.

Gram-positive Infections

Gram-positive cocci (GPC) infections were recently reported to represent most nosocomial infections, predominantly *S aureus* and *Enterococcus* spp, many of them MRSA or vancomycin-resistant *Enterococcus*.[41] Therapeutic options for drug-resistant GPC include vancomycin, daptomycin, linezolid, ceftaroline, tigecycline, and telavancin. Each has its own advantages and disadvantages, and they have recently been reviewed by Vazquez-Guillamet and Kollef.[42]

In the past, vancomycin has been regarded as the treatment of choice for GPC infections caused by MRSA, including bloodstream infections, pneumonia, skin and soft tissue infections (SSTI), and central nervous system (CNS) infections. With increased use, the susceptibility of MRSA to vancomycin has been shifting toward higher MICs, termed MIC creep, which has been associated with increased mortality. Woods and colleagues[43] reported that the prevalence of MRSA with an MIC of 2 mg/L in their patients in ICUs with bacteremia was 5.1%. They noted an escalation of mortality as MIC increased, up to 80% when reaching an MIC of 2 mg/L. Selective pressure from repeated vancomycin exposure has allowed staphylococci to adapt, with the emergence of vancomycin-intermediate *S aureus* (VISA) or heterogeneous resistant VISA (hVISA). hVISA refers to organisms reported as vancomycin susceptible but that contain a subpopulation with a thicker cell wall and that expresses resistance to vancomycin.[44] Less commonly, horizontal transfer of *vanA* from vancomycin-resistant enterococci has resulted in the emergence of highly resistant vancomycin-resistant *S aureus* (VRSA).

Linezolid is indicated in MRSA nosocomial pneumonia and SSTI, especially when it involves strains secreting Panton-Valentine leukocidin virulence factor given its ability to inhibit toxin production (as in necrotizing pneumonia).[45] In the setting of MRSA nosocomial pneumonia or when the vancomycin MIC is greater than 1 mg/L, linezolid seems to be of greatest utility and may be a superior agent.[46,47] It has been successfully used off label for secondary MRSA bacteremia, endocarditis, and CNS infections. Its adverse effects are limited to myelosuppression, peripheral and optic neuropathy, lactic acidosis, and serotonin syndrome. It retains activity against VISA and VRSA, but, like all other antibiotics, resistance has been reported with increased use.[48] Tedizolid is a newer oxazolidinone that is US Food and Drug Administration (FDA) approved for SSTI with activity against linezolid-resistant isolates and dosed once a day. At this time, it is too early to be recommended for other indications.

Daptomycin is an alternative in the treatment of MRSA infections, including when vancomycin has failed. It is indicated for SSTI and bloodstream infections at doses of 6 mg/kg and 8 mg/kg respectively. Falcone and colleagues[49] observed high daptomycin clearance in critically ill patients and suggested a minimum dose of 750 mg/d. The Infectious Diseases Society of America (IDSA) also recommends a dose of 10 mg/kg for persistent bacteremia or vancomycin failure.[50] Emergence of daptomycin resistance when used as salvage therapy after vancomycin failure is common and should be suspected, but might be avoided if used in combination with a β-lactam, trimethoprim/sulfamethoxazole, rifampin, or an aminoglycoside.[51]

Ceftaroline is an anti-MRSA cephalosporin approved by the FDA in 2010 for community-acquired pneumonia and SSTI. At present, only clinical evidence in the form of case series exists supporting its use in severe MRSA infections such as endocarditis and osteomyelitis.[52] Although limited clinical data support the use of ceftaroline for hVISA, VISA, and daptomycin non-susceptible MRSA infections, there are positive in vitro data to support such off-label use.[53,54]

Telavancin is FDA approved for SSTI and hospital-acquired infections by gram-positive organisms, including MRSA. It has more rapid concentration-dependent killing activity than vancomycin and maintains antimicrobial activity against VISA and hVISA strains. In 2 clinical trials for hospital-acquired pneumonia, it produced similar cure, mortality, and renal failure rates than vancomycin.[55] Caution is needed when used in patients with moderate to severe renal failure because this group of patients had lower survival in the same trials, and this treatment should be reserved for when no other options are available.

Tigecycline is a tetracycline analogue with broad-spectrum activity including MRSA and MDROs such as ESBL Enterobacteriaceae and A baumannii. It is approved for complicated intra-abdominal infections, SSTI, and community-acquired pneumonia. It has been used off label for nosocomial pneumonia, diabetic foot infection, and urinary tract infections. Several meta-analyses have found the incidence of death to be greater with tigecycline than with alternative antibiotics, especially in nosocomial pneumonia studies. This

excess mortality seems to be driven by gram-negative bacteria and could possibly be caused by serum concentrations less than the MICs achieved with currently recommended standard doses. Thus, caution is needed when using this antimicrobial in the ICU setting.

Fungal Infections

In the United States, candida BSIs are the third leading cause of BSI in ICUs.[56] Recently, an analysis of the Extended Prevalence of Infection in the ICU (EPIC II) study reported the prevalence of candida BSIs in the ICU.[57] The study included 14,414 patients and the prevalence of candida BSI was 6.9 per 1000 patients. Candidemia had the highest crude mortality (42.6%) compared with gram-negative (29.1%) or gram-positive BSI (25.3%), although this was not statistically significant. Risk factors for developing invasive candida infections in the ICU have been described, providing a specific population that might benefit from empiric or prophylactic antifungal therapy. Benefit from antifungal prophylaxis in critically ill patients has been described in single-centers studies[58] and a meta-analysis.[59] Most recently, Ostrosky-Zeichner and colleagues[60] reported the results of a multicenter, randomized, double-blind, placebo-controlled trial of caspofungin prophylaxis in high-risk patients. Patients considered high risk for this study were those in the ICU for at least 3 days requiring mechanical ventilation, receiving antibiotics, and with 1 additional risk factor (parenteral nutrition, dialysis, surgery, pancreatitis, systemic steroids, or other immunosuppressants). Patients were randomized to receive caspofungin or placebo. There was a numerical benefit with lower incidence of probable/proven invasive candidiasis in the prophylactic caspofungin arm, but this was not statistically significant (16.9% vs 9.8%; $P = .14$). An important limitation is that it included a highly selective population, recruiting only 222 patients out of 16,000 screened in 15 ICUs in the United States, resulting in an underpowered study. Although caspofungin is a safe drug, the lack of proven benefit along with the emergence of resistance to echinocandins (in already fluconazole-resistant isolates of Candida glabrata) reported to be as high as 12.3%,[61] argues against prophylactic antifungals in the general ICU population.

Empiric antifungal therapy has also been studied in the critical care setting. Schuster and colleagues[62] reported that there was no benefit of empiric fluconazole compared with placebo in ICU patients who had persistent fever despite broad-spectrum antibiotics. The Incidence

Table 2
Rapid diagnostic technology available

Test	Technology	Time to Identification (h)	Application	Susceptibilities	Trade Product
MAIDI-TOFMS	MALDI-TOFMS	0.2–1	Rapidly identify multiple bacterial and fungal pathogens from a variety of sources	No	MALDI Biotyper, Vitek MS system
PCR/multiplex PCR	PCR	1–2.5	Real-time automated PCR. Probe with 1 or multiple primers to amplify a piece of target DNA specific for an organism (bacterial or yeast) or a marker of resistance	Yes, identification of markers of resistance: *mecA*, *vanA/B*, KPC	Life Cycler Septifast *mecA*, FilmArray BCID, Expert MRSA/SA BC, and SSTI
Nanoparticle probe technology	Nucleic acid extraction and PCR amplification	1–2.5	Rapid identification of the presence of multiple gram-positive and gram-negative bacteria in positive blood cultures	Yes, identification of markers of resistance: *mecA*, *vanA/B*, CTX-M (ESBL), and carbapenemases (KPC, NDM, VIM, IMP, OXA)	Verigene Gram-Positive Blood Culture (BC-GP), Verigene Gram-Negative Blood Culture (BC-GN)
PNA FISH/QuickFISH	PNA FISH	0.5–3	Uses approved probes for rapid identification of certain gram-positive, gram-negative, and *Candida* spp organisms in positive blood cultures	No	*Staphylococcus* QuickFISH, *Enterococcus* QuickFISH, gram-negative QuickFISH, *Candida* QuickFISH

Abbreviations: FISH, fluorescent in situ hybridization; MAIDI-TOFMS, matrix-assisted laser desorption/ionization time-of-flight mass spectrometry; PCR, polymerase chain reaction; PNA, peptide nucleic acid.

of invasive candidiasis was only 9% in the placebo group, suggesting that the population selected was not at high enough risk. The increased mortality associated with delayed therapy and the safety profile of echinocandins and fluconazole support that empiric therapy should be considered in a highly selective group of patients with risk factors for invasive candidiasis.

DIAGNOSTICS

Establishing an early diagnosis through appropriate diagnostic testing allows for more rapid institution of appropriate antimicrobial therapy. Equally important is controlling the source of infection and determining the identification and susceptibility profile of the pathogen so that targeted therapy may be commenced. Traditionally, standard microbiology laboratories require 48 to 72 hours to provide final culture results when the specimens submitted are positive. During that waiting period, clinicians rely on surrogate data (eg, risk factors for MDRO infections, prior infections, prior antimicrobial exposure, suspected site of infection, antibiograms) to make an educated guess to select the appropriate empiric antibiotic regimen, following a 2-tier thought process: (1) the most likely pathogen involved, and (2) the antimicrobial susceptibility of the organism. Selecting a standard regimen of broader spectrum antimicrobials for empiric therapy used to be enough, but in the era of MDROs and XDROs this results in the delay of appropriate therapy for many patients. Multiple strategies exist to aid in this process. One possibility that has been suggested is the concept of unit-specific combination antibiograms in the ICU to aid in selecting the optimal antibiotic combination and increasing the probabilities of achieving IAAT for gram-negative pneumonia.[63] This concept still entails using historical surrogate data to assume an organism's susceptibility. The development of rapid molecular methods for organism identification provides objective data and results within minutes to a few hours.[64] Rapid diagnostic tests can identify organisms and, in certain cases, ascertain the presence of genetic resistance markers, providing a result that aids the clinician in selecting the appropriate antibiotic in a timelier manner. **Table 2** includes the technology currently available for rapid diagnostic tests. Strategies that integrate the implementation of rapid diagnostic tests (which include rapid reporting and antimicrobial stewardship) have been reported to have a positive impact on multiple outcomes, including time to appropriate therapy, length of hospital stay, duration of antibiotic therapy, hospital costs, and most importantly mortality.[65–69] At present, most of the tests require the growth of the organism in standard culture media, limiting their benefit. Tests performed directly on clinical specimens are being developed, and are already available for blood culture specimens.

SUMMARY

Clinicians treating critically ill patients with infection should always focus on providing timely appropriate antibiotic treatment and minimizing the use of unnecessary antibiotics. Although challenging, the availability of new antibiotics targeting MDROs as well as the availability of rapid diagnostic methods offers a real opportunity to strike this important balance. ICU physicians should promote the tenets of antimicrobial stewardship in their daily practice, which include optimizing patient outcomes, reducing the emergence of antibiotic resistance, and minimizing health care costs.

REFERENCES

1. Kumar A, Roberts D, Wood KE, et al. Duration of hypotension before initiation of effective antimicrobial therapy is the critical determinant of survival in human septic shock. Crit Care Med 2006;34(6): 1589–96.
2. Zilberberg MD, Shorr AF, Micek ST, et al. Antimicrobial therapy escalation and hospital mortality among patients with health-care-associated pneumonia: a single-center experience. Chest 2008;134(5):963–8.
3. Ibrahim EH, Sherman G, Ward S, et al. The influence of inadequate antimicrobial treatment of bloodstream infections on patient outcomes in the ICU setting. Chest 2000;118(1):146–55.
4. Hranjec T, Sherman G, Ward S, et al. Aggressive versus conservative initiation of antimicrobial treatment in critically ill surgical patients with suspected intensive-care-unit-acquired infection: a quasi-experimental, before and after observational cohort study. Lancet Infect Dis 2012;12(10):774–80.
5. Udy AA, Baptista JP, Lim NL, et al. Augmented renal clearance in the ICU: results of a multicenter observational study of renal function in critically ill patients with normal plasma creatinine concentrations. Crit Care Med 2014;42(3):520–7.
6. Udy AA, Jarrett P, Stuart J, et al. Determining the mechanisms underlying augmented renal drug clearance in the critically ill: use of exogenous marker compounds. Crit Care 2014;18(6):657.
7. Roberts JA, Paul SK, Akova M, et al. DALI: defining antibiotic levels in intensive care unit patients: are current beta-lactam antibiotic doses sufficient for critically ill patients? Clin Infect Dis 2014;58(8): 1072–83.

8. American Thoracic Society, Infectious Diseases Society of America. Guidelines for the management of adults with hospital-acquired, ventilator-associated, and healthcare-associated pneumonia. Am J Respir Crit Care Med 2005;171(4):388–416.

9. Kett DH, Cano E, Quartin AA, et al. Implementation of guidelines for management of possible multidrug-resistant pneumonia in intensive care: an observational, multicentre cohort study. Lancet Infect Dis 2011;11(3):181–9.

10. Heyland DK, Dodek P, Muscedere J, et al. Randomized trial of combination versus monotherapy for the empiric treatment of suspected ventilator-associated pneumonia. Crit Care Med 2008;36(3): 737–44.

11. Siedner MJ, Galar A, Guzmán-Suarez BB, et al. Cefepime vs other antibacterial agents for the treatment of Enterobacter species bacteremia. Clin Infect Dis 2014;58(11):1554–63.

12. Lee NY, Lee CC, Huang WH, et al. Cefepime therapy for monomicrobial bacteremia caused by cefepime-susceptible extended-spectrum beta-lactamase-producing Enterobacteriaceae: MIC matters. Clin Infect Dis 2013;56(4):488–95.

13. Chopra T, Marchaim D, Veltman J, et al. Impact of cefepime therapy on mortality among patients with bloodstream infections caused by extended-spectrum-beta-lactamase-producing Klebsiella pneumoniae and Escherichia coli. Antimicrob Agents Chemother 2012;56(7):3936–42.

14. Centers for Disease Control and Prevention. Vital signs: carbapenem-resistant Enterobacteriaceae. MMWR Morb Mortal Wkly Rep 2013; 62(9):165–70.

15. Falagas ME, Lourida P, Poulikakos P, et al. Antibiotic treatment of infections due to carbapenem-resistant Enterobacteriaceae: systematic evaluation of the available evidence. Antimicrob Agents Chemother 2014;58(2):654–63.

16. Rafailidis PI, Falagas ME. Options for treating carbapenem-resistant Enterobacteriaceae. Curr Opin Infect Dis 2014;27(6):479–83.

17. Tzouvelekis LS, Markogiannakis A, Piperaki E, et al. Treating infections caused by carbapenemase-producing Enterobacteriaceae. Clin Microbiol Infect 2014;20(9):862–72.

18. Tumbarello M, Viale P, Viscoli C, et al. Predictors of mortality in bloodstream infections caused by Klebsiella pneumoniae carbapenemase-producing K. pneumoniae: importance of combination therapy. Clin Infect Dis 2012;55(7):943–50.

19. Daikos GL, Tsaousi S, Tzouvelekis LS, et al. Carbapenemase-producing Klebsiella pneumoniae bloodstream infections: lowering mortality by antibiotic combination schemes and the role of carbapenems. Antimicrob Agents Chemother 2014;58(4): 2322–8.

20. Plachouras D, Karvanen M, Friberg LE, et al. Population pharmacokinetic analysis of colistin methanesulfonate and colistin after intravenous administration in critically ill patients with infections caused by gram-negative bacteria. Antimicrob Agents Chemother 2009;53(8):3430–6.

21. Ramirez J, Dartois N, Gandjini H, et al. Randomized phase 2 trial to evaluate the clinical efficacy of two high-dosage tigecycline regimens versus imipenem-cilastatin for treatment of hospital-acquired pneumonia. Antimicrob Agents Chemother 2013;57(4):1756–62.

22. Cunha BA. Pharmacokinetic considerations regarding tigecycline for multidrug-resistant (MDR) Klebsiella pneumoniae or MDR Acinetobacter baumannii urosepsis. J Clin Microbiol 2009;47(5):1613.

23. Le J, McKee B, Srisupha-Olarn W, et al. In vitro activity of carbapenems alone and in combination with amikacin against KPC-producing Klebsiella pneumoniae. J Clin Med Res 2011;3(3):106–10.

24. Lodise TP Jr, Lomaestro B, Drusano GL. Piperacillin-tazobactam for Pseudomonas aeruginosa infection: clinical implications of an extended-infusion dosing strategy. Clin Infect Dis 2007;44(3):357–63.

25. Yost RJ, Cappelletty DM, RECEIPT Study Group. The retrospective cohort of extended-infusion piperacillin-tazobactam (RECEIPT) study: a multicenter study. Pharmacotherapy 2011;31(8):767–75.

26. Dulhunty JM, Roberts JA, Davis JS, et al. Continuous infusion of beta-lactam antibiotics in severe sepsis: a multicenter double-blind, randomized controlled trial. Clin Infect Dis 2013;56(2):236–44.

27. Falagas ME, Kastoris AC, Kapaskelis AM, et al. Fosfomycin for the treatment of multidrug-resistant, including extended-spectrum beta-lactamase producing, Enterobacteriaceae infections: a systematic review. Lancet Infect Dis 2010;10(1):43–50.

28. Falagas ME, Giannopoulou KP, Kokolakis GN, et al. Fosfomycin: use beyond urinary tract and gastrointestinal infections. Clin Infect Dis 2008;46(7):1069–77.

29. Reina R, Estenssoro E, Sáenz G, et al. Safety and efficacy of colistin in Acinetobacter and Pseudomonas infections: a prospective cohort study. Intensive Care Med 2005;31(8):1058–65.

30. Hachem RY, Chemaly RF, Ahmar CA, et al. Colistin is effective in treatment of infections caused by multidrug-resistant Pseudomonas aeruginosa in cancer patients. Antimicrob Agents Chemother 2007;51(6):1905–11.

31. Rios FG, Luna CM, Maskin B, et al. Ventilator-associated pneumonia due to colistin susceptible-only microorganisms. Eur Respir J 2007;30(2):307–13.

32. Kallel H, Hergafi L, Bahloul M, et al. Safety and efficacy of colistin compared with imipenem in the treatment of ventilator-associated pneumonia: a matched case-control study. Intensive Care Med 2007;33(7): 1162–7.

33. Zavascki AP, Li J. Intravenous colistimethate for multidrug-resistant Gram-negative bacteria. Lancet Infect Dis 2008;8(7):403–5.

34. Shorr AF, Zilberberg MD, Micek ST, et al. Predictors of hospital mortality among septic ICU patients with *Acinetobacter* spp. bacteremia: a cohort study. BMC Infect Dis 2014;14(1):572.

35. Lee SY, Shin JH, Park KH, et al. Identification, genotypic relation, and clinical features of colistin-resistant isolates of *Acinetobacter* genomic species 13BJ/14TU from bloodstreams of patients in a university hospital. J Clin Microbiol 2014;52(3): 931–9.

36. Poulikakos P, Tansarli GS, Falagas ME. Combination antibiotic treatment versus monotherapy for multidrug-resistant, extensively drug-resistant, and pandrug-resistant *Acinetobacter* infections: a systematic review. Eur J Clin Microbiol Infect Dis 2014;33(10):1675–85.

37. Tumbarello M, De Pascale G, Trecarichi EM, et al. Effect of aerosolized colistin as adjunctive treatment on the outcomes of microbiologically documented ventilator-associated pneumonia caused by colistin-only susceptible gram-negative bacteria. Chest 2013;144(6):1768–75.

38. Michalopoulos AS, Falagas ME. Inhaled antibiotics in mechanically ventilated patients. Minerva Anestesiol 2014;80(2):236–44.

39. Montgomery AB, Rhomberg PR, Abuan T, et al. Potentiation effects of amikacin and fosfomycin against selected amikacin-nonsusceptible Gram-negative respiratory tract pathogens. Antimicrob Agents Chemother 2014;58(7):3714–9.

40. Athanassa ZE, Myrianthefs PM, Boutzouka EG, et al. Monotherapy with inhaled colistin for the treatment of patients with ventilator-associated tracheobronchitis due to polymyxin-only-susceptible Gram-negative bacteria. J Hosp Infect 2011;78(4): 335–6.

41. Sievert DM, Ricks P, Edwards JR, et al. Antimicrobial-resistant pathogens associated with healthcare-associated infections: summary of data reported to the National Healthcare Safety Network at the Centers for Disease Control and Prevention, 2009–2010. Infect Control Hosp Epidemiol 2013; 34(1):1–14.

42. Vazquez-Guillamet C, Kollef MH. Treatment of gram-positive infections in critically ill patients. BMC Infect Dis 2014;14:92.

43. Woods CJ, Chowdhury A, Patel VM, et al. Impact of vancomycin minimum inhibitory concentration on mortality among critically ill patients with methicillin-resistant *Staphylococcus aureus* bacteremia. Infect Control Hosp Epidemiol 2012;33(12): 1246–9.

44. Pitz AM, Yu F, Hermsen ED, et al. Vancomycin susceptibility trends and prevalence of heterogeneous vancomycin-intermediate *Staphylococcus aureus* in clinical methicillin-resistant *S. aureus* isolates. J Clin Microbiol 2011;49(1):269–74.

45. Micek ST, Dunne M, Kollef MH. Pleuropulmonary complications of Panton-Valentine leukocidin-positive community-acquired methicillin-resistant *Staphylococcus aureus*: importance of treatment with antimicrobials inhibiting exotoxin production. Chest 2005;128(4):2732–8.

46. Wunderink RG, Niederman MS, Kollef MH, et al. Linezolid in methicillin-resistant *Staphylococcus aureus* nosocomial pneumonia: a randomized, controlled study. Clin Infect Dis 2012;54(5):621–9.

47. Choi EY, Huh JW, Lim CM, et al. Relationship between the MIC of vancomycin and clinical outcome in patients with MRSA nosocomial pneumonia. Intensive Care Med 2011;37(4):639–47.

48. Morales G, Picazo JJ, Baos E, et al. Resistance to linezolid is mediated by the CFR gene in the first report of an outbreak of linezolid-resistant *Staphylococcus aureus*. Clin Infect Dis 2010;50(6): 821–5.

49. Falcone M, Russo A, Venditti M, et al. Considerations for higher doses of daptomycin in critically ill patients with methicillin-resistant *Staphylococcus aureus* bacteremia. Clin Infect Dis 2013;57(11): 1568–76.

50. Liu C, Bayer A, Cosgrove SE, et al. Clinical practice guidelines by the Infectious Diseases Society of America for the treatment of methicillin-resistant *Staphylococcus aureus* infections in adults and children. Clin Infect Dis 2011;52(3):e18–55.

51. Rybak JM, Barber KE, Rybak MJ. Current and prospective treatments for multidrug-resistant gram-positive infections. Expert Opin Pharmacother 2013;14(14):1919–32.

52. Lin JC, Aung G, Thomas A, et al. The use of ceftaroline fosamil in methicillin-resistant *Staphylococcus aureus* endocarditis and deep-seated MRSA infections: a retrospective case series of 10 patients. J Infect Chemother 2013;19(1):42–9.

53. Werth BJ, Steed ME, Kaatz GW, et al. Evaluation of ceftaroline activity against heteroresistant vancomycin-intermediate *Staphylococcus aureus* and vancomycin-intermediate methicillin-resistant *S. aureus* strains in an in vitro pharmacokinetic/ pharmacodynamic model: exploring the "seesaw effect". Antimicrob Agents Chemother 2013;57(6): 2664–8.

54. Steed M, Vidaillac C, Rybak MJ. Evaluation of ceftaroline activity versus daptomycin (DAP) against DAP-nonsusceptible methicillin-resistant *Staphylococcus aureus* strains in an in vitro pharmacokinetic/pharmacodynamic model. Antimicrob Agents Chemother 2011;55(7):3522–6.

55. Corey GR, Kollef MH, Shorr AF, et al. Telavancin for hospital-acquired pneumonia: clinical response and

28-day survival. Antimicrob Agents Chemother 2014;58(4):2030–7.

56. Wisplinghoff H, Bischoff T, Tallent SM, et al. Nosocomial bloodstream infections in US hospitals: analysis of 24,179 cases from a prospective nationwide surveillance study. Clin Infect Dis 2004;39(3):309–17.

57. Kett DH, Azoulay E, Echeverria PM, et al. Candida bloodstream infections in intensive care units: analysis of the extended prevalence of infection in intensive care unit study. Crit Care Med 2011; 39(4):665–70.

58. Pelz RK, Hendrix CW, Swoboda SM, et al. Double-blind placebo-controlled trial of fluconazole to prevent candidal infections in critically ill surgical patients. Ann Surg 2001;233(4):542–8.

59. Shorr AF, Chung K, Jackson WL, et al. Fluconazole prophylaxis in critically ill surgical patients: a meta-analysis. Crit Care Med 2005;33(9):1928–35 [quiz: 1936].

60. Ostrosky-Zeichner L, Shoham S, Vazquez J, et al. MSG-01: a randomized, double-blind, placebo-controlled trial of caspofungin prophylaxis followed by preemptive therapy for invasive candidiasis in high-risk adults in the critical care setting. Clin Infect Dis 2014;58(9):1219–26.

61. Alexander BD, Johnson MD, Pfeiffer CD, et al. Increasing echinocandin resistance in Candida glabrata: clinical failure correlates with presence of FKS mutations and elevated minimum inhibitory concentrations. Clin Infect Dis 2013;56(12):1724–32.

62. Schuster MG, Edwards JE Jr, Sobel JD, et al. Empirical fluconazole versus placebo for intensive care unit patients: a randomized trial. Ann Intern Med 2008;149(2):83–90.

63. Pogue JM, Alaniz C, Carver PL, et al. Role of unit-specific combination antibiograms for improving the selection of appropriate empiric therapy for gram-negative pneumonia. Infect Control Hosp Epidemiol 2011;32(3):289–92.

64. Bauer KA, Perez KK, Forrest GN, et al. Review of rapid diagnostic tests used by antimicrobial stewardship programs. Clin Infect Dis 2014;59(Suppl 3): S134–45.

65. Huang AM, Newton D, Kunapuli A, et al. Impact of rapid organism identification via matrix-assisted laser desorption/ionization time-of-flight combined with antimicrobial stewardship team intervention in adult patients with bacteremia and candidemia. Clin Infect Dis 2013;57(9):1237–45.

66. Perez KK, Olsen RJ, Musick WL, et al. Integrating rapid diagnostics and antimicrobial stewardship improves outcomes in patients with antibiotic-resistant Gram-negative bacteremia. J Infect 2014;69(3): 216–25.

67. Sango A, McCarter YS, Johnson D, et al. Stewardship approach for optimizing antimicrobial therapy through use of a rapid microarray assay on blood cultures positive for Enterococcus species. J Clin Microbiol 2013;51(12):4008–11.

68. Perez KK, Olsen RJ, Musick WL, et al. Integrating rapid pathogen identification and antimicrobial stewardship significantly decreases hospital costs. Arch Pathol Lab Med 2013;137(9):1247–54.

69. Parta M, Goebel M, Thomas J, et al. Impact of an assay that enables rapid determination of Staphylococcus species and their drug susceptibility on the treatment of patients with positive blood culture results. Infect Control Hosp Epidemiol 2010;31(10): 1043–8.

Index

Clin Chest Med 36 (2015) 543–548
http://dx.doi.org/10.1016/S0272-5231(15)00096-9
0272-5231/15/$ – see front matter © 2015 Elsevier Inc. All rights reserved.

Printed and bound by CPI Group (UK) Ltd, Croydon, CR0 4YY

03/10/2024

01040375-0010